Halberdier, Johnny

BASIC CLINICAL PARASITOLOGY

BROWN
BASIC CLINICAL

APPLETON-CENTURY-CROFTS
Educational Division
MEREDITH CORPORATION

New York

PARASITOLOGY
THIRD EDITION

HAROLD W. BROWN, M.D.

Sc.D., Dr. P.H., L.H.D. (Hon.), LL.D. (Hon.);
Professor of Parasitology, Columbia University
College of Physicians and Surgeons; Parasitol-
ogist, Presbyterian Hospital, New York

Thou shall have a place also without the camp whither thou shall go forth abroad.
And thou shalt have a paddle upon thy weapon and it shall be where thou wilt ease thyself abroad, thou shalt dig therewith and shall turn back and cover that which cometh from thee.

Deuteronomy, Chapter 23: 12, 13

Preface

The third edition has been extensively revised and rewritten to include recent important additions in knowledge. The needs of medicine have dictated the selection of subject matter and the placing of emphasis upon the medical aspects of parasitology, such as pathology, symptomatology, diagnosis, and prevention. Therefore, discussion of the morphologic and biologic characteristics of the various parasites has been restricted to those that are essential for diagnosis. Treatment of the various diseases has been considered briefly, and only established methods of treatment and chemotherapeutic agents of proven value are presented. A number of new chemotherapeutic agents used abroad but not yet approved by the Food and Drug Administration for use in the United States have been included. In the chapter on diagnostic methods, only those technical methods that are commonly used by students or hospital laboratory technicians are given. As parasitic diseases are largely preventable, pictorial life cycles have been included to make clear their vulnerable sites.

I should like to acknowledge the helpful suggestions for the preparation of the first edition of Dr. Edgar E. Baker, Dr. Alice T. Marston, Dr. Matthew A. Derow, and Dr. Manson Meads. I am indebted to Miss Florence Turner for bibliographic assistance.

Dr. Louis H. Miller was most helpful in organizing material on the serologic diagnosis of parasitic diseases. Mr. Armand Miranda and Miss Meredith Behr were of great assistance in photographing the pictorial material.

Dr. Kathleen L. Hussey reviewed the manuscript, made many useful suggestions, and contributed numerous drawings to the second edition. Dr. Roger Williams contributed advice and drawings for the entomological section. I am grateful to the many investigators in the field of parasitology, whose original contributions have provided the material for this book, and to the Medical Editorial Department of Appleton-Century-Crofts for guidance throughout publication.

Finally, it is my pleasant duty to acknowledge my indebtedness to David Belding who prepared the first edition of *Basic Clinical Parasitology* to meet the needs of medical students and busy physicians. It has served this purpose admirably. His long experience in teaching medical students is reflected in the clarity and conciseness of presentation.

Following are several references on parasitology and tropical medicine to which the student is referred for a more thorough study. The extensive textbooks of Belding, and also Faust and Russell should be consulted for detail, and for their extensive bibliographies. The monthly annotated bibliography of the Tropical Disease Bulletin is invaluable for its summary of current literature on tropical diseases.

HAROLD W. BROWN

Adams, and Maegraith. Clinical Tropical Diseases, 3rd ed. Philadelphia, F. A. Davis Co., 1964.

Anderson, Bostick, and Johnstone. Amebiasis. Springfield, Ill., Charles C Thomas, Publisher, 1953.

Ash, and Spitz. Pathology of Tropical Diseases. Philadelphia, W. B. Saunders Company, 1945.

Belding. Textbook of Clinical Parasitology, 3rd. ed. New York, Appleton-Century-Crofts, Inc., 1965.

Bowesman. Surgery and Clinical Pathology in the Tropics. Baltimore, The Williams & Wilkins Co., 1960.

Faust, and Russell. Craig and Faust's Clinical Parasitology, 7th ed., Philadelphia, Lea & Febiger, 1964.

Garnham. Malaria Parasites and other haemosparidia. Oxford, Blackwell Scientific Publications, 1966.

Herms, and James. Medical Entomology, 5th ed. New York, The Macmillan Company, 1961.

Hunter, Frye, and Swartzwelder. A Manual of Tropical Medicine, 4th ed. W. B. Saunders Company, 1966.

Manson-Bahr. Manson's Tropical Diseases, 16th ed. Baltimore, The Williams & Wilkins Co., 1966.

Russell, West, Manwell, and MacDonald. Practical Malariology, 2nd ed. London, Oxford University Press, 1963.

Spencer, and Monroe. The Color Atlas of Intestinal Parasites. Springfield, Ill., Charles C Thomas, Publisher, 1961.

Strong. Stitt's *Diagnosis,* Prevention and Treatment of Tropical Diseases, 7th ed., 2 vols. Philadelphia, The Blakiston Company, 1944.

Trowell, and Jelliffe. Diseases of Children in the Subtropics and Tropics. London, Edward Arnold, Ltd., 1958.

Acknowledgments

Life cycle plate figures are original or from the following various sources.

Figure 16, Winterbottom's sign, after Koch, from Strong: Stitt's *Diagnosis, Prevention and Treatment of Tropical Diseases,* 7th Edition, courtesy of the McGraw-Hill Book Co. Figure 16, later stage of sleeping sickness, and Figure 96, severe cirrhosis, courtesy of Dr. E. R. Kellersberger. Figure 17, megacolon, courtesy of Dr. F. Köberle, published in *Journal of Tropical Medicine and Hygiene,* 61, 1958. Figure 17, primitive house, Chile, courtesy of Dr. R. Donckaster. Figure 36, clinical figures from S. E. Gould, *Trichinosis,* 1st edition, courtesy of Charles C Thomas, Publisher. Figure 38, rectal prolapse, and Figure 46, pinworm and perianal region, courtesy of Dr. Ralph Platou, Department of Pediatrics, Tulane Medical School. Figure 43, adult hookworms, and Figure 46, adult pinworms, from *Helmintologia Humana,* 1949, Habana, Cuba, courtesy of Drs. Pedro Kouri and José G. Basnuevo. Figure 43, cardiac enlargement, from A. W. Hill and J. Andrews, courtesy of *American Journal of Tropical Medicine.* Figure 46, Scotch tape swab technic, adapted from Brooke, Donaldson, and Mitchell, 1949. Figure 53, developmental stages of filaria in mosquito, courtesy of E. Francis, *Filariasis in Southern United States,* Government Printing Office, 1919. Figure 67, coracidium, procercoid, plerocercoid, scolex from the film, *The Life Cycle of Diphyllobothrium latum,* U. S. Public Health Service, 1950. Figure 80, brain containing cysts, Figure 96, liver pathology, and Figure 130, lesions, from J. E. Ash and S. Spitz, *Pathology of Tropical Diseases,* courtesy of The Armed Forces Institute of Pathology, Washington, D.C. Figure 80, cysts in muscles, from H. B. Dixon and W. H. Hargreaves, 1944, *Quarterly Journal of Medicine.*

Figure 86, family picture, courtesy of Drs. E. H. Sadun and C. Maiphoom, *American Journal of Tropical Medicine and Hygiene,* 1953; water nuts from E. C. Faust, *Human Helminthology,* 3rd edition, courtesy of Lea & Febiger, metacercaria, from C. H. Barlow, *American Journal of Hygiene,* Monographic Series, 1925. Figure 102, lesions on child, courtesy of Michigan Department of Health, from 1939 Progress Report of the Division of Water Itch Control, Stream Control Commission. Figure 106, head lesions and nit, from McCarthy, *Diseases of the Hair,* The C. V. Mosby Company; body louse lesions after J. B. and B. Shelmire, from G. C. Andrews, *Diseases of the Skin,* 4th edition, courtesy of W. B. Saunders Co. Figure 106, nymphal stages, and Figure 109, egg, larva, and pupa from *Arthropods of Medical Importance,* Naval Medical School. Figure 112, bites, from B. W. Becker and M. E. Obermayer, *Modern Dermatology and Syphilology,* courtesy of J. B. Lippincott Co., Philadelphia.

Figure 125, adult and pupa, and Figure 130, female depositing eggs, from Metcalf, Flint and Metcalf, *Destructive and Useful Insects,* 4th edition, courtesy of McGraw-Hill Book Company. Figure 130, adult, from N. I. H. Bulletin No. 171, 1938. Figure 132, life cycle figures, from H. E. Ewing, *Journal of Parasitology,* 1944; lesions from Dr. G. W. Wharton, chigger attached from Dr. C. B. Philip, chigger bite, all courtesy of Dr. R. W. Williams, Columbia University. Figure 133, life cycle stages and skin burrow, from K. Mellanby, *Scabies,* courtesy of Oxford University Press; lesions from O. S. Ormsby and H. Montgomery, *Diseases of the Skin,* 7th edition, courtesy of Lea & Febiger Co.

Color plates of malaria (Figures 25, 26, 27) from A. Wilcox, *Manual for the Microscopical Diagnosis of Malaria in Man,* Bulletin No. 180, N. I. H., Washington, D.C., 1943, in G. C. Shattuck, *Diseases of the Tropics,* courtesy of Appleton-Century-Crofts.

Unacknowledged figures are from earlier editions of Belding, from old pictures we have been unable to trace, or from the personal collections of H. W. Brown and K. L. Hussey.

Contents

BASIC CLINICAL PARASITOLOGY

1

General Parasitology

Parasitology is the science which deals with organisms that take up their abodes, temporarily or permanently, on or within other living organisms for the purpose of procuring food, and with the relationship of these organisms to their hosts. In the restricted sense employed here the term is applied only to animal parasites belonging to the protozoa, helminths, and arthropods.

PARASITES AND PARASITISM

Parasitism includes any reciprocal association in which a species depends upon another for its existence. This association may be temporary or permanent. In *symbiosis* there is a permanent association of two organisms that cannot exist independently; in *mutualism* both organisms are benefited; and in *commensalism* one partner is benefited and the other is unaffected. The term *parasite,* however, is ordinarily applied to a weaker organism that obtains food and shelter from another organism and derives all the benefit from the association. The harboring species, known as the *host,* may show no harmful effects or may suffer from various functional and organic disorders.

Various descriptive names denote special types or functions of parasites. An *ectoparasite* lives on the outside (infestation) and an *endoparasite* within the body of the host (infection). Parasites are termed *facultative* when they are capable of leading both a free and parasitic existence, and *obligate* when they take up a permanent residence in and are completely dependent upon the host. An *incidental* parasite is one that establishes itself in a host in which it does not ordinarily live. A *temporary* parasite is free-living during part of its existence and seeks its host intermittently to obtain nourishment. A *permanent* parasite remains on or in the body of the host from early life until maturity, sometimes for its entire life. A *pathogenic* parasite causes injury to the host by its mechanical, traumatic, or toxic activities. A *pseudoparasite* is an artifact mistaken for a parasite. A *coprozoic* or spurious parasite is a foreign species that has passed through the alimentary tract without infecting man.

Parasites often lack the necessary organs for assimilating raw food materials and depend upon the host for predigested food. An adequate supply of moisture is assured inside the host, but during the free-living existence of the parasite inadequate moisture may either prove fatal or prevent larval development. Temperature is, likewise, important. Each species has an optimal temperature range for its existence and development. Both high and low temperatures are detrimental and even lethal.

Scientific Nomenclature.   Animal parasites are classified according to the International Code of Zoological Nomenclature. Each parasite belongs to a phylum, class, order, family, genus, and species. At times the further divisions of suborder, superfamily, subfamily, and subspecies are employed. The family name ends in "idæ," the superfamily in "oidea" and the subfamily in "inæ." The names are Latinized, and the scientific designation is binomial for species, and trinomial for subspecies.

The law of priority obtains as to the oldest available specific name, even if only a portion of the parasite or its larva has been described. To be valid a generic name must not have been given previously to another genus of animals. The names of genera and species are printed in italics; the generic name begins with a capital and the specific name with a small letter—*Ascaris lumbricoides.*

Geographic Distribution.   The endemicity of a parasite depends upon the presence and habits of a suitable host, upon easy escape from the host, and upon environmental conditions favoring survival outside the host. Parasites with simple life cycles are more likely to have a cosmopolitan distribution than those with complicated life cycles. Economic and social conditions affect the distribution of the parasites of man. Thus, irrigation projects and the use of night soil in agriculture provide facilities for parasitic infection. Inadequate individual and community sanitation, low standards of living, and ignorance favor the spread of parasitic diseases. Religious rites such as ablution and immersion in heavily contaminated water may be responsible for their transmission. Migrations of populations have spread parasitic disease throughout the world. The importation of the Negro to the Western Hemisphere was accompanied by hookworm disease and schistosomiasis. Immigrants from the Baltic countries introduced the fish tapeworm into North America.

Although many important species of parasites have a worldwide distribution, tropical countries where optimal conditions of temperature and humidity are present are most favorable for the survival, larval development, and transmission of parasites. The short summer season in the temperate zones prevents the development of many species that require high temperatures during their larval stages. Intense dry heat or direct sunlight may destroy the larval forms. On the other hand, low temperatures arrest the development of eggs and larvae and may even destroy them. Freezing temperatures and snow force man to use privies and prevent general soil pollution. Moisture is essential for the development of free-living larvae, and it is also necessary for the propagation of intermediate hosts such as arthropods, snails, and fishes. Even in the tropics, dry plateaus, because of lack of humidity, are practically free from parasites except resistant species or those that are transferred directly from host to host.

Life Cycle.   Parasites have developed more or less complicated life cycles through adaptation to their hosts and external environment. Most parasites of man attain sexual maturity in him. Some spend their entire lives within the host, one generation following another; others, on leaving the host, are exposed to the vicissitudes of an external environment. During their extracorporeal life they may remain quiescent in the form of resistant cysts, eggs, or larvae, or they may undergo active growth and metamorphosis. Furthermore, the larval parasite may pass through developmental stages in an intermediate host before it reaches a final host.

The *final* or *definitive* host harbors the adult or sexually mature parasite.

Man may be the only definitive host, the most important source of human disease; one of several animal hosts; or merely an incidental host of a parasite prevalent in other animals. Animals that harbor the same species of parasites as man are known as *reservoir* hosts. Such hosts ensure the continuity of the parasite's life cycle and act as additional sources of human infection. Part or all of the larval stage may be passed in another animal, known as the *intermediate* host. Certain species of trematodes and cestodes have two such hosts, known as primary and secondary intermediate hosts. At times man may serve as an intermediate host. From a medical standpoint, knowledge of the life cycle of a parasite is important, since it indicates how man becomes infected and the stages at which preventive measures can be most effectively applied. The more complicated the life cycle, the less the chance of survival, but overdeveloped reproductive organs and larval multiplication tend to offset the increased hazards of a complex life history.

PARASITIC DISEASES

The transmission of parasitic diseases involves 3 factors: (1) the source of the infection, (2) the mode of transmission, and (3) the presence of a susceptible host. The combined effect of these factors determines the dispersibility and prevalence of the parasite at any given time and place.

Since parasitic diseases often tend to run a chronic course with few or no symptoms, an infected individual may become a carrier without showing clinical evidence of infection, thus serving as a potential source of infection to others. In other words, the conditions in the carrier represent the normal state of infection in which there is an equilibrium between the host and the parasite.

The methods whereby parasites reach susceptible hosts from their primary sources are varied. Some parasites require only direct contact; others with more complicated life cycles must pass through various developmental stages—either as free-living forms or in intermediate hosts—before becoming infective. Transmission is effected through direct and indirect contact, food, water, soil, vertebrate and arthropod vectors, and, rarely, from mother to offspring. The chances of infection are increased by environmental conditions favoring the extracorporeal existence of the parasite and by lack of sanitation and communal hygiene. Man, when infected by a parasite, may serve as: (1) its only host, (2) its principal host with other animals also infected, or (3) its incidental host with one or several other animals as principal hosts. In addition to the natural adaptability of the parasite in respect to its host, the ease of transmission depends upon the habits and communal associations, as well as the resistance, of the host.

Pathology and Symptomatology. Various distinctions have been made between the terms infection and infestation, although they are often used indiscriminately to denote parasitic invasion. In this textbook *infection* is applied to invasion by endoparasites and *infestation* to the external parasitism of ectoparasites such as arthropods or to the presence of parasites in soil or plants. Distinction should be made also between parasitic infection with few, slight, or no symptoms and parasitic disease with definite clinical evidence of pathologic changes. Injury to the host is caused by the mechanical and irritative activities or by the toxic products of the parasite. The degree of injury depends upon the number, size, activity, and toxicity of the parasites and their location in the host.

After entering the host the parasite migrates to that part of the body which serves as its permanent residence, tissue specificity being one of the most striking characteristics of parasitic infections. Under certain conditions some parasites may

Table 1. Helminth

	COMMON NAME OF PARASITE OR DISEASE	LENGTH OF PARASITE	SITE IN HOST	PORTAL OF ENTRY
NEMATHELMINTHES	ROUNDWORMS			
Necator americanus	New world or tropical hook- worm Uncinariasis	to 1.1 cm	Small intestine, attached	Skin, usually feet
Ancylostoma duodenale	Old world hook- worm Ancylostomiasis	to 1.3 cm		
Ancylostoma braziliense	Creeping eruption, cutaneous larva migrans (hook- worm larva)	to 0.3 mm (larva)	Intradermal	Skin
Ascaris lumbricoides	Large roundworm	to 35 cm	Small intestine	Mouth
Toxocara canis T. cati	Visceral larva migrans	0.3 mm (larva)	Liver, lung, brain, eye	Mouth
Enterobius vermicularis	Pinworm, seat- worm, Oxyuris	to 1.3 cm	Large intestine, appendix	Mouth
Trichuris trichiura	Whipworm, threadworm	to 5.0 cm	Caecum, large intestine, ileum	Mouth
Trichinella spiralis	Trichinosis	to 0.4 cm	Adult: small intestine wall. Encysted larva: striated muscle	Mouth
Strongyloides stercoralis	Cochin China diarrhea	to 0.2 cm	In wall of small intestine	Skin
Wuchereria bancrofti	Filariasis	to 10 cm	Lymphatics	Skin
Brugia malayi	Filariasis	to 6 cm	Lymphatics	Skin
Acanthocheilonema perstans	Persistent filaria	to 8 cm	Body cavities	Skin
Mansonella ozzardi		to 8 cm	Body cavities	Skin

Infections of Man

Source of Infection, Intermediate Host or Vector	Most Common Clinical Symptoms	Laboratory Diagnosis	Therapeutic Agents	Remarks
Infective filariform larvae in soil	Anemia, growth retardation, G.I. symptoms	Eggs in stool	Tetrachlorethylene Bephenium-hydroxynaphthoate Thiabendazole	Prophylaxis by excreta disposal. Iron therapy important in blood regeneration.
Dog & cat hookworm larvae in soil	Serpiginous skin lesions, itch	History & physical examination	Freezing, x-ray Thiabendazole	Infection of bathers, plumbers, "Sandbox" babies
Eggs from soil or vegetables	Vague abdominal distress	Eggs in stool	Piperazine Hexylresorcinol Bephenium-hydroxynaphthoate Thiabendazole	Worms migrate into bile, pancreatic ducts & peritoneum. Intestinal obstruction.
Eggs from soil	Pneumonitis, eosinophilia	Hemagglutination, flocculation tests	Steroids Antibiotics	Eosinophilia, anemia, hyperglobulinemia.
Eggs in environment; autoinfection	Anal pruritis	Eggs in perianal region. Scotch tape swab	Pyrvinium pamoate Piperazine Thiabendazole Stilbazium	Entire family frequently infected. Personal hygiene important
Eggs from soil or vegetables	Abdominal discomfort, anemia, bloody stools	Eggs in stool	Hexylresorcinol enema Stilbazium Thiabendazole	Worm lives many years. Frequently with hookworm & Ascaris.
Infected pork, cyst (rarely bear)	Orbital edema, muscle pain, eosinophilia	Skin test, comp. fix., flocculation, biopsy	Cortisone gives symptomatic relief Thiabendazole	Thorough cooking of pork & pork products kills encysted larvae.
Larva in soil	Abdominal discomfort, diarrhea	Larvae in stool	Thiabendazole Pyrvinium pamoate	Autoinfection occurs.
Mosquitoes	Lymphangitis, fever	Blood smear, night	Hetrazan,* antibiotics, sulfonamides, surgery	Elephantiasis of leg, arms, scrotum, breasts.
Mosquitoes	Lymphangitis, fever	Blood smear, night	Sulfonamides, surgery, Diethylcarbamazine, antibiotics	Elephantiasis.
Culicoides (fly)	Abdominal pain due to liver invasion?	Blood smear	Diethylcarbamazine	
Culicoides (fly)	Asymptomatic?	Blood smear		

* Diethylcarbamazine

Table 1. Helminth

	COMMON NAME OF PARASITE OR DISEASE	LENGTH OF PARASITE	SITE IN HOST	PORTAL OF ENTRY
Loa loa	Eyeworm	to 7 cm	Subcutaneous	Skin
Onchocerca volvulus	Blinding filariasis	to 50 cm	Subcutaneous	Skin
Dracunculus medinensis	Fiery serpent Guinea worm	to 120 cm	Subcutaneous	Mouth
PLATYHELMINTHES	TAPEWORMS			
Taenia saginata	Beef tapeworm	to 12 meters	Small intestine	Mouth
Hymenolepis nana	Dwarf tapeworm	to 4 cm	Adults & cysts in small intestine	Mouth
Hymenolepis diminuta	Rat tapeworm	to 60 cm	Small intestine	Mouth
Diphyllobothrium latum	Fish or broad tapeworm	to 10 meters	Small intestine	Mouth
Taenia solium	Pork tapeworm	to 7 meters	Small intestine	Mouth
T. solium (cysts)	Cysticercosis Verminous epilepsy	to 0.8 cm Brain, to 2.5 cm	Muscles, brain, eye	Mouth
Echinococcus granulosus	Hydatid cyst	to 15 cm	Liver, lungs, brain, bones	Mouth

take up secondary locations in other organs, producing a more generalized infection. The location of the parasite in a vital organ, its toxic action, and the intensity of the infection determine the presence, time of appearance, and severity of the local and systemic symptoms. Such a symptomatic response results in a typical clinical syndrome; when the maladjustment between parasite and host is less marked, mild or atypical disease is produced; and when there is an equilibrium, a carrier state with slight or no clinical evidence of disease is created.

Parasitic infections produce a wide range of clinical signs and symptoms, depending upon the species of the parasite, the condition of the host, the organs affected, and the number of parasites. Likewise, symptoms may be induced by supersensitivity of the host to the parasite or its products; an infection that nor-

Infections of Man (cont.)

Source of Infection, Intermediate Host or Vector	Most Common Clinical Symptoms	Laboratory Diagnosis	Therapeutic Agents	Remarks
Chrysops (fly)	Local inflammation, transient tumor	Blood smear, day	Diethyl-carbamazine, surgical removal	Calabar swelling.
Simulium (fly)	Subcutaneous nodules, loss of vision	Skin biopsy, nodule aspirate	Hetrazan,* Suramin, surgical removal	Nodules on head and body
Cyclops	Inflammation & ulcers of legs & feet	Lesions, x-ray of calcified worm	Niridazole, worm extraction	Boil or filter drinking water
Cysts in beef	Usually none	Eggs and segments in stool, Scotch tape swab	Quinacrine	Usually only 1 worm.
Eggs from feces	Abdominal discomfort	Eggs in stool	Quinacrine	Numerous worms, infection of children
Cysts from insects	Usually none	Eggs in stool	Oleoresin of Aspidium	Primarily a rat parasite
Plerocercoid in fresh-water fish	Anemia very rare	Eggs in stool	Amodiaquine	Prophylaxis by excreta disposal. Cook fish well.
Cyst in pork	Usually none	Eggs & segments in stool, Scotch tape swab	Niclosamide * (Yomesan) T. solium: prochlorperazine (compazine)	Uncommon in U.S. Frequent in Mexico, Central, South America
Eggs from feces regurgitation of eggs	Intracranial pressure. Epilepsy	Skin test, x-ray of calcified cysts	Surgery	Uncommon in U.S. Autoinfection possible.
Eggs from dog feces	Pressure symptoms in various organs	Skin, comp. fix., hemagglutination tests, x-ray	Surgery	Uncommon in untraveled natives of U.S.

* Not advocated for *T. solium*.

mally elicits no response may result in a pronounced reaction in a sensitized host.

The resistance of the host to animal parasites depends upon the barrier it presents to the invading parasite, and upon its cellular and humoral immunity. External factors, such as habits, nutrition, occupation, associations, and climatic environment of the host, may influence infection. Parasitic infections are particularly dependent upon the extrasystemic conditions that favor the spread of infection in a community. Resistance is a relative affair of varying degrees. Absolute immunity, except in the natural resistance of unsuitable hosts, is rarely found. The host may be able to withstand invasion by the parasite, establish an equilibrium with it, curtail its pathogenic activities, or even destroy it.

Immunity may be a natural heritage of species, race, or individual against para-

Table 2. Helminth and

	COMMON NAME OF PARASITE OR DISEASE	LENGTH OF PARASITE	SITE IN HOST	PORTAL OF ENTRY
PLATYHELMINTHES	FLUKES			
Schistosoma mansoni	Schistosomiasis "Bilharzia"	to 1.4 cm	Veins of large intestine	Skin
Schistosoma haematobium	"	2.0 cm	Veins of urinary bladder	Skin
Schistosoma japonicum	"	2.6 cm	Veins of small intestine	Skin
Fasciolopsis buski	Intestinal fluke	2-7 cm	Small intestine	Mouth
Clonorchis sinensis	Human liver fluke	1-2.5 cm	Bile ducts	Mouth
Paragonimus westermani	Lung fluke	1.0 cm	Lungs	Mouth
PROTOZOA				
Plasmodium vivax	Benign tertian malaria			
Plasmodium falciparum	Malignant tertian malaria	Intracellular	Liver parenchyma, red blood cells	Skin
Plasmodium malariae	Quartan malaria			
Plasmodium ovale				
Leishmania donovani	Visceral leish-maniasis, Kala-azar	Intracellular 2 μ	Monocytes, P.M.N., endo-thelial cells	Skin
Leishmania tropica	Cutaneous leish-maniasis	"	In histiocytes of skin & mucosa	Skin
Leishmania braziliensis	Espundia, mucocu-taneous leish-maniasis	"	"	Skin
Trypanosoma gambiense / *Trypanosoma rhodesiense*	African sleeping sickness	14-33 μ	Lymph glands, blood stream, brain	Skin

Protozoan Infections of Man

Source of Infection Intermediate Host or Vector	Most Common Clinical Symptoms	Laboratory Diagnosis	Therapeutic Agents	Remarks
Cercaria in fresh water, from snail	Chronic dysentery, cirrhosis of liver	Eggs in stool, rectal or liver biopsy	Antimony (Sb^{111}) Stibophen Tartar emetic Lucanthone Miracil D Nilodin Niridazole Ambilhar	Africa, South America. Common in Puerto Ricans.
"	Urinary disturbances, hematuria	Eggs in urine, cystoscopy		Africa, Middle East
"	Dysentery, hepatic cirrhosis	Eggs in stool, liver biopsy		China, Japan, Philippines.
Water nuts & vegetables	Diarrhea, edema, abdominal pain	Eggs in stool	Bephenium hydroxynaphthoate Tetrachlorethylene Hexylresorcinol	
Fresh-water fish	Indigestion, diarrhea, hepatomegaly	Eggs in stool	Chloroquine	Usually in Orientals.
Fresh-water crustaceans (crabs)	Hemoptysis, cough, abdominal pain, fever	Eggs in sputum & stool	Thiobis-dichlorophenol (Bithionol) Chloroquine	Wandering worms in brain and other organs.
Anopheles mosquito	Fever, chill, sweat, enlarged spleen Hemoglobinuria in "Black water fever"	Repeated blood smears	Chloroquine Primaquine Chloroguanide Pyrimethamine Quinacrine Quinine	Fever irregular in early disease. Incubation long after drug suppression.
Phlebotomus (fly)	Fever, enlarged liver and spleen, leukopenia	Liver biopsy, sternal puncture, comp. fix. test, F.A.T.	Sb^{V} compounds Stilbamidine Pentamidine	Signs and symptoms resemble malaria.
Phlebotomus	Chronic ulceration of exposed skin areas	Skin scrapings	Sb^{111}, Sb^{V} compounds X-ray Quinacrine	Immunity following lesion.
Phlebotomus	Ulceration of naso-oral region	Scrape lesions	Sb^{111}, Sb^{V} Antibiotics Cycloguanil pamoate Pyrimethamine	
Tsetse fly	Fever, rash, headache; spleen & liver enlarge	Blood smear, gland puncture, cerebrospinal fluid for trypanosomes	Tryparsamide Suramin (Bayer 205), Mel B Pentamidine Stilbamidine	Enlargement of posterior cervical lymph nodes, Winterbottom's sign.

Table 2. Helminth and

	COMMON NAME OF PARASITE OR DISEASE	LENGTH OF PARASITE	SITE IN HOST	PORTAL OF ENTRY
PROTOZOA				
Trypanosoma cruzi	South American trypanosomiasis	Intracellular stages Tryp. 20 μ	Tissues—heart Blood	Skin
Entamoeba histolytica	Intestinal amebiasis	15–60 μ	Lumen & wall of large intestine	Mouth
" "	Amebic hepatitis Amebic liver abscess		Liver	Mouth
Dientamoeba fragilis		5–12 μ	Large intestine	Mouth
Balantidium coli		50–100 μ	Large intestine	Mouth
Giardia lamblia	Flagellate diarrhea	11–18 μ	Upper small intestine	Mouth
Trichomonas vaginalis		10–30 μ	Vagina, prostate	Genitalia
Toxoplasma gondii	Toxoplasmosis	4–6 μ	All organs	Mouth
Pneumocystis carinii	Pneumonia	0.5–1.0 μ	Lungs	Respiratory

sites in general or more commonly against a specific parasite. It may be absolute, but more often is partial. Differences in resistance have been observed in certain races—e.g., Negroes are more resistant than whites to hookworm disease and vivax malaria. Likewise, individuals vary in their resistance, and resistance usually tends to increase with age. It is difficult, however, in many instances to eliminate the possibility of acquired immunity.

Active immunity is acquired naturally by previous infection with parasites. It is often difficult to differentiate between *premunition,* a concomitant immunity due to an existing latent infection that prevents superinfection, and a true residual immunity. Parasites that are intimately associated with the tissue of the host produce the most vigorous and lasting immunity, especially after repeated or intense infections. The duration of the immunity varies with the parasite and the individual host.

Systematic immunity depends upon the production of specific antibodies, the phagocytic activity of corpuscular elements, tissue resistance, and other factors, such as body temperature, action of digestive juices, impenetrability of the skin, and physical well-being. Specific antibodies are induced by the parenteral introduction of antigens in the form of parasites or their products. The skin and reticuloendothelial

Protozoan Infections of Man (cont.)

Source of Infection, Intermediate, Host or Vector	Most Common Clinical Symptoms	Laboratory Diagnosis	Therapeutic Agents	Remarks
Kissing bug Triatomidae	Fever; spleen & liver enlarge Myocarditis	Blood smear, comp. fix., rat inoculation, F.A.T.	Primaquine Amphotericin B	Unilateral peri-orbital edema, Romaña's sign. Megaesophagus
Cysts in food & water, from feces	Mild to severe G.I. distress, dysentery	Cysts in cold stool. Trophs in purged stool	Diodoquin Paramomycin Emetine, Niri-dazole Tetracyclines Metronidazole	Consider possi-bility of hepatic infection.
"	Enlarged tender liver, fever, leukocytosis	X-ray, comp. fix., cysts or trophs in stool	Chloroquine Emetine, Niri-dazole Metronidazole	Treat intestinal amebic infec-tion.
Stool (trophs)	Abdominal dis-comfort Diarrhea	Stool exam, trophs	Diodoquin	
Stool (cyst)	Diarrhea Dysentery	Cysts & trophs in stool	Diodoquin Tetracyclines	Porcine source.
Cysts in food & water, from feces	Mild G.I. dis-tress & diar-rhea	Cysts & trophs in stool	Quinacrine Metronidazole (Flagyl)	More common in children than adults.
Trophs in va-ginal & prostatic secretion	Frothy vaginal discharge	Trophs in va-ginal & pro-static fluid	Metronidazole (Flagyl)	Treat both sex-ual partners.
Congenital, stool Infected meat? Respiratory?	Chorioretinitis Hydrocephalus Convulsions Mimics infect. mono.	Biopsy, methyl-ene blue dye test, comp. fix.	Pyrimethamine with sulfona-mides	Cerebral calcifi-cation. Asymp-tomatic infec-tions.
Respiratory?	Pneumonia	Sputum exam, comp. fix.?	Pentamidine isethionate	Premature babies. Moribund adults.

system are intimately concerned with the production of antibodies, which may re-main in the tissue cells or enter the circulation as part of the serum globulin. The complex antigenic structure of parasites gives rise to many distinct antibodies, among which are agglutinins, precipitins, lysins, antitoxins, and complement-fixing and pro-tective antibodies.

The mechanism of immunity in the host varies with the different parasites. Thus, parasitic immunity, according to the predominating type, may be classed as humoral or cellular and general or local. In humoral immunity the body fluids contain anti-bodies that destroy parasites, inhibit their development, or more rarely neutralize their toxic products. Cellular immunity comprises phagocytosis by leukocytes and by mobile or sessile cells. Opsonins, tropins, and other immune bodies stimulate the phagocytic aciton of these cells or alter the parasites so that they are susceptible to phagocytosis. Local immunity, evidently a phase of general immunity, presents a barrier to the spread and development of the parasite through an inflammatory reaction of the tissues. In man supersensitivity to a parasite may be interpreted as evidence of previous infection or contact with a parasite, and its presence may be demonstrated by intracutaneous and serologic tests.

So far, immunization against parasitic diseases has not been particularly successful, except in a few protozoan infections—such as oriental sore and animal helminth
infections—nor has it been of practical importance.

Diagnosis.   The clinical manifestations of parasitic diseases are so general that
in most instances diagnosis based upon symptomatology alone is inadequate. Although the experienced clinician may recognize the characteristic signs and symptoms of certain parasitic disease, the symptoms in atypical cases may be so confusing
that no clear clinical picture is presented. Likewise, many infections, chiefly of
helminthic origin, give few and indefinite symptoms and often are clinically indistinguishable. Final diagnosis and proper methods of treatment require the identification of the parasite in the laboratory.

Treatment.   The successful treatment of the infected patient includes medical
and surgical measures, adequate nutrition to build up general resistance, and specific
chemotherapy. The physician should also be familiar with the patient's ability to
cooperate intelligently, the sanitary environment, the epidemiology of the disease,
and the best methods of controlling the spread of the infection. No efficient antipara-
sitic drug is entirely nontoxic to man. Successful chemotherapy depends upon the
use of a drug that has a minimal toxic effect upon the tissues of the host and a lethal
action upon the parasite. New chemotherapeutic agents, largely synthetic, are being
constantly developed, and therapeutic methods are continually undergoing revision.

Prevention.   The prevention of parasitic diseases depends upon the erection of
barriers to the spread of parasites through the practical application of biologic and
epidemiologic knowledge. Almost every parasite at some time in its life cycle is susceptible to special exterminative measures. Thus, barriers may be established by
breaking such weak links in the life cycle as may exist at the departure of the parasite or its eggs from its host, during its extracorporeal existence, or at the time of its
invasion of man. The control of parasitic diseases includes the following procedures:
(1) reduction of the sources of infection in man by therapeutic measures, (2) education in personal prophylaxis to prevent dissemination of infection and to reduce
opportunities for exposure, (3) sanitary control of water, food, living and working
conditions, and waste disposal, (4) destruction or control of reservoir hosts and
vectors, and (5) erection of biologic barriers to the transmission of parasites.

The therapeutic reduction of human sources of infection is a practical measure,
but usually it is not applicable to animal reservoir hosts. Education of the general
public in personal prophylaxis and knowledge of the precautions necessary to escape
infection and to prevent its transmission to others is an effective means of combating
parasitic diseases. Public health education, however, is a slow process, particularly
in countries with limited educational facilities. Sanitary measures of waste disposal
include the establishment of sewage systems, the installation of screened sanitary
latrines, and the prohibition of untreated night soil as garden fertilizer. Food handlers, who may be carriers, require careful supervision and training in personal
hygiene. The reduction in number of intermediate hosts or vectors has made possible
the control of many parasitic diseases. Insect vectors may be controlled by the destruction of their breeding grounds, the application of insecticides, and the protection of the susceptible host by screens and repellents. Snails, the intermediate hosts
of trematodes, may be destroyed, if sufficiently segregated, by chemical and physical agents, but the destruction of such intermediate hosts as mammals and fishes is
usually impractical.

THE PROTOZOA

2

Parasitic Protozoa

BIOLOGY OF THE PROTOZOA

Protozoa are unicellular animals that occur singly or in colony formation. Each protozoon is a complete unit capable of performing the physiologic functions which in higher organisms are carried on by specialized cells. For the most part they are free living, but some are parasitic, having adapted themselves to an altered existence inside the host.

Morphology. The vital functions of the protozoa are carried out by the protoplasm, a coarsely or finely granular substance, differentiated into nucleoplasm and cytoplasm, which often consists of a thin outer ectoplasm and a voluminous inner endoplasm.

The ectoplasm functions in movement, ingestion of food, excretion, respiration, and protection. The organs of locomotion are prolongations of ectoplasm known as pseudopodia, cilia, flagella, or undulating membranes. Food may be taken in at any place in the cytoplasm or ingested at a particular point. In some species there is a definite area, the *peristome*, through which food passes directly into the *cytostome* and then through a tubelike *cytopharynx* to the endoplasm. The INFUSORIA, MASTIGOPHORA, and SPOROZOA have a cell membrane, whereas in the SARCODINA, except for the resistant cysts, there is only an ectoplastic covering.

The granular endoplasm is concerned with nutrition and, since it contains the nucleus, with reproduction. It may also contain food vacuoles, food reserves, foreign bodies, contractile vacuoles, and chromatoidal bodies. *Contractile vacuoles* function in the regulation of osmotic pressure and the elimination of waste material. In the MASTIGOPHORA there may be present a *kinetoplast* consisting of two parts, the *parabasal body* and the *blepharoplast*, from which the flagellum arises.

The nucleus is essential for maintaining and reproducing life. A nuclear membrane enevolps a fine reticulum filled with nuclear sap and chromatin. In the vesicular nucleus the chromatin is concentrated in a single mass; in the granular type it is distributed diffusely. Near the center of the nucleus is a deeply staining *karyosome*, which plays a part in promitosis. In many protozoa a *centrosome* is also present. The structure of the nucleus, particularly the arrangement of the chromatin and karyosome, helps to differentiate species. In the INFUSORIA a *macronucleus* and one or more *micronuclei* may be present. The former is believed to be concerned with the vegetative activities of the cell and the latter with the reproductive functions.

Physiology. All essential metabolic, reproductive, and protective functions are carried on either by specialized properties of the protoplasm or by structural and functional adaptations known as *organelles*.

13

Movement is employed to obtain food and to react to physical and chemical stimuli. It ranges from marked activity in the flagellates and ciliates to almost negligible action in the SPOROZOA, except during certain stages of their life cycles. Pseudopodia produce ameboid movements in the SARCODINA; cilia rhythmically propel the INFUSORIA; and flagella assisted by the undulating membrane permit the MASTIGOPHORA to move in all directions.

Protozoa respire either directly by taking in oxygen and expelling carbon dioxide or indirectly by utilizing the oxygen liberated from complex substances by the action of enzymes. Because free oxygen is rarely available in the intestine and certain tissues of the host, most parasitic protozoa have an anaerobic metabolism.

Nutrition may be affected by the absorption of liquid food, the ingestion of solid particles, or by both methods. The solid material after ingestion through the ectoplasm or cytosome is surrounded by a food vacuole, where it is converted by digestive enzymes into forms suitable for assimilation. Inorganic salts, carbohydrates, fats, proteins, vitamins, and growth accessory substances are required. The undigested particles are extruded at the surface of the body or through a specialized opening, the *cytopyge*. Some species maintain a reserve food supply.

Excretion is effected through osmotic pressure, diffusion, and precipitation. The solid and liquid wastes are discharged from the general surface or at definite locations. In some species contractile vacuoles act as excretory organs.

Protozoa secrete digestive ferments, pigments, and material for the cyst wall. Pathogenic protozoa also secrete proteolytic enzymes, hemolysins, cytolysins, and various toxic and antigenic substances.

Certain protozoa at times enter an inactive cystic state, in which they secrete a resistant membranous wall and usually undergo nuclear division. In the parasitic intestinal species, encystment is usually necessary for survival outside the body and for protection against the digestive juices of the upper gastrointestinal tract. Thus, the cyst is closely associated with passage from host to host and constitutes the infectious stage of most of the parasitic amebas, ciliates, and intestinal flagellates that are transmitted through food or water. The trophozoites or vegetative forms are easily destroyed by an unfavorable environment, but the cysts show considerable resistance.

The survival of protozoa is largely due to their highly developed reproductive powers. Reproduction in the parasitic protozoa may be asexual or sexual. In the asexual or simple fission type, characteristic of the SARCODINA, INFUSORIA, and MASTIGOPHORA, the division of the nucleus may be amitotic, mitotic, or so modified that it is not characteristic of either type. Certain species may also reproduce in the encysted state, the nucleus dividing so that upon excystation each cyst may give rise to several new trophozoites. The sexual union of two cells, *syngamy,* may precede some form of division and may be temporary or permanent. Temporary union or conjugation is a rejuvenation process in some species and a reproductive process in others.

All the intestinal parasitic amebas and ciliates, and most of the intestinal, atrial, and blood and tissue flagellates of man have been cultivated on artificial noncellular mediums usually enriched with blood, serum, and growth accessory substances. None of the parasitic SPOROZOA of man have been so cultivated, except for the slight growth of the malarial parasites in an elaborate and complex medium.

Transmission.   The life cycle and transmission of the intestinal and atrial protozoa are relatively simple. The parasites pass from host to host directly or through food and water after an extracorporeal existence. In most instances the cyst, which is capable of resisting adverse environmental conditions and the digestive juices of the upper gastrointestinal tract, is the infective form. The spore containing the sporozoites is the infective form of the intestinal SPOROZOA. Its resistant covering provides greater protection than is required by the sporozoites that are passed directly from insect vectors to man.

Most blood and tissue parasites pass an alternate existence in a vertebrate (man) and an invertebrate (insect) host, the latter acting as the transmitting agent or vector. Even when the life history involves two hosts, direct transmission without cyclic development may take place by contact or by biting and nonbiting insects. In indirect transmission the parasite undergoes cyclic development in a bloodsucking insect before it attains the infective stage. Temperature and humidity, by affecting the abundance of insect vectors and the development cycle of the parasite in the insect, are important factors in the transmission of insect-borne diseases.

Pathology and Symptomatology. Pathogenic protozoa affect the host by their multiplication, invasion, and destruction of cells, and by their toxic or enzymatic activities. The infection passes through an acute primary stage that either leads to death or develops into a chronic latent stage, at times interspersed with relapses before eventual recovery. On the other hand, from the onset it may remain at a subclinical level with or without occasional exacerbations.

Diagnosis. The clinical diagnosis of certain diseases—e.g., malaria, trypanosomiasis, and visceral leishmaniasis—may be made from characteristic symptoms, but it is difficult in atypical cases. The more important laboratory diagnosis entails obtaining and identifying the parasite by the examination of material from the intestinal tract (amebiasis) and from the blood and tissues (malaria and trypanosomiasis) by direct smears, concentration methods, cultures, and animal inoculation, as well as by indirect cutaneous and serologic tests (toxoplasmosis).

Immunity. Immunity is presented under each disease or group of diseases. Man has an innate natural resistance, independent of present or past infections, to the intestinal invasion of *Entamoeba histolytica* and *Balantidium coli* and, perhaps to a lesser degree, to the blood and tissue protozoa. For instance, a high percentage of amebic and toxoplasmic infections are on a subclinical level. Age is a factor; young children or infants are more susceptible than adults. Races and individuals show different degrees of natural resistance—e.g., the Negro is more resistant than the white race to vivax malaria. Natural resistance may be lowered by malnutrition, or concurrent bacterial or debilitating diseases.

The parasitic protozoa of the intestinal tract, as a rule, give rise to little acquired immunity as compared with that evoked by the parasites of the blood and tissues. Active immunity, which inhibits the reproductive activities of the parasite and ultimately destroys it, is acquired by a previous natural infection or by immunization with an attenuated strain. It may be dependent on a continuing low grade infection, premunition, or it may be a true residual immunity, although it is often impossible to distinguish between these types. Immunity is usually specific against a particular species or strain. The degree of immunity is a relative affair; absolute immunity is seldom found. Its duration is variable, from a few to many years depending upon the parasite. An attack of visceral or cutaneous leishmaniasis apparently gives a lasting immunity.

Prevention. The usual methods of reducing the sources of infection, blocking the channels of transmission, and protecting the susceptible host are employed. Each important disease presents problems that call for special methods. In general, the prevention of intestinal protozoan infection is largely a problem of sanitation and hygiene, and that of the blood and tissue protozoa the control of the insect vector.

3

Intestinal and Atrial Protozoa of Man

PARASITIC AMEBAS OF MAN

Members of this group of protozoa, which includes many free-living and parasitic amebas, are probably the most primitive of animal forms. Presumably, they are the close relatives of man's ancestors, many phyla removed, which lived in the mud millions of years ago. They are the conservative side of the protozoa family—not changing or participating in the evolution and ascent of man.

At least six species of amebas belonging to four genera have been definitely established as parasites of man: (1) *Entamoeba histolytica,* (2) *E. coli,* (3) *E. gingivalis,* (4) *Dientamoeba fragilis,* (5) *Endolimax nana,* and (6) *Iodamoeba bütschlii.* All live in the large intestine, except *E. gingivalis* which is found in the mouth. Only one species, *Entamoeba histolytica,* is an important pathogenic parasite of man. The differential characteristics of the six species parasitic in man are given in Table 3 and are represented graphically in Figure 1.

Commensal Amebas of Man

The identification of *E. histolytica* requires differentiation from other parasitic species, of which only *Dientamoeba fragilis* is credited with possessing any pathogenic powers. *Entamoeba polecki,* a rare incidental parasite of man, and the free-living *E. moshkovskii* and the reptilian *E. invadens,* which may be fecal contaminants, closely resemble *E. histolytica* morphologically.

Dientamoeba fragilis is a small parasitic ameba of the intestinal tract that is found only as a trophozoite. It differs from the other intestinal amebas in that it has, generally, two nuclei (in about two-thirds of the these organisms). It can be recognized only in fresh liquid or soft stools; identification is based on its small size, two nuclei, circular appearance at rest, rapid action of the multiple leaf-shaped pseudopodia that give it a stellate appearance, and its explosive disintegration in water. Some may engorge red blood cells. Its incidence is variable, averaging about 4 percent. In some individuals it produces a moderate persistent diarrhea and gastrointestinal symptoms, but in most persons there is no apparent harmful effect.

Endolimax nana, an intestinal commensal, has an incidence of 10 to 20 percent throughout the world. It is identified by its small size, sluggish movements, characteristic nuclei, and quadrinucleated cyst of irregular shape.

Iodamoeba bütschlii is an intestinal commensal with an incidence of about 8 percent. It is identified by the characteristic nucleus, irregular shape, and large glycogen body of its uninucleated cyst.

Entamoeba coli is a parasite of the large intestine with a cosmopolitan incidence of 10 to 30 percent. Its life cycle is similar to that of *E. histolytica.* It is of medical

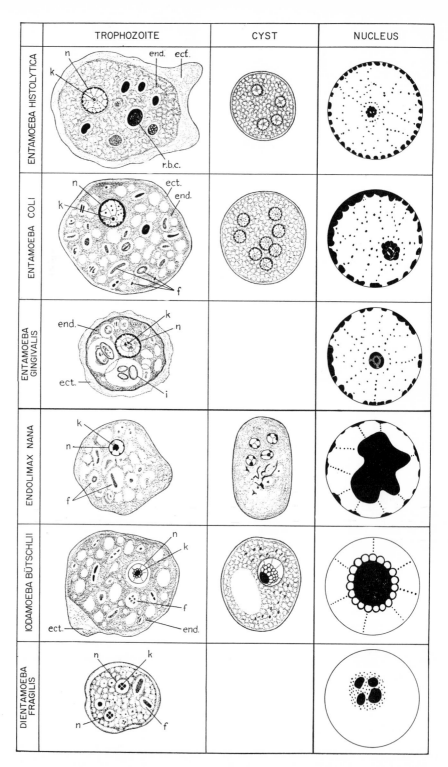

Fig. 1. Comparative morphology of the amebas of man and schematic representation of their nuclei. Trophozoites and cysts of *Entamoeba histolytica, E. coli,* and *E. gingivalis* and of *Endolimax nana, Iodamoeba bütschlii,* and *Dientamoeba fragilis.*

ect., ectoplasm; end., endoplasm; f, food vacuoles; i, inclusion nuclei; k, karyosome; n, nucleus; r.b.c., red blood cells.

Table 3. Differential Characteristics of Amebas Living in Man

Characteristics	Entamoeba histolytica	Entamoeba coli	Entamoeba gingivalis	Endolimax nana	Iodamoeba bütschlii	Dientamoeba fragilis
TROPHOZOITE						
Size (microns) Average	20	25	15	8	11	9
Range	10–60	10–50	5–35	6–15	6–20	5–12
Inclusions Red blood cells	Present	Absent	Present at times	Absent	Absent	Usually absent
Bacteria & other material	Absent in fresh specimens	Present, abundant	Present, abundant	Present	Present	Present
Vacuoles	Scanty	Numerous	Numerous	Numerous	Numerous	Numerous
Pseudopodia	Blade or finger-shaped, hyaline, formed rapidly	Blunt, usually granular, formed slowly	Usually blunt, hyaline, often formed rapidly	Blunt, hyaline, usually formed slowly	Blunt or finger-like, hyaline, formed slowly	Leaf-like, hyaline, formed rapidly, multiple
Motility	Active progression in definite direction	Sluggish, usually not progressive	Moderately active, progressive	Sluggish, moderately progressive	Sluggish, slightly progressive	Active, progressive
CYST						
Size (microns) Average	Variable	17	No cysts demonstrated	9	10	No cysts demonstrated
Range	5–20	10–33		5–14	5–18	
Glycogen in young cysts (iodine treated)	Diffuse, mahogany brown	Large mass, ill-defined, dark brown		Usually absent, diffuse, ill-defined, brownish	Usually present, large mass, compact, dark brown	
Chromatoid bodies	Often present, large bars or thick rod-like masses	Sometimes present, splinter-like with square or pointed ends		Occasionally small spherical or elongated granules	Usually absent, small granules	
Nuclei (No.)	1–4 rarely more	1–8 rarely more		1–4 rarely more	1, rarely 2	

importance only because it may be mistaken for *E. histolytica*. Certain differential characteristics from *E. histolytica* (Table 3) should be emphasized. *Entamoeba coli* has (1) a more granular endoplasm containing ingested bacteria and debris; it rarely, if ever, contains red blood cells; (2) a narrower, less differentiated ectoplasm; (3) broader and blunter pseudopodia; (4) more sluggish indeterminate movements; (5) heavier, irregular peripheral chromatin and a large eccentric karyosome in the nucleus; and (6) larger cysts with more granular cytoplasm, slender, splinter-like chromatoidal bodies, and as many as eight nuclei.

Entamoeba gingivalis is a nonpathogenic inhabitant of the mouth, being present chiefly in the tartar of the teeth and gingival pockets. Its most striking characteristic is the large number of food vacuoles and dark-staining bodies derived from the nuclei of degenerated cells in the cytoplasm. Its incidence ranges from 10 percent in persons with healthy mouths to 95 percent in those with diseased teeth and gums.

Soil-Water Amebas Causing Meningoencephalitis in Man

A species of amebas of the genus *Naegleria* has been isolated and cultured from patients who died of meningoencephalitis. *Naegleria* is a free-living organism, which has both an ameboid and a flagellate stage. It is found in stagnant water and often is coprozoic. Twenty cases of amebic encephalitis due to *Naegleria* and *Hartmanella* (*Acanthamoeba*) have been reported from Florida, Virginia, Texas, and Australia since 1964, when the first infection was described. The symptoms frequently developed soon after the victim had been swimming in warm, still waters of lakes, ponds, or backwater bays. The ameba has been isolated and cultured from some of these waters. From the nasal mucosa, the amebas presumably penetrate the cribiform plate and multiply in the gray matter of the brain. Severe frontal headache, fever, sore throat, and blocked nose were followed by the central nervous system involvement. Altered taste and smell may be present, as well as a stiff neck and Kernig's sign. The white blood cell count may be as high

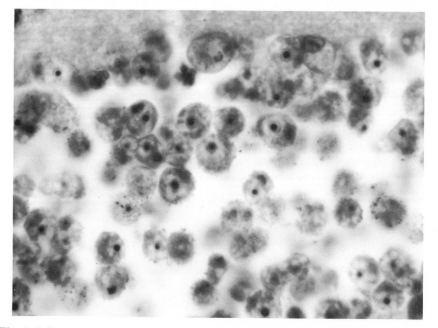

Fig. 2. Soil amebas (*Naegleria*) showing characteristic large karyosomes and sharp cytoplasmic outlines, from olfactory trigone in 16 year old white male. (Courtesy of Dr. Cecil G. Butt.)

as 24,000/cu mm with 92 percent neutrophils and 7 percent lymphocytes. The spinal fluid is purulent and may contain many red blood cells and motile amebas. Death of the patient usually follows within 4 to 5 days after the onset of symptoms. At autopsy the amebas are abundant in the purulent exudate, the necrotic areas, and in the perivascular spaces (Fig. 2). In 1968, 16 cases of acute purulent meningo-encephalitis occurring between 1962 and 1965 in Bohemia were reported. Death came in 2 to 7 days after onset of the illness and *Acanthamebae* were found in the brain at autopsy. Seven days before the onset of illness all 16 patients had bathed in an indoor swimming pool.

Treatment with sulfadiazine, chloroquine, emetine and antibiotics has proven ineffective.

Hartmanella amebae have been cultured from the spinal fluid of a child with fever, stiff neck, and lethargy, who subsequently recovered. This suggests that the soil-water group of amebas may be the cause of unrecognized infections. In view of the widespread geographic distribution of the soil-water amebas, it is not un-likely that their infection of man is worldwide.

Entamoeba histolytica

Disease.   Amebiasis, amebic dysentery, amebic hepatitis.

In 1875 Lösch discovered *E. histolytica* in the feces of a Russian with severe dysentery; he also experimentally produced intestinal lesions in a dog. However, the association of the parasite with dysentery was not definitely established until the investigations of Kartulis in 1887. In 1901 Councilman and Lafleur made their important study of the pathology of amebic dysentery and hepatic abscess. Schaudinn, of spirochete fame, differentiated *E. histolytica* from *E. coli* in 1903. In 1913 Walker and Sellards definitely established the pathogenicity of *E. histolytica* by feeding cysts to volunteers, thus furnishing the basis of our present concept of its host-parasite relation in respect to clinical infection.

Morphology and Physiology.   *E. histolytica* may be observed in the feces as: (1) trophozoite, (2) precyst, and (3) cyst (Table 3, Fig. 3).

The trophozoite or active vegetative *E. histolytica* (Fig. 3) is distinguished from the other intestinal amebas by morphologic characteristics of diagnostic importance. It ranges in size from 10 to 60 μ, but the majority are from 15 to 30 μ. The wide, clear, refractile, hyaline ectoplasm, sharply separated from the endoplasm, constitutes about one-third of the entire animal. The thin, finger-like, ectoplasmic pseudopodia are extended rapidly. The finely granular endoplasm usually contains no bacteria or foreign particles, but sometimes includes red blood cells in various stages of disintegration. The single eccentric nucleus may be faintly discerned as a finely granular ring in the unstained ameba. Hematoxylin staining reveals a clearly defined nuclear membrane, the inner surface of which is lined with uniform and closely packed fine granules of chromatin (Fig. 3). The small, deeply staining, centrally located karyosome consists of several granules in a halo-like capsule, from which a linin network of fine fibrils radiates toward the periphery of the nucleus. De-generating trophozoites show sluggish motility, a fading line of demarcation between ectoplasm and endoplasm, a more granular cytoplasm, and a more distinct nucleus.

The precystic amebas (Fig. 3) are colorless, round or oval cells that are smaller than the trophozoite, but larger than the cyst; they are devoid of food inclusions. Pseudopodial action is sluggish, and there is no progressive movement.

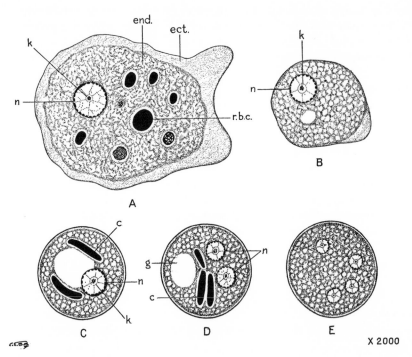

Fig. 3. Schematic representation of *Entamœba histolytica*. A, trophozoite containing red blood cells undergoing digestion B, precystic ameba devoid of cytoplasmic inclusions; C, young uninucleate cyst; D, binucleate cyst; E, mature quadrinucleate cyst.

c, chromatoid bodies; ect., ectoplasm; end., endoplasm; g, glycogen vacuole; k, karyosome; n, nucleus; r.b.c., red blood cells.

The cysts (Fig. 3 and 140) are round or oval, slightly asymmetrical hyaline bodies with a smooth, refractile, nonstaining wall about 0.5 μ thick. The great variation in size, from 5 to 20 μ, has been attributed to the existence of large and small cyst races. The cytoplasm of the young cysts contains vacuoles with glycogen and dark-staining, refractive, sausage-shaped bars with rounded ends. These chromatoid bodies, which are reported to contain ribonucleic and desoxyribonucleic acid and phosphates, tend to disappear as the cyst matures, so that they may be absent in about one-half of the cysts. Both types of cytoplasmic inclusions are believed to represent stored food. The immature cyst has a single nucleus, about one-third of its diameter, while the mature infective cyst contains four smaller nuclei, rarely more. Thus, cysts containing from one to four nuclei may be passed in the feces.

The habitat of the trophozoite is the wall and lumen of the colon, especially in the cecal and sigmoidorectal regions. It multiplies by binary fission, the nucleus dividing by a modified mitosis. Reproduction also takes place through cyst formation, eight amebulae being produced by the metacystic amebas after excystation. Encystment is essential for transmission, since only the mature cyst is infectious. *E. histolytica* grows best in an anaerobic environment or under reduced oxygen tension. It synthesizes protoplasmic compounds from nutritional substances by the action of various enzymes, such as alkaline phosphatase. It produces a glutaminase which is activated by phosphate but not chloride, but it does not produce collagenase in vitro. The organism may be capable of utilizing extracellular dextrose. Amylolytic activity has been demonstrated in cultures. Waste products in soluble or granular form are eliminated in excretory vacuoles at the surface, while undigested particles are egested through ectoplasmic protuberances.

The ameba absorbs nourishment from the tissues dissolved by its cytolytic enzymes and ingests red blood cells, hemoglobin, substances partially synthesized by the host, and fragments of tissues through pseudopodial encirclement. It can ingest bacterial and particulate fecal elements from the intestine. Improved methods of cultivation have increased our knowledge of the biologic characteristics, nutritive requirements, viability, life cycle, and pathogenicity of *E. histolytica*. As a rule, the rich, complex mediums foster the best growth; optimal growth occurs at 37° C, at pH 7.0, and under anaerobic conditions.

In cultures amebas obtain their nourishment mostly from the soluble ingredients of the medium and from the material synthesized by the bacteria. The mechanism of the symbiotic association with bacteria is not fully understood, but the bacterial associates furnish many growth factors for the complex nutritional requirements of the ameba. The best growth is obtained with a mixed flora, but single species—e.g., *Streptobacillus*—promotes the growth of certain strains. Penicillin and streptomycin are useful in reducing bacterial overgrowth and in increasing the percentage of positive diagnostic cultures. In metabolic studies of *E. histolytica,* bacteria have been successfully replaced by *Trypanosoma cruzi* which led to axenic cultures. Growth in tissue cultures using chick embryo cells and frequent transplants has been successful.

Trophozoites are more easily destroyed than cysts. In feces they can survive for 5 hours at 37° C, 16 hours at 25° C, and 96 hours at 5° C. The resistant cysts die in 5 minutes at 50° C. They withstand freezing temperatures, but succumb to desiccation and putrefaction. They survive in feces or in feces diluted with water for 2 days at 37° C, 9 days at 22° C, and 60 days at O° C. Below freezing the survival time decreases rapidly; at −28° C it is less than 7 hours, death probably resulting from crystallization of the water molecules in the protoplasm.

The cysticidal action of physical and chemical agents, particularly chlorine, has received the attention of epidemiologists. Under ideal conditions, 4 ppm of free chlorine will destroy cysts in from 15 to 30 minutes, but length of exposure, number of cysts, temperature, hydrogen-ion concentration, and organic material in the water modify its cysticidal action, which is dependent upon the combination of the chlorine with the cellular proteins. Thus, the difficulty in standardizing environmental conditions precludes dependence upon chlorination for the protection of water supplies, since even 2 ppm of residual chlorine at times may be insufficient to destroy cysts. Cysts are killed by 0.04 percent mercuric chloride, 1 percent phenol, and 5 percent formalin.

Strains.   The small (under 10 μ) and large (over 10 μ) cyst races or strains have been designated as *minuta* and *magna* varieties, respectively. The proportion of the small strain, sometimes known as *E. hartmanni,* is reported to be higher in the temperate zones than in the tropics. *E. hartmanni* is considered by some authorities to be a separate species. The trophozoites of the small strain ingest bacteria rather than red blood cells and are more uniform in size, less actively motile, have a more distinct nucleus, and are less pathogenic than those of the large strains. On the basis of nonpathogenicity to animals, symptomless carriers, and the ingestion of bacteria, the idea has been advanced that *E. histolytica* has a commensal phase and that most healthy carriers harbor the *minuta* variety. On the other hand, size and pathogenicity are insecure criteria for the establishment of races: small strains have been reported to change to large during cultivation or animal passage; some small strains have produced intestinal ulcers in laboratory animals; and both strains have been observed in the same person. Strains often show little correlation in size, virulence, invasiveness, and cultivability. Pathogenicity depends not merely upon the strain but also upon accessory factors, such as bacteria, diet, and resistance of the host.

Life Cycle.   The life history of *E. histolytica* is comparatively simple. The resistant infective cysts, formed in the lumen of the large intestine, pass out in the feces, and after an extracorporeal existence are ingested by a new host (Fig. 4). Few if any cysts are voided in acute dysentery, but they predominate in chronic infections and carriers. Man is the principal host and source of infection; other mammals are a negligible source. Spontaneous natural infections with amebas indistinguishable from *E. histolytica* have been reported in monkeys, dogs, hogs, and rats, and experimental infections have been established in kittens, puppies, monkeys, and laboratory rodents. On ingestion only the mature cysts, which are resistant to the acidic digestive juices of the stomach, pass to the lower part of the small intestine. Here, under the influence of the neutral or alkaline digestive juices and the activity of the ameba, the cyst wall disintegrates, liberating a four-nucleated metacystic ameba that ultimately divides into eight small trophozoites. These small immature amebas move downward to the large intestine. Intestinal stasis often enables the amebas to establish a site of infection in the cecal region of the colon, but they may be swept along to the sigmoidorectal region or even out of the body. The chances of establishing a foothold in the intestinal epithelium are reduced when the organisms are few, the volume of food large, or there is intestinal hypermotility. Thus, the massive and frequent doses acquired in endemic areas are of epidemiologic importance.

Epidemiology.   The actual incidence of amebiasis throughout the world, especially in the temperate zone, remains unknown. Surveys indicate that the incidence of infection throughout the world varies from 0.2 to 50 percent and is directly correlated with sanitary conditions, which are especially poor in tropical and subtropical

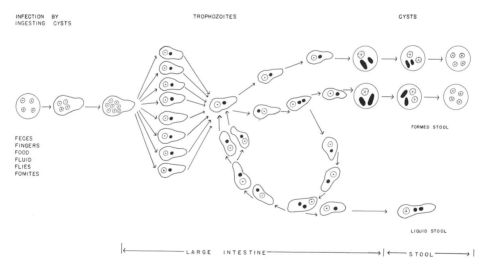

Fig. 4. Life cycle of *Entamœba histolytica*.

areas. It is endemic in civilian and military groups and is particularly prevalent in mental hospitals, children's homes, and prisons. The lower economic classes show a high incidence, probably because of malnutrition, overcrowding, and insanitary environment.

The main source of infection is the cyst-passing chronic patient or asymptomatic carrier. Acutely ill patients are not important, and reservoir hosts play a negligible role. Cysts reach man through water and vegetables contaminated with infective feces, through food contaminated by flies or the hands of infected food handlers, or by direct transmission by cyst carriers. Examination for fingerprints of pats of butter served at home or in public gives evidence of the amount of contact human hands have with our food. The artistically arranged fruit salads can only result from human hand contact. Circumstantial evidence overwhelmingly incriminates water as a vehicle of transmission. In 1933 two Chicago, Ill., hotels experienced inadvertent connections between their water supply and sewage which resulted in 1,400 clinical infections and over 100 deaths from amebiasis. Wells and springs, which in small rural communities are often exposed to contamination with local sewage, may serve to spread the infection. Contaminated food is the most satisfactory explanation for the widespread distribution of amebic infection. Vegetables and fruits may be contaminated by night soil or polluted water, and other foods and utensils by flies and foodhandlers. Viable cysts have been recovered from the vomitus, feces, and bodies of flies. Small epidemics in the tropics have been attributed to flies or other insects, particularly in military or civilian camps. The connection between foodhandlers and infected food is difficult to prove. Infection may be transmitted by direct contact where there is close association in home and institutional groups under insanitary and unhygienic conditions. Intrafamilial transmission in the average home environment in the United States is minimal. However, an infected mother who prepares her family's food is a potential source of infection. There appears to be a correlation between the presence of *E. histolytica, E. nana, G. lamblia,* and viral infectious hepatitis in missionaries abroad. The chief factor in the transmission of amebiasis is the cyst passer, who is either a known chronic, relapsing or latent convalescent patient, or an unrecognized asymptomatic carrier. The latter presents a perplexing public health problem. The carrier is a potential danger, and his detection and treatment is of epidemiologic importance. Surveys to detect the numerous carriers are economically impracticable, but known convalescent patients and carriers should be treated.

Pathology The lesions produced by *E. histolytica* are primarily intestinal and secondarily extraintestinal. The intestinal lesions, except for a few in the terminal portion of the ileum, are confined to the large intestine. The most frequent primary sites are the cecal and sigmoidorectal region, where the colonic flow is slow; less frequently the site is the ascending colon, rectum, sigmoid, or appendix. As the infection progresses, additional colonic sites of invasion develop. Secondary systemic invasion may occur in patients with clinical dysentery or in those with mild or latent infections. As would be expected, the liver is most frequently involved, but nearly every organ of the body may be affected.

It has been postulated that *E. histolytica,* particularly the *minuta* variety, is normally a harmless, lumen-inhabiting commensal which, under certain circumstances, becomes a tissue-invading pathogen. In the temperate zone, in at least 90 percent of the infections the equilibrium between parasite and host is so well balanced that there is an absence of definite clinical symptoms.

The pathogenic activities of *E. histolytica* depend upon: (1) the resistance of the host, (2) the virulence and invasiveness of the amebic strain, and (3) the conditions in the intestinal tract. Resistance depends on innate immunity, state of nutrition, and freedom from infectious and debilitating diseases. There is considerable evidence that virulence varies with the strain. In culture it declines, but may be restored or enhanced by serial passage in animals. Virulence, invasiveness, the number of the amebas, and local conditions in the intestinal tract—where invasion is facilitated by a carbohydrate diet, physical or chemical injury of the mucosa, stasis, and particularly the bacterial flora—are important in determining the extent of the intestinal ulceration. The importance of concomitant bacteria in producing pathogenic infections has been demonstrated repeatedly both in animals and man. Germ-free guinea pigs fail to develop lesions, while a high percentage of control animals show ulcerations. The associated bacteria may stimulate the invasive powers of the ameba or produce favorable conditions for invasion.

The early lesion is a tiny area of necrosis in the superficial mucosa or a small nodular elevation with a minute opening that leads to a flask-shaped cavity containing cytolyzed cells, mucus, and amebas. In most infections the early lesions develop into small, round or oval ulcers that are formed in the mucosa by erosion or the discharge of a small abscess. In the infected individuals who develop acute or chronic dysentery, there is rapid lateral and downward extension of the ulcerative processes to both the superficial and deep layers of the intestine. The lesions vary from small, punctate, crateriform ulcers, distributed over the mucosa like craters in a bombed field; to large, irregular ulcers with undermined edges and necrotic gelatinous bases, often covered with a yellow, purulent, leathery membrane; and even to large areas of necrosis, which at times encircle the bowel. The typical flask-like primary ulcer has a crateriform appearance with a wide base and narrow opening with irregular, slightly elevated, overhanging edges (Fig. 5). As the process invades the submucosa and extends laterally along the axis of the intestine, the dissolution of the tissues may become so extensive that communicating sinuses produce honey-combed areas beneath apparently intact mucosa that may eventually slough off, exposing large necrotic areas. Destruction of tissue is followed by regenerative proliferation of connective tissue, which, in cases of extensive damage, may ultimately cause a fibrous thickening of the intestinal wall.

The histologic changes include histolysis, thrombosis of the capillaries, petechial hemorrhages, round-cell infiltration, and necrosis. The process is regenerative rather

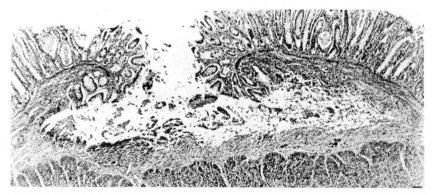

Fig. 5. *Entamœba histolytica* in the large intestine. Notice the flask-shaped ulcer.

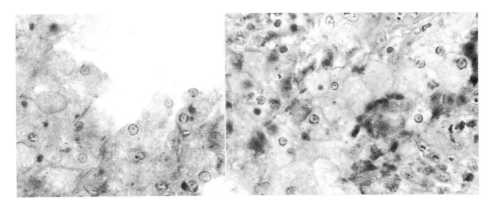

Fig. 6. *Entamœba histolytica* in intestinal mucosa.

than inflammatory; signs of inflammation other than hyperemia and edema are usually absent unless secondary bacterial infection supervenes. Red blood cells are abundant because of the destruction of small blood vessels. The amebas may be found in the floor of the ulcer, particularly at the base of the intestinal glands, or scattered through the tissues (Fig. 6). Extensive ulceration is invariably accompanied by secondary bacterial infection, which tends to confuse the histologic picture as well as to intensify the destructive process.

The complications of intestinal amebiasis include appendicitis, perforation, hemorrhage, stricture, granulomas, and pseudopolyposes. In amebic appendicitis, the appendix is nongangrenous, slightly thickened, and has irregular superficial ulcers in the mucosa. Amebic appendicitis or typhlitis contraindicates surgical interference without antiamebic treatment. Intestinal perforations occur most frequently in the cecum, and the erosion of a large blood vessel may produce a massive hemorrhage. Strictures are usually confined to the cecum or sigmoid and occasionally the rectum, but complete stenosis is rare. Amebic granulomas (ameboma) are firm, painful, movable, nodular, inflammatory thickenings of the intestinal wall around an ulcer, occurring most commonly in the cecum or sigmoid in a small percentage of infections. Histologically they show collagen, fibroblasts, and chronic inflammatory and granulation elements. They may be confused with neoplastic growths, or tuberculous or actinomycotic granulomas, but may be diagnosed by biopsy, serologically or antiamebic treatment.

In systemic amebiasis the liver is invaded chiefly and other organs less frequently (Fig. 7A). Dissemination from the primary intestinal focus is chiefly metastatic, but at times occurs by direct extension. There are authentic records of amebiasis of lung, brain, spleen, genitalia, and skin, and more questionable reports of involvement of kidneys, urinary bladder, testes, and other tissues. The syndrome known as "diffuse amebic hepatitis," characterized by a large tender liver and once considered a phase preliminary to abscess formation, is now regarded by several investigators as not indicative solely of amebic invasion but also as representing a nonspecific reaction of the liver to the bacteria, debris, toxins, and other noxious material resulting from intestinal ulceration. A very high percentage of persons with chronic amebic colitis showed impaired metabolic and secretory activity of the liver.

The early liver abscess is a small, oval or rounded mass with a grayish-brown matrix of necrosed hepatic cells. As it increases in size the center liquefies, the wall

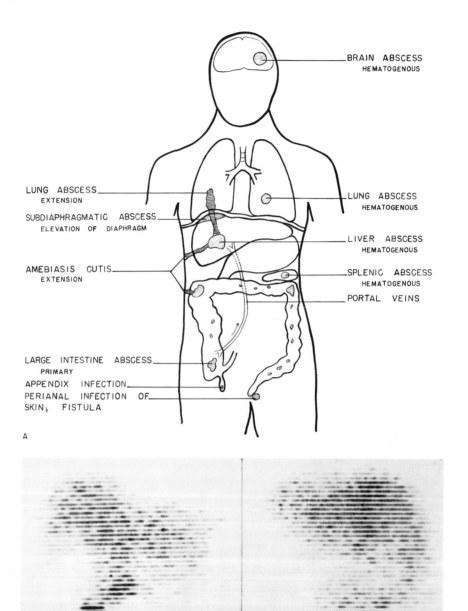

Fig. 7. Amebiasis. A, Sites of leisons; B and C, Liver abscess and photoscan of liver using Rose Bengal I[131]. B, Anterior scan: area of diminished uptake of radioactive material. C, lateral scan: shows abscess lies posteriorly. (*J.A.M.A.,* 187: 709, fig. 1, 1964. Courtesy of B. M. Schuman, M. A. Block, R. E. Eyler, and L. DuSault.)

thickens, and the contents become a viscid chocolate, reddish, or cream-colored mass of autolyzed hepatic cells, red blood cells, bile, fat, and other products of tissue disintegration, interspersed with strands of connective tissue. Occasionally, it becomes inspissated and is absorbed or calcified. Hepatic abscesses may be single or multiple and acute or chronic. The condition may arise from subclinical, as well as symptomatic, intestinal amebiasis. Amebas have been demonstrated in the stool of approximately one-third of the patients with hepatic amebiasis; careful search would probably disclose more. Approximately 85 percent of the abscesses are confined to the right lobe of the liver with a predilection for the posterior portion of the dome, thus causing an upward bulging of the diaphragm. Males are chiefly affected. At times there is secondary bacterial invasion. Multiple hepatic amebic abscesses are not uncommon, even in children, and left lobe involvement facilitates pericardial invasion.

Pulmonary amebiasis, although infrequent, ranks next to liver abscess in rate of occurrence. It usually results from direct extension of an hepatic abscess, and less frequently from emboli. The pulmonary abscess, often secondarily infected with bacteria, appears as a pneumonic consolidation in the lower right lung. Abscess of the brain is a rare complication usually associated with hepatic and pulmonary amebiasis; splenic abscess is even more rare. Ulcerative vaginitis and cervicitis, involvement of the penis and prostate, and questionable urinary infections are due chiefly to spread from the rectal area.

Secondary cutaneous lesions in the form of indolent indurated ulcers with overhanging edges occur in the perianal region or at the sites of intestinal or hepatic fistulas. Chronic ulcers of the rectum may cause hemorrhoids, fissures, fistulas, and anorectal abscesses.

Symptomatology. The clinical response is exceedingly variable, depending upon the location and intensity of the infection. Outright dysenteric disease develops in but a small proportion of infected individuals. Secondary bacterial invasion may account for a considerable proportion of the symptoms, which may be vague and unlocalized despite extensive lesions. Subclinical chronic infections may persist for years with or without occasional exacerbations, at times leaving in their wake an irritable colon or postdysenteric colitis (Fig. 8)

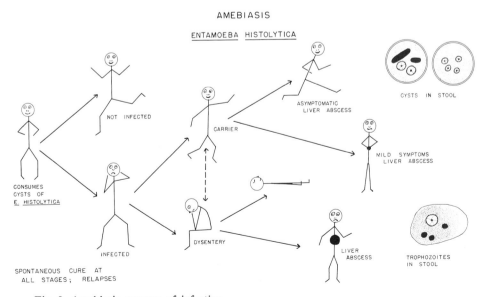

Fig. 8. Amebiasis, courses of infection.

Asymptomatic infections are most common, especially in the temperate zone. These so-called healthy carriers may be passing millions of cysts per day, presumably from trophozoite multiplication in the intestinal lumen. The vague abdominal discomfort, weakness, and neurasthenia reported by some patients may be related to the infection. The next stage of the infection is characterized by a syndrome which lacks specificity. These patients have moderate, though definite, malaise. Constipation may alternate with mild diarrhea. Irregular colicky abdominal pain with or without local abdominal tenderness is present, indicating mucosal invasion by the parasite.

Acute intestinal amebiasis has an incubation period of from 1 to 14 weeks. There is severe dysentery with numerous small stools containing blood, mucus, and shreds of necrotic mucosa, and accompanied by acute abdominal pain and tenderness, and fever of 100 to 102° F. Dehydration, toxemia, and prostration may be marked. A leukocytosis of 7,000 to 20,000/cu mm is not uncommon and may be a reflection of superimposed bacterial infection. Trophozoites of *E. histolytica* are found in the stools.

Chronic amebiasis is characterized by recurrent attacks of dysentery with intervening periods of mild or moderate gastrointestinal disturbances and constipation. Localized abdominal tenderness is present, and the liver may be enlarged. In longstanding infections, psychoneurotic disturbances may be present. This chronic debilitating disease leads to marked weight loss and cachexia. Ulcerative colitis, carcinoma of the large intestine, and diverticulitis must be considered in the differential diagnosis.

Hepatic amebiasis which includes amebic hepatitis and abscess of the liver is the most common and a grave complication of intestinal amebiasis. Hepatic amebiasis is due to metastasis of the infection from the intestinal mucosa by way of the portal blood stream. Amebic hepatitis is characterized by an enlarged, tender liver with pain in the upper right hypochondrium which may radiate to the right shoulder. The signs and symptoms of amebic abscess of the liver are very similar to, though usually more severe than, those of amebic hepatitis. Leukocytosis of 10,000 to 16,000/cu mm with 78 to 80 percent polymorphonuclear neutrophils helps distinguish it from viral hepatitis. The erythrocyte sedimentation rate may be elevated. Fever is common and chills may occur. The thymol turbidity test is often normal, but the bromsulfalein test and alkaline phosphatase determination may show some elevation. Mild jaundice is present in an occasional patient. Elevation and relative immobility of the right diaphragm and severe pain referred to the right shoulder are often present. The abscess may extend through the diaphragm into the lungs or rupture through the abdominal wall.

Hepatic amebiasis occasionally is present for a considerable time without the classic signs and symptoms and may be very difficult to diagnose.

Pulmonary amebiasis is characterized by chills, fever, leukocytosis, and evidence of pulmonary consolidation.

Amebic infections of the brain give the usual signs and symptoms of brain abscess or tumor. Unfortunately, these infections have only been diagnosed at autopsy.

Prognosis depends upon early and efficient treatment, and the duration and type of the disease. It is good with early treatment, but is less favorable if there have been recurrent attacks. Modern therapeutics yields a high percentage of cures, but irrespective of the type of treatment, relapses occur. Persons subject to continuous exposure and secondary bacterial infections in an endemic environment have little chance of permanent cure. The prognosis for patients with hepatic abscess is less favorable, and is grave for those with pulmonary and cerebral abscesses.

Diagnosis.   The final diagnosis of amebiasis rests upon the identification of the parasite in the feces or tissues. All available methods should be exhausted before accepting a clinical diagnosis. On the other hand, diagnosis by therapy must be resorted to occasionally.

The clinical diagnosis of intestinal amebiasis requires differentiation from other dysenteries and intestinal diseases, and that of hepatic abscess from hydatid cyst, gallbladder infection, malignancy, and pulmonary disease. Clinical diagnosis is based on a history of residence in an endemic area, typical gastrointestinal and general signs and symptoms on physical examination, sigmoidoscopy, and roentgenology. With the sigmoidoscope it is possible to recognize the classic ulcerative or congestive granular petechial lesions; however, the picture is not always pathognomonic, and sigmoidoscopic diagnosis should always be supplemented by the microscopic examination of aspirated or biopsied specimens. Roentgenology is useful in detecting the shagginess of localized areas in colitis, cecal deformities, inflammatory amebomas, and strictures in intestinal amebiasis, and in defining abnormalities above and below the right diaphragm in hepatic and pulmonary abscesses (Figs. 7B and C). Bacillary dysentery may be distinguished by its acute onset, short incubation, fever, leukocytosis, epidemic character, lack of response to antiamebic drugs, and type of stool.

Laboratory diagnosis (See Chap. 18 for details) may be made by the microscopic or cultural identification of the parasite in the feces or tissues. Its microscopic detection depends upon the proper collection of material and the diligent examination of carefully prepared smears or sections. Diagnosis is not always easy and requires repeated examinations, especially in chronic cases. Failure may result from faulty technic, inadequate search, or confusion of *E. histolytica* with other protozoa, cells, or artifacts.

The following schedule outlines the usual diagnostic procedures in the order in which they should be undertaken. In intestinal amebiasis no one method is superior, and the best results are obtained by their combination (Page 321).

Intestinal Amebiasis
  Examination of feces by direct smears
    Diarrheic or fluid feces for trophozoites
      Examine material from fresh warm feces in saline mount
      Feces obtained after magnesium sulfate or phosphosoda purge given in the morning on an empty stomach. Examine both formed and liquid specimens. Do not purge pregnant women or patients with right lower quadrant pain.
      Permanent mounts with trichrome, Lawless, or iron hematoxylin stains
    Solid or formed feces for cysts (carriers or chronic patients)
      Examine in saline or iodine mounts, especially shreds of mucus or flecks of blood on formed feces
      Concentration methods (See Page 323)
    If local laboratory facilities are not available, feces may be preserved in P.V.A. or M.I.F. fixative and sent to the nearest laboratory (See Page 321)
  Sigmoidoscope examination (one-third of the lesions are in sigmoidorectal region)
    Visual for lesions
    Material aspirated with plastic tube examined immediately for trophozoites

    Biopsy specimens
Culture
    Trophozoites or cysts from feces
    Material collected through sigmoidoscope
Hemagglutination, precipitin tests
Hepatic Amebiasis
    Determine presence of intestinal amebiasis
    Leukocyte count
    Hemagglutination test, precipitin tests
    Roentgenology, an important aid in clinical diagnosis; liver scintillation scan
    Liver function tests, especially bromsulfalein and alkaline phosphatase
    Chemotherapeutic trial
    Aspiration of abscess
        Characteristic chocolate-colored contents
        Trophozoites recovered in about one-third of cases, best obtained from wall
            of abcess if surgical drainage is employed

    The character of the feces in intestinal amebiasis is sometimes of confirmatory value, particularly in differentiating from bacillary dysentery. The typical amebic stool is acidic, and consists of copious fecal material, scanty cellular exudate, blood from small amounts to actual hemorrhage with degenerated erythrocytes often in adhesive masses, few polymorphonuclear neutrophils or epithelial cells, numerous pyknotic residues, Charcot-Leyden crystals, few bacteria, and amebas. The typical bacillary dysentery stool is offensive, alkaline, and consists of scant fecal material, massive cellular exudate, varying amounts of blood, erythrocytes usually unaltered, numerous polymorphonuclear neutrophils and epithelial cells, few pyknotic residues, no Charcot-Leyden crystals, no pathogenic amebas, and numerous bacteria.

    The parasite may be identified as trophozoites in the liquid stools of patients with acute dysentery and in aspirated material, and as cysts in the formed stools of chronic patients and carriers. *E. histolytica* requires differentiation from free-living amebas contaminating feces and from *E. coli* and the other parasitic amebas of man (Table 3). In fresh, warm feces the trophozoites are identified by their active, progressive, directional movements, sharply defined ectoplasm, blade-like hyaline pseudopodia, indistinct nucleus, and partly disintegrated ingested red blood cells. The cysts are distinguished by the presence of one to four nuclei, diffuse glycogen mass, and large chromatoidal bodies. Failure to find cysts is not conclusive evidence of the absence of infection, since their number may fluctuate from day to day, from none to 6,000,000 per gram of feces. Positive results can only be obtained, even after four or more examinations, in a minority of persons who pass less than 100,000 cysts per day. The chances of finding cysts in infected persons by direct smears of formed stools are about 20 percent for one examination, and 50 percent for three; six or more tests may be required to establish a reliable diagnosis. When combined with concentration methods, the chances are increased to 30 to 50 percent for one examination.

    Cultural methods frequently reveal the presence of *E. histolytica* when microscopic examination has failed. The number of positive cultures is increased by the addition of penicillin and streptomycin to reduce bacterial overgrowth, the use of fresh fecal specimens, and by the examination of the culture sediment after fixation in polyvinyl alcohol (P.V.A.). The precipitin test is of supportive value in hepatic amebiasis. The indirect hemagglutination test is positive in 96 percent of those patients with hepatic abscesses, and it is usually positive in those with clinically recognized intestinal infections, and remains so for several months after successful therapy. Asymptomatic infections often give a negative reaction.

Treatment. In severe dysenteric infections with fever and prostration, patients should remain in bed and receive a bland high-protein and high-vitamin diet with adequate fluids. Sedation will ensure rest. The effect of chemotherapy includes (1) the relief of the acute attack, (2) destruction of the trophozoites in the intestinal mucosa and lumen, and (3) control of secondary bacterial infection.

For acute amebic dysentery, three to five days of emetine hydrochloride (cardiotoxic) therapy given subcutaneously is usually effective in controlling the dysentery but generally does not eliminate the infection. Therefore diiodohydroxyquinoline (Diodoquin) is given concurrently to completely cure the infection. This may be followed by a course of paromomycin or a tetracycline. Recently, metronidazole (Flagyl) 800 mg t.i.d. for 10 days has proven curative in acute amebic dysentery and liver abscess. Niridazole (Ambilhar) is also effective. Corticosteroids are contraindicated.

Chronic, severe infections, which may be refractory to the above treatment, benefit from a 5-day course of an antibiotic such as penicillin 500,000 units I.M. daily, a tetracycline 0.25 g q.i.d., or succinylsulfathiazole 1 g q.i.d., to control bacterial infection. This should be given immediately after the course of emetine.

For the multitude of patients who are asymptomatic carriers or who present mild symptoms and moderate diarrhea, diiodohydroxyquinoline or oxytetracycline are curative in a high percentage of infections. One should suspect the accuracy of diagnosis when amebiasis resists thorough treatment. If the patient has laboratory-confirmed amebiasis that recurs, a check on his environment and family for sources of reinfection should be made.

A large number of oral amebacides are available and can replace those given above. Some are less effective and may produce more side effects. When one drug fails to cure, another may be successful.

Bismuth glycolylarsanilate (Milibis, Wintodon), 0.5 g t.i.d. for 8 days
Diloxanide furoate (Furamide), 0.5 g t.i.d. for 10 days
Emetine bismuth iodide, 0.2 g daily for 10 days
Iodochlorhydroxyquine (Vioform), 0.25 g q.i.d. for 10 days
Paromomycin (Humatin), 1.0 to 2.0 g daily for 5 to 10 days
Carbamylaminophenylarsonic acid (Carbarsone), 0.25 g 2 times daily for 10 days

Hepatic amebiasis is best treated with emetine and chloroquine. Emetine gives a significantly higher cure rate in amebic abscess than does chloroquine. These two drugs can be used consecutively or concurrently. Dihydroemetine apparently has no great advantage over emetine. Metronidazole (Flagyl) and Niridazole (Ambilhar) are also effective in hepatic infections. Aspiration or surgical drainage of the abscess may be necessary. The intestinal infection which is also present must be treated.

CARBARSONE. Carbarsone, a pentavalent arsenical, is a substituted phenylarsenite with an arsenical content of 29 percent. Used in intestinal amebiasis and balantidiasis. Administered orally in gelatin capsules containing 0.25 g twice a day for 10 days; total daily dose, 0.5 g. It may be given as a 1 percent enema in a 2 percent sodium bicarbonate solution. Occasionally the patient may experience nausea, vomiting, diarrhea, and abdominal distress, and very rarely may develop an exfoliative dermatitis. Contraindications are renal or hepatic disease or super-sensitivity to arsenic.

CHLOROQUINE. Chloroquine (Aralen, Resoquine, Resochin, Tanakan) is a 4-aminoquinoline derivative. It is administered orally as chloroquine diphosphate (62 percent chloroquine base). For hepatic amebiasis 1.0 g chloroquine is given daily for 2 days, then 0.5 or 0.75 g daily for 14 to 28 days or a total dose of 15.0 to 20.0 g. The course may be repeated after 1 month. Chloroquine is rapidly absorbed, has a high concentration in the liver, and is slowly excreted. The rare toxic symptoms include pruritus, transient headache, nausea, disturbances of visual accommodation, bleaching of the hair, and diminution of the T wave of the ECG.

DIODOQUIN. Diodoquin is an iodohydroxyquinoline drug with an iodine content of 64 percent. Effective in patients with mild chronic intestinal amebiasis. Administered orally in enteric-coated tablets at a daily dosage of 1.95 g in three divided doses for 20 days. A few patients show minor intolerance in the form of headache, malaise, abdominal pain, diarrhea, rash, and pruritus. Contraindications are severe thyroid, hepatic, and renal disease, and iodine sensitivity.

EMETINE. Emetine is an alkaloid of *Cephaelis ipecacuanha*. Used chiefly in acute intestinal amebiasis for the control of dysentery and in hepatic and other extraintestinal amebiasis. Administered deep subcutaneously as emetine hydrochloride or dihydrochloride. Patients should remain in bed during treatment and for several days after and should avoid strenuous exercise for several weeks during convalescence. For intestinal amebiasis the adult daily dose should not exceed 0.065 g for 3-6 days, and for hepatic amebiasis up to 10 days. The maximal safe dose is 1 mg/kg per day. Cutaneous amebiasis usually responds to 0.03 g daily for 7 days.

Emetine is a general irritant, especially to the mucous membranes, and a protoplasmic poison with predilection for the cardiac muscles, gastrointestinal tract, and skeletal system. The most serious toxic effects of emetine are on the cardiovascular system, and include hypotension, tachycardia, precordial pain, dyspnea, and ECG changes. The patient should have an ECG before emetine therapy, and it should be repeated during therapy. The pulse rate and blood pressure should be recorded several times daily, and the patient carefully examined and questioned concerning symptoms. Upon the appearance of tachycardia the drug should be stopped.

Emetine toxicity is also manifested by diarrhea, nausea, and vomiting; the neuromuscular manifestations of emetine toxicity are varied and consist of weakness, aching, tenderness and stiffness of muscles of the neck and extremities, and fatigability—all due presumably to myositis caused by the drug.

Fortunately, most of the untoward effects are mild and transient; they may disappear while treatment is continued and disappear on cessation of therapy. Emetine is contraindicated in patients with renal or cardiac disease and during pregnancy, except when severe dysentery or liver abscess is uncontrolled by other drugs.

Paromomycin (Humatin) is an antibiotic obtained from culture filtrates of a *Streptomyces*. It is effective against amebic intestinal infections. The adult dose is 1.0 to 2.0 g daily in divided doses at mealtime for 5 to 10 days, depending upon the severity of the infection. Excessive doses may produce diarrhea; and abdominal cramps and pruritis ani have been reported as side effects.

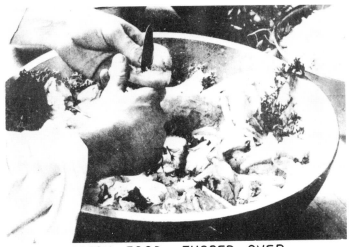

FRESH FOOD, FUSSED OVER
WITH "FECALED" FINGERS

Fig. 9. Transmission of amebiasis. (From S. A. Tydskrif vir Geneeskunde, 1944.)

MILIBIS.   Milibis (Wintodon, Wia) is a bismuth derivative of *p*-N-glycolylar-sanilic acid, containing 15 percent arsenic and 42 percent bismuth, administered orally to adults at a daily dosage of 1.5 g in three divided doses for 8 days. It is tolerated as well or better than carbarsone. Patients occasionally show slight nausea, epigastric discomfort, intestinal colic, or diarrhea; and in persons sensitive to arsenic, rarely an exfoliative dermatitis or encephalitis. Supersensitivity to arsenic is a contraindication.

Prevention.   Since man is the chief source of infection, all infections should be treated and contacts examined. Carriers should be removed from food-handling occupations, instructed in personal hygiene, and treated (Fig. 9). Effective environmental sanitation is necessary to prevent water and food contamination. Sanitary methods of sewage disposal should be instituted, latrines should be screened, and feces used as fertilizer should be stored an appropriate length of time. A properly safeguarded, filtered water supply is important since chlorination is not wholly effective. In areas where potable water is not available, special care must be taken. Boiling water is a safe, effective method of producing pleasant tasting drinking water. Ice should be made from boiled water. Small quantities of drinking water may be treated with iodine-compound tablets. Residual free iodine, 6 to 7 ppm, is cysticidal in 10 minutes at 23° C in water below pH 7.5 in the presence of 5 ppm of urea nitrogen. Tablets that release 8 ppm iodine have been compounded with an acidic excipient to reduce the pH of highly alkaline waters. Stable tablets, which are used as a disinfectant of water in canteens by the U.S. Army, contain 20 mg tetraglycine hydroperiodide, 90 mg disodium dihydrogen pyrophosphate, and 5 mg talc (Globaline *).

Insects may be controlled by insecticides. Food should be screened and protected from dust contamination. Uncooked vegetables from areas where night soil is used as fertilizer should be thoroughly washed in water treated with iodine tablets or scalded at 80° C for at least 30 seconds. The public should be informed regarding methods of avoiding infection.

* Globaline, Maltbie Laboratories Division, Wallace & Tiernan, Inc., Belleville, N. J.

Balantidium coli

Disease.   Balantidiasis, balantidiosis, balantidial dysentery.

Morphology and Physiology.   *B. coli* is the largest intestinal protozoon of man and his only pathogenic ciliate (Fig. 10). The grayish-green unstained, ovoid trophozoite, averaging 60 μ (30 to 150) by 45 μ (25 to 120), is shaped like a sac (balantidium means little bag) and is enclosed in a delicate protective pellicle covered with spiral longitudinal rows of cilia. The narrow triangular peristome and cytostome at the anterior end are lined with long cilia adapted for procuring food. At the posterior end is an indistinct excretory opening, the cytopyge, through which the solid waste material is discharged. Within the granular cytoplasm are two contractile vacuoles, a large, elongated, kidney-shaped macronucleus, a small subspherical micronucleus, and numerous food vacuoles. The trophozoites form a protective resistant cyst by secreting a double wall. The unstained, greenish-yellow subspherical or oval cyst (Fig. 10), averaging about 55 by 52 μ and ranging from 45 to 65 μ, shows only the macronucleus, contractile vacuoles, and cilia.

The trophozoite lives in the mucosa and submucosa of the large intestine, chiefly the cecal region, and in the terminal portion of the ileum. It moves actively by the rhythmic motion of its cilia. Its extreme plasticity and its rotary boring action enable it to penetrate the intestinal mucosa. Erythrocytes, leukocytes, tissue fragments, oil globules, starch granules, and other debris are carried through the cytopharynx into the endoplasm, where, enclosed in vacuoles, the materials are digested by enzymes. The trophozoite divides by transverse binary fission to form two new individuals, each containing a daughter macro- and micronucleus. Rapid division may produce nests of balantidia in the tissues. Trophozoites do not survive long

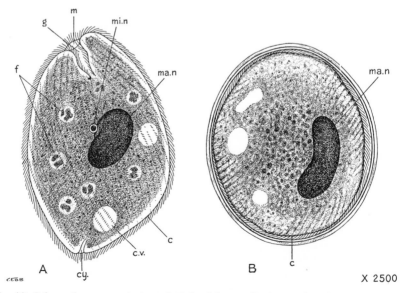

Fig. 10. Schematic representation of *Balantidium coli*. A, trophozoite; B, cyst. c, cilia; cy., cytopyge; c.v., contractile vacuole; f, food vacuole; g, gullet; m, mouth; ma.n, macronucleus mi.n, micronucleus. (Modified from Dobell and O'Connor, 1921.)

extracorporeally, but cysts may remain viable for several weeks. *B. coli* may be cultivated on the noncellular mediums used for intestinal protozoa, but only trophozoites are formed.

Life Cycle. The life cycle of *B. coli* is similar to that of *E. histolytica,* except that there is no multiplication in the cyst. Cysts, which are capable of surviving outside the body for several weeks in a moist environment, are the infective forms. When ingested by a new host the cyst wall dissolves, and the liberated trophozoite invades and multiplies in the intestinal wall.

Epidemiology. The incidence of *B. coli* in man is low. On the other hand the incidence is high in hogs (63 to 91 percent). Hogs harbor *B. coli* and *B. suis.* The former is infectious for man, while the latter, the more common species, apparently does not infect man. There is considerable epidemiologic evidence against the hog being the important source of human infection, as formerly considered. The incidence of infection in man engaged in occupations and living in areas where he is closely associated with hogs is low, and man is refractory to infection with porcine strains. During outbreaks, man appears to be the chief source of infection through hand-to-mouth transmission and food contamination.

Pathology and Symptomatology. The mucosa and submucosa of the large intestine are invaded and destroyed by the multiplying organisms. Invasion is effected by cytolytic ferments and mechanical penetration. The multiplying parasites form nests and small abscesses that break down into oval, irregular ulcers with red undermined edges. All degrees of severity, from simple catarrhal hyperemia to marked ulceration, occur. The individual ulcers may be discrete with normal or hyperemic intervening mucosa, or they may coalesce with communicating sinuses. In fatal cases there is multiple and diffuse ulceration and gangrene. Histologic sections show hemorrhagic areas, round-cell infiltration, abscesses, necrotic ulcers, and invading parasites, the predominating reaction being mononuclear unless secondary bacterial invasion is present (Fig. 11). In chronic infections during exacerbations the ulcers are small and discrete, the mucosa diffusely inflamed, and small membranous patches with raw underlying areas may be present. In moderately acute infections there may be 6 to 15 liquid stools per day with mucus, blood, and pus. In the chronic disease there may be intermittent diarrhea alternating with constipation, tender colon, anemia, and cachexia. Many infections are asymptomatic. Prognosis depends upon the severity of the infection and the response to treatment. It is good in asymptomatic and chronic infections. *Balantidium* does not successfully invade the liver. The low incidence of infection and the failure of experimental infection indicates that man has a high natural resistance.

Diagnosis. Balantidiasis may be confused clinically with other dysenteries and enteric fevers. Diagnosis depends upon the identification of trophozoites in diarrheic stools and, less frequently, of cysts in formed stools. Several stools should be examined, since the discharge of parasites is variable. In patients with sigmoidorectal infection, the sigmoidoscope is useful in obtaining material for examination.

Treatment. See Page 33. Diiodohydroxyquinoline (Diodoquin), Carbarsone, chlortetracycline, and oxytetracycline have all produced favorable results when used in the same dosage as for amebiasis.

Prevention. The same prophylactic measures used in amebic dysentery with respect to carriers and sanitary control of food and water should be employed. Until more knowledge is available, it is well to consider the hog as a potential source of infection.

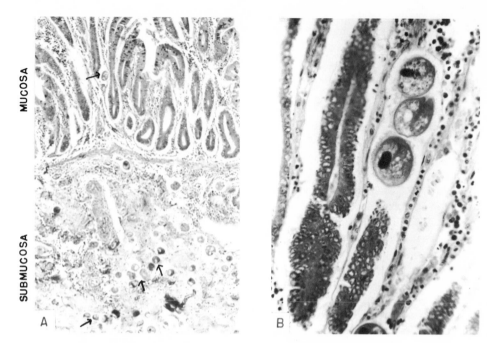

Fig. 11. *Balantidium coli* in large intestine.
A. Note that trophozoites have invaded both the mucosa and submucosa.
B. Trophozoites in mucosal crypts.

INTESTINAL AND ATRIAL FLAGELLATES OF MAN

Almost every species of vertebrate may serve as host to intestinal and atrial flagellates, and a single host may harbor several species. Special organs such as sucking disc, axostyle, and undulating membrane have been developed to withstand the peristaltic action of the intestine. Transmission from host to host is through the formation of resistant cysts in many species, but in others infection apparently is transmitted through the less hardy trophozoites. Owing to morphologic variation, it is difficult to determine whether the species infecting man and lower animals are identical.

Man is the host of seven species, including five intestinal and two atrial parasites. The five nonpathogenic cosmopolitan species are: (1) *Chilomastix mesnili;* (2) *Enteromonas hominis;* (3) *Embadomonas intestinalis;* (4) *Trichomonas hominis* of the intestine; and (5) *Trichomonas tenax* of the mouth. The differential characteristics of these and the pathogenic (6) *Giardia lamblia* and (7) *Trichomonas vaginalis* are given in Figure 12. All have been cultivated on artificial mediums.

Giardia lamblia

Disease. Giardiasis, lambliasis.

The trophozoite (Fig. 12) is a bilaterally symmetrical, pear-shaped flagellate, 12 to 15 μ, with a broad, rounded anterior and a tapering posterior extremity. The dorsal surface is convex. An ovoid concave sucking disc occupies about three-fourths of the flat ventral surface. There are two nuclei with large central karyo-

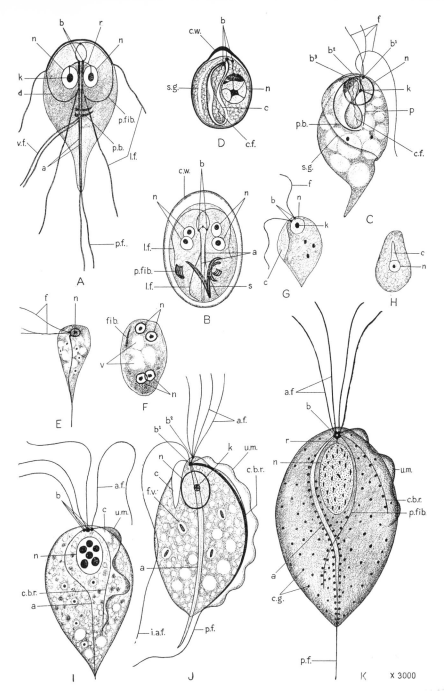

Fig. 12. The intestinal and atrial flagellates of man. A, *Giardia lamblia* trophozoite viewed from dorsal surface; B, *Giardia lamblia* cyst; C, *Chilomastix mesnili* trophozoite ventral view; D, *Chilomastix mesnili* cyst ventral view, showing thickening of anterior wall; E, *Enteromonas hominis* trophozoite, showing characteristic caudal protuberance; F, *Enteromonas hominis* quadrinucleated cyst; G, *Embadomonas intestinalis* trophozoite; H, *Embadomonas intestinalis* cyst; I, *Trichomonas tenax* trophozoite; J, *Trichomonas hominis* trophozoite; K, *Trichomonas vaginalis* trophozoite.

a, axostyle; a.f., anterior flagella; b, b¹, b², b³, blepharoplasts; c, cytostome, c.b.r., chromatoid basal rod; c.f., cytostomal flagella; c.g., chromatin granules; c.w., cyst wall; d, sucking disc; f, flagella; f.v., food vacuole; fib., fibril; i.a.f., inferior anterior flagellum; k, karyosome; l.f., lateral flagella; n, nucleus; p, parastyle; p.b., parabasal body; p.f., posterior flagellum; p.fib., parabasal fiber; r, rhizoplast; s, shield; s.g., spiral groove; u.m., undulating membrane; v, vacuole; v.f., ventral flagella.

39

somes, two axostyles, two blepharoplasts, two deeply staining bars considered to be parabasal bodies, and four pairs of flagella, although five have been demonstrated. The ellipsoidal cyst (Fig. 12 and Fig. 140), 9 to 12 μ, has a smooth well-defined wall, and contains two to four nuclei and many of the structures of the trophozoite. The flagellate inhabits the duodenum and upper jejunum, and at times, possibly the bile ducts and gallbladder. The lashing flagella propel the trophozoite with a rapid, jerky, twisting motion. The sucking disc enables the trophozoites to resist ordinary peristalsis; hence, they are rarely found except in fluid stools. Food is absorbed from the intestinal contents, although the parasite possibly may obtain nourishment from the epithelial cells through its sucking disc. Multiplication occurs by mitotic division during encystment, followed by separation into daughter trophozoites after excystation. Longitudinal binary fission has been observed in trophozoites. An alkaline environment, increased by achlorhydria and a rich carbohydrate diet, favors multiplication. Under moist conditions cysts may remain viable for months outside the host.

Man is the natural host of *G. lamblia,* but rats occasionally may be temporarily infected. *G. lamblia* is three times more common in children than adults, particularly in the 6- to 10-year group. Transmission is through food and water contaminated by sewage, flies, or foodhandlers, and by hand-to-mouth. The recent epidemic of giardiasis among adult winter visitors at a Colorado resort town was probably water-borne, aided by a cross-connection with the sewage system. Numerous *Giardia* cysts were present in the sewage. Thus, the athletic, the affluent, and the well fed are not immune to this infection. Large numbers of cysts are passed intermittently in the feces, but relatively few trophozoites except in diarrheic stools. When ingested by a new host the cysts pass unharmed through the gastric juices and undergo excystation in the duodenum. The ingestion of 100 or more cysts produces infection in all volunteers; of 10 to 25 cysts, in one-third; and 1 cyst in none.

Opinions differ as to the role of *G. lamblia* as a primary pathogen. Clinical evidence indicates that the attachment of the parasites to the intestinal mucosa may produce a low-grade catarrhal inflammation, and that their mechanical and toxic action may interfere with the absorption of vitamin A and fats. Definite pathologic lesions other than reaction to irritation rarely occur. Giardial infections in animals produce no lesions. Functional and anatomic changes in the duodenum may be demonstrated radiologically in some of the infected persons, and diarrhea is not infrequently observed, particularly in children. Extensive ulceration of the upper small intestine has been found at autopsy in a patient with a rare fulminating case.

In adults the asymptomatic carrier predominates and, except in a few cases, the infection is of little clinical importance. Experimental infection of adults with cysts has demonstrated that there is a prepatent period of 6 to 15 days, a duration of infection of from 5 to 41 days, no clinical illness attributable to giardiasis, and slight changes in the stool pattern in two-thirds of the infected persons. Some adults may show a diarrheic syndrome like that in children, or symptoms simulating biliary disease.

Children, more frequently than adults, show an acute or chronic enteritis, with varied gastrointestinal symptoms accompanied by general and nervous manifestations associated with disordered nutrition and intestinal irritation. In the more advanced infections the important symptom complex is a chronic steatorrheal diarrhea alternating with constipation, but at times becoming acute with frequent watery stools. Abdominal pain, epigastric distress, and abdominal distention also may be present.

Diagnosis may be made by finding cysts in formed stools, and trophozoites and cysts in diarrheic feces. Its distinctive morphology in saline and iodine mounts and in stained films, distinguishes *G. lamblia* from other intestinal protozoa. Concentration methods increase the chances of detection. Examination of the duodenal content gives a slightly higher percentage of positive findings than that of the feces. Fresh material is advisable for the examination of trophozoites.

Treatment. As treatment with quinacrine (Page 93) is safe and effective, we routinely treat all infections with the following doses: adults, 100 mg, thrice daily for 5 days; children, 8 mg/kg daily for 5 days. Maximum daily dose is 300 mg.

Metronidazole (Page 42) treatment is as follows: adults, 250 mg twice daily for 5 days; children: less than 2 years, 125 mg daily for 5 days; 2 to 4 years, 250 mg daily for 5 days; 4 to 8 years, 375 mg daily for 5 days; and over 9 years, 500 mg daily for 5 days.

Measures similar to those employed for *E. histolytica* are used in prevention.

Trichomonas vaginalis

The genus *Trichomonas* comprises flagellates that have three to five anterior flagella, an undulating membrane, an axostyle, and usually a cytosome. Trichomonads are widely distributed and infect nearly every mammal associated with man. There are three species in man: *T. vaginalis* of the vagina, *T. hominis* of the intestine, and *T. tenax* of the mouth. They may be differentiated by morphology (Fig. 12), cultural characteristics, and failure to cross infect. *T. vaginalis,* the largest and most robust, is the only pathogen.

Disease. Trichomonad vaginitis, urethritis, prostatovesiculitis.

T. vaginalis (Fig. 2) is a colorless pyriform flagellate, 15 to 18 μ in fresh preparations but smaller in fixed. No cysts have been found. Its habitat is the vagina of the female and the urethra, epididymis, and prostate of the male; hence, it is frequently found in the urine. It may cause a "nonspecific" urethritis. *T. vaginalis* advances rapidly, rotating through debris by the lashing of the anterior flagella and by the action of the undulating membrane.

In cultures it has been observed to ingest bacteria, starch, and even erythrocytes. Dextrose, maltose, and other carbohydrates stimulate growth. Reproduction takes place by binary longitudinal fission with mitotic division of the nucleus.

The trophozoite is one of the most resistant of the parasitic protozoa. It is killed in 4 minutes at 50° C, but survives for 5 days at 0° C. In cultures it loses its vitality below pH 4.9; hence it cannot live in the acid vaginal secretions (pH 3.8 to 4.4) of young healthy adults. It is susceptible to a large number of disinfectants, dyes, and antibiotics.

Epidemiology. The incidence of infection is about 25 percent in women. It is higher in groups in which feminine hygiene is deficient. Only about one-seventh of the women with trichomonad infection complain of symptoms, although the vaginal secretions are invariably altered. The detected infection rate in husbands of infected wives is surprisingly low, but this may be due to technical difficulties in securing adequate specimens for diagnosis. Evidently there are several modes of transmission. Sexual intercourse, especially by asymptomatic infected males is probably most important. However, as young virgins are found infected, it appears that direct contact with infected females, contaminated toilet articles and toilet seats transmit the infection. Infections acquired while passing through the birth canal probably account for some infections in babies.

Pathology and Symptomatology.   Clinicians generally regard *T. vaginalis* as the causative agent of a persistent vaginitis. Clinical evidence supports the view that the flagellate is responsible for a low grade inflammation, although it is possible that the trichomonad as a secondary invader may merely aggravate a pre-existing condition. Additional evidence is furnished by its toxic action on cells in tissue cultures and the production of vaginitis in women by bacteria-free cultures. The size of the dose, the bacterial flora, and the physiologic status of the vagina are among the factors that determine infection, although the parasite appears capable of inducing vaginitis in the normal vaginal mucosa even without an abnormal bacterial flora.

In trichomonad vaginitis the vaginal walls are injected and tender, in some instances showing hyperemia and petechial hemorrhages, and in advanced cases, granular areas. The vaginal and cervical mucosa is highly injected with a bright or dark red punctate mottling and is infiltrated with lymphocytes, a few polymorphonuclear neutrophils, and occasionally plasma cells. The surface is covered with a frothy, seropurulent, creamy or yellowish discharge, frequently forming a pool in the posterior fornix. Patients present signs of vaginal and cervical inflammation, complain of itching and burning, and have a profuse irritating leukorrheic discharge. At times erosion and necrosis are observed. In the male there may be a urethritis and prostatovesiculitis.

Diagnosis.   Clinical diagnosis is based on symptoms of burning, a frothy creamy discharge, and punctate lesions and hyperemia of the vagina. The microscopic examination in a drop of saline for motile trichomonads of the fresh vaginal discharge, preferably obtained with a speculum, is the most practical method of diagnosis. Occasionally, cultures will reveal the organism when the microscopic examination is negative. Prostatic secretions following prostatic massage and urine of the male should be examined.

Treatment.   The basis of treatment is the restoration of normal conditions in the vagina by local cleansing of the vaginal mucosa, and the oral and topical application of chemotherapeutic agents.

Metronidazole (Flagyl) is the drug of choice for the treatment of trichomoniasis, both in the male and female. The therapeutic regimen for women consists of 250 mg three times a day orally for 10 days. Vaginal inserts containing 500 mg of the drug are available for local therapy. The recommended dosage for men is 250 mg twice daily for 10 days. Temporary leukopenia may occur which may be due to an accelerated disappearance of the elements from the blood which temporarily exceeds the bone marrow release rather than a bone marrow suppression. A white blood cell count should be done before and after therapy. Metronidazole should not be given to pregnant patients until further studies on its effect on the fetus are fully evaluated. A *Trichomonas* infection may be uncomfortable to the mother, but it is not serious and can wait a few months for therapy. Side effects are reported to be infrequent and minor; they include nausea, metallic taste, furry tongue, and headache. Other effects, all reported in an incidence of less than 1 percent, are diarrhea, dizziness, vaginal dryness and burning, dry mouth, rash, urticaria, gastritis, drowsiness, insomnia, pruritus, sore tongue, darkened urine, anorexia, vomiting, epigastric distress, dysuria, depression, vertigo, incoordination, ataxia, abdominal cramping, constipation, stomatitis, numbness of an extremity, joint pains, confusion, irritability, weakness, flushing, cystitis, pelvic pressure, dyspareunia, fever, polyuria, incontinence, decreased libido, nasal congestion, proctitis, and pyuria. Elimination of trichomonads may aggravate candidiasis. The desire for alcoholic drinks may be decreased.

Vaginal treatment with iodoquinolines (Floroquin tablets) or pentavalent arsenicals (acetarsone powder) in the form of insufflation powders or suppositories, followed by acid douches, has been used with more or less success.

Prevention. Attention to personal hygiene. The detection and treatment of infected males should help in reducing infections.

Isospora belli and *Isospora hominis*

Isospora belli and *I. hominis,* the principal intestinal species in man, have been repeatedly confused in the literature, so that it is necessary to consider them together. The only clear-cut differential characteristic is the larger size of the oocyst of *I. belli,* which apparently is the more common parasite. The parasites, though rare, have a wide distribution. Endemic areas have been found in South Africa, South America (Brazil, Chile, and Venezuela), China, India, Japan, the Philippines, Indonesia, and the islands of the South Pacific. Of the 91 cases reported in the United States up to 1956, only seven were definitely autochthonous. Occasionally other species have been reported—e.g., *I. rivolta* and the closely similar *I. natalensis* of South Africa.

Morphology. Only the elongated ovoid oocysts are known, 25 to 33 μ by 12 to 16 μ for *I. belli* and 16 by 10 μ for *I. hominis*. In fresh feces the granular cytoplasm, contained within a smooth, colorless, two-layered wall, is usually unsegmented and contains a single nucleus (Fig. 13). Division takes place into two sporoblasts that secrete a cystic wall. Within each spore further division produces four elongated nucleated sporozoites. The oocyst of *I. belli* differs from that of *I.*

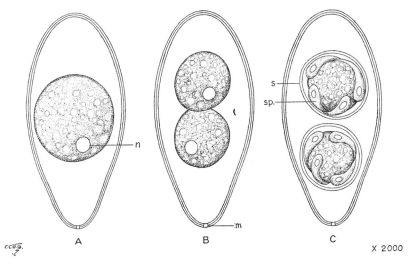

Fig. 13. *Isospora hominis.* A, unicellular oocyst; B, oocyst with two sporoblasts; C, oocyst with two spores, each containing four sporozoites.

m, micropyle; n, nucleus; s, spore; sp., sporozoite. (Modified from Dobell and O'Connor, 1921.)

hominis in its larger size, harder cyst wall, and less advanced development, two sporoblasts rarely being present in specimens from fresh feces. The parasites inhabit the small intestine, but the exact site is in doubt. Oocysts of *I. belli* have been obtained by intubation from the duodenum and jejunum. The parasites have not been cultivated.

Life Cycle.   The life cycle is unknown, but it is doubtless similar to that of comparable species in dogs and cats, in which schizogonic development takes place in the intestinal epithelial cells. In sporogony the fertilized ovum is enclosed in the oocyst, which is passed in the feces. A new host is infected by the ingestion of mature oocysts or spores. In the intestine the freed sporozoites enter the epithelial cells. The incidence of human infection is low, which suggests that man may be an incidental host, but no animal reservoir hosts have been incriminated. Transmission evidently takes place through contaminated food or water, or by hand-to-mouth.

Pathology and Symptomatology.   Pathogenicity is slight. Oocysts have been found in apparently healthy individuals, as well as in those with diarrhea, which is often due to a concomitant bacterial or parasitic infection. The pathologic lesions have not been observed in man. Uncomplicated infections may show a self-limited diarrhea, loose stools with undigested food, steatorrhea, some abdominal pain and discomfort, fever, and lassitude. In experimentally infected persons, the discharge of the oocysts in the feces begins 9 to 16 days after infection and lasts for 21 days. An initial stage of 7 days is followed by fever and malaise, then diarrhea with abdominal pains and general debility.

Diagnosis depends upon finding the easily overlooked oocysts in unstained cover-glass mounts. Zinc sulfate concentration is helpful.

Herring, sardine, and sprat harbor their own *Eimeria,* and their oocysts may be found in the stool of man, an example of spurious parasitism.

Treatment.   Rest and bland diet. Chemotherapy is unnecessary, since the disease is self-limited.

Prevention.   Similar to that of *E. histolytica.*

4

Blood and Tissue Protozoa of Man

PARASITIC TRYPANOSOMES OF MAN

Trypanosoma and *Leishmania* have species pathogenic to man and other mammals. Their transitional forms in insects and cultures resemble species of the genera *Leptomonas* and *Crithidia,* which are found in invertebrates (Table 4). The widely distributed members of the genus *Trypanosoma* spend part of the life cycle in vertebrates and, with few exceptions, part in invertebrates. Numerous species, mostly nonpathogenic, are found in the blood and tissues of mammals, birds, reptiles, amphibians, and fishes. The three pathogenic species of man are *T. gambiense* and *T. rhodesiense* in Africa, and *T. cruzi* in America.

Morphology. Trypanosomes are minute, actively motile, fusiform protozoa, flattened from side to side (Fig. 14). The long sinuous body has a tapering anterior and a blunt posterior end. Even in the same species the shape varies. The electron microscope reveals surface striations due to spiral bundles of longitudinal contractile fibrils beneath the enveloping pellicle. The flagellum, which consists of five to nine striated parallel fibrils in a cytoplasmic sheath, projects from the anterior end after passing along the margin of the undulating membrane, a wavy fold of the periplast on the convex border of the trypanosome. A large oval nucleus, which has a central

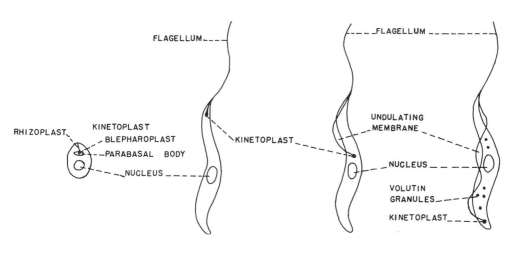

LEISHMANIA   LEPTOMONAS   CRITHIDIA   TRYPANOSOMA

Fig. 14. Developmental forms of Trypanosomidae.

45

Table 4. Developmental Forms of Trypanosomidae Pathogenic for Man

Species	Developmental forms				Transmission	Insect vectors	Reservoir hosts other than man
	Leishmania	Leptomonas	Crithidia	Trypanosoma			
Trypanosoma							
T. gambiense	None	None	1. Salivary glands of insects 2. Culture	1. Blood, lymphatic glands, & spinal fluid of mammals 2. Intestine & salivary glands of insects	Anterior station, bite	Tsetse flies (Glossina)	Hog, goat, & cattle
T. rhodesiense	None	None	1. Salivary glands of insects 2. Culture	1. Blood, lymphatic glands, & spinal fluid of mammals 2. Intestine & salivary glands of insects	Anterior station, bite	Tsetse flies (Glossina)	Wild game animals & cattle
T. cruzi	1. Intracellular in viscera, particularly myocardium & brain, of mammals 2. Tissue culture	Intracellular in mammals but transitional	1. Intracellular in mammals but transitional 2. Intestine of insects 3. Culture	1. Blood & tissues of mammals 2. Intestine & rectum of insects 3. Culture	Posterior station, feces	Reduviid bugs (TRIATOMINAE)	Dog, cat armadillos, & small wild mammals
Leishmania							
L. donovani	1. Intracellular in reticuloendothelial system, lymphatic glands, spleen, liver, bone marrow, & phagocytes 2. Tissue culture	1. Midgut & pharynx of insects 2. Culture	None	None	None	Sandflies (Phlebotomus)	Dog
L. tropica and L. braziliensis	1. Intra- and extracellular in skin & mucous membranes of mammals 2. Tissue culture	1. Midgut & pharynx of insects 2. Culture	None	None	None	Sandflies (Phlebotomus)	Wild rodents & dog (?)

karyosome, is situated toward the middle of the body. Near the posterior end there is a kinetoplast, consisting of a spherical or rod-shaped parabasal body of variable size and an anterior connecting basal granule, the blepharoplast. At times, minute refractile volutin granules and vacuoles may be seen in the cytoplasm. Trypanosomes travel with a wavy spiral motion produced by the contractile flagellum and undulating membrane. Changes in body form are probably effected by the contractile fibers in the periplast. Reproduction takes place by binary longitudinal fission. Variations in the metabolism and respiration of the different species apparently are dependent on different enzyme systems. Trypanosomes fail to store carbohydrates and thus require as sources of energy the readily available supplies of their hosts. In the blood, dextrose is utilized by *T. gambiense* and *T. rhodesiense* at a high rate, but by *T. cruzi* at a negligible rate. In cultures *T. cruzi* can use proteins in the absence of available carbohydrates. Nourishment is obtained from the blood plasma, lymph, cerebrospinal fluid, and products of cellular disintegration. *T. cruzi* grows readily on noncellular mediums that contain serum and blood, passing through stages resembling those in the invertebrate host, while *T. gambiense* and *T. rhodesiense* are cultivated with difficulty. The original Novy-MacNeal-Nicolle (N.N.N.) medium with its various modifications is still popular. Tissue cultures of various organs of chick and rat embryos have been used in studying the intracellular leishmanian forms of *T. cruzi*.

Life Cycle. The life cycle of most mammalian trypanosomes involves alternate existence in vertebrate and invertebrate hosts. Transmission of infection in vertebrates may be direct or indirect. The direct method involves the mechanical transmission of the infective trypanosomes: *T. equiperdum* by coitus, *T. hippicum* by nonbiting flies, and *T. evansi* and *T. equinum* by the contaminated proboscis of biting flies. In indirect transmission the trypanosome must undergo a cyclic development in a bloodsucking insect before it becomes infective. There are two types of cyclic development. With *T. cruzi*, the ingested trypanosomes in the midgut of the reduviid bug first become stumpy, and then long crithidial forms, which are transformed in 8 to 20 days into infective metacyclic trypanosomes in the hindgut and rectum. They are then ready for extrusion in the feces, which contaminates the small lesion made by the insect while biting. In the second type, which includes species transmitted by tsetse flies, the trypanosomes develop first in the digestive tract and become infective on reaching the salivary glands. When the insect feeds, the infective forms are injected with the saliva. Multiplication in the mid- and hindgut produces numerous broad forms, which develop into long slender forms in the proventriculus. These migrate through the esophagus, hypopharynx, and salivary ducts to the salivary glands, where they become crithidial flagellates; after multiplying they are transformed into infective metacyclic trypanosomes. Successful transmission depends upon the number of trypanosomes ejected by the tsetse fly; experimentally, a minimal dose of 350 trypanosomes is necessary to infect man.

Classification. Classifications of trypanosomes have been based on morphology, natural hosts, method of transmission, and pathogenicity. It has been postulated that *T. gambiense* and *T. rhodesiense*, which are common to man, are varieties or mutants of *T. brucei* of equidae and ruminants because of morphologic similarity and common group antigens. *T. brucei* differs from the species that infect humans, in its inability to infect man and its production of a highly fatal infection in equidae; it differs from *T. gambiense* in its greater virulence for laboratory animals. Of the three human species, *T. rhodesiense* morphologically resembles *T. gambiense* but differs in various biologic characteristics, while *T. cruzi* is distinct.

The heterogenicity of strains in the polymorphic trypanosomes presents perplexing problems. Strains vary in morphology, hostal characteristics, antigenicity, pathogenicity, and resistance to chemotherapy. Strains vary in virulence and in their ability to infect their vertebrate hosts and insect vectors.

Pathogenicity.   Most species are not injurious to their natural hosts, but some produce marked pathologic changes. Man and domesticated animals, apparently more recent hosts, are more susceptible than wild animals. The three trypanosomes of man are pathogenic for man and laboratory animals, but as a rule they do not produce disease in large domesticated or wild animals.

Both species and strains vary in virulence and in their ability to invade a host, multiply, and produce tissue damage. Strains of *T. cruzi* differ in virulence, tissue selectivity, and the number of trypanosomes in the peripheral blood of mice. Virulence is usually diminished by serial cultures and restored by animal passage. It is possible that mutant strains of increased virulence may be produced in nature by passage through susceptible young hosts.

The species pathogenic for the large domesticated mammals are not only of veterinary importance, but also, by their close resemblance to those of man, complicate the epidemiologic problem of reservoir hosts. The names, geographic distribution, disease produced, and method of transmission of the more important pathogenic trypanosomes of domesticated animals are: (1) *T. equiperdum* of cosmopolitan distribution, produces dourine in horses and donkeys, by coitus; (2) *T. brucei* of tropical Africa, causes nagana in equidae and ruminants, by tsetse flies; (3) *T. congolense* of tropical Africa; a wasting disease in equidae, ruminants, and dogs, by tsetse flies; (4) *T. simiae* of East Africa, unnamed disease in hogs, sheep, cattle, horses, and monkeys, by tsetse flies; (5) *T. vivax* of tropical Africa, causes souma in equidae and ruminants, by tsetse flies; (6) *T. evansi* of Asia, Australia, and Madagascar, causes surra in equidae, ruminants, and dogs, by *Tabanus* and *Stomoxys* flies; (7) *T. equinum* of South America, produces mal de caderas in equidae and ruminants, by *Tabanus* and *Stomoxys* flies; and (8) *T. hippicum* of Central America, produces murina de caderas in horses and mules, by nonbiting flies.

Man possesses a natural resistance against the pathogenic trypanosomes of domesticated animals, and, conversely, these animals show only transitory, chronic, or latent infections with the pathogenic African trypanosomes of man. Certain breeds of cattle are more resistant than others to the pathogenic *T. vivax* and *T. congolense*. Individuals vary in resistance, and young animals are more susceptible than old.

Immunity against *T. gambiense* in man and experimental animals is slight and of short duration. Immunity depends on both the trypanocidal properties of the serum and phagocytic activity. In *T. cruzi* infections the trypanosomal forms are phagocytosed by the mobilized cells of the reticuloendothelial system, but the infection is maintained by the protected intracellular leishmanian forms. Lysins, agglutinins, precipitins, and complement-fixing protective, immobilizing, and sensitizing antibodies have been demonstrated in infected or immunized animals. At present there is no practical method of active or passive immunization against the pathogenic mammalian African trypanosomes.

Trypanosoma gambiense

Disease. Gambian trypanosomiasis, Mid-African sleeping sickness.

Morphology (Fig. 15). In the blood *T. gambiense* is polymorphic, ranging from typical, long, slender trypanosomes to short, blunt forms without free flagella, or even to bizarre degenerate types. In the cerebrospinal fluid all sizes and shapes occur, including multiple and even involuted round or pear-shaped forms. Its length ranges from 15 to 30 μ and its breadth from 1.5 to 3.5 μ.

Life Cycle (Fig. 6). The vertebrate host is man. No reservoir host among wild or domesticated animals is known, but hogs, cattle, and goats are under suspicion. The principal invertebrate hosts are riverine tsetse flies of the palpalis group, *Glossina palpalis, G. palpalis fuscipes,* and *G. tachinoides,* but other species occasionally may serve as hosts (Page 282).

Epidemiology. This disease is limited to tropical West and Central Africa, and to the range of vectors—the palpalis group of tsetse flies. In the past the incidence of Gambian trypanosomiasis has varied from 3 to 43 percent in endemic areas. At times the infection has reached epidemic proportions with devastating reductions in population. In recent years the incidence has fallen notably as the result of preventive measures. Likewise, the disease has disappeared from some old areas and has spread to new ones.

The highest incidence is in the 20- to 40-year group of males because of greater occupational exposure, but in epidemics the proportion of infected women and children increases. The seasonal incidence is correlated with the distribution of prevalence of the insect vectors. The infection rate is affected by the proximity of villages, watering places, and trade routes to the habitat of the tsetse flies. Ambulatory carriers in the early stages of the disease provide abundant opportunity for the infection of tsetse flies along trade routes and permanent waterways.

T. gambiense is ordinarily transmitted to man by the bite of an infected tsetse fly after the cyclic development of the parasite. From a practical standpoint, the disease is spread by a man-fly-man transmission, since reservoir hosts are relatively unimportant. Infection by mechanical transmission may occur during epidemics when infected individuals and flies are numerous. Occasionally, the disease may be transmitted by coitus and, rarely, congenitally. The percentage of infected flies in endemic areas is only 2 to 4 percent. Their abundance and seasonal incidence are affected by humidity and temperature (optimal 24 to 30° C), and their dispersal is determined by the food supply and length of life (Page 282).

Pathology and Symptomatology. In man the disease varies in severity from a mild type—with few trypanosomes in the blood and which may be slowly progressive, self-limited, or may revert to serious manifestations—to a severe fulminating type resembling that of *T. rhodesiense.* In the typical case the disease progresses from the acute stage with trypanosomes multiplying in the blood and lymphatics during the first year, to the chronic sleeping sickness stage with invasion of the central nervous system, which starts at the end of the first or the beginning of the second year, and terminates fatally during the second or third year.

At the site of the bite there may be transient inflammation. The incubation period is usually about 14 days, but may be delayed for months. The acute disease lasts a year and is characterized by irregular fever, headache, joint and muscle

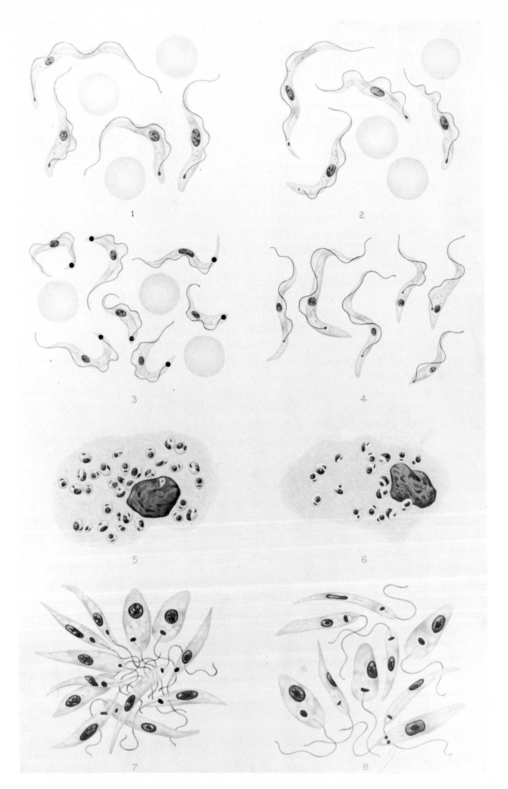

Fig. 15. Blood and tissue flagellates of man ($\times$ 1500). 1, *Trypanosoma gambiense* in blood; 2, *Trypanosoma rhodesiense* in blood; 3, *Trypanosoma cruzi* in blood; 4, *Trypanosoma gambiense,* developmental forms in *Glossina palpalis;* 5, *Leishmania donovani* in endothelial cell; 6, *Leishmania tropica* in large mononuclear cell; 7, *Leishmania donovani,* flagellated forms from culture; 8, *Leishmania tropica,* flagellated forms from culture.

TRYPANOSOMA GAMBIENSE   TRYPANOSOMA RHODESIENSE

AFRICAN SLEEPING SICKNESS

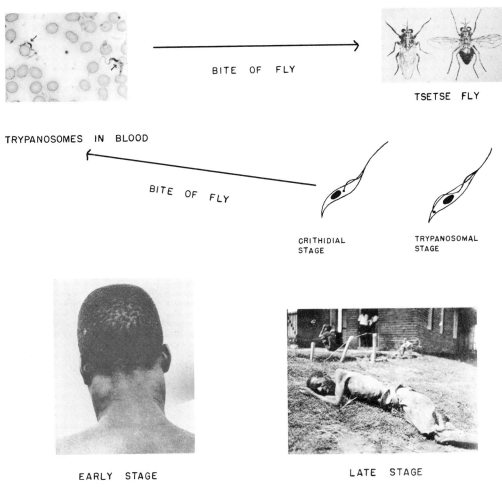

TRYPANOSOMES IN BLOOD

BITE OF FLY

TSETSE FLY

BITE OF FLY

CRITHIDIAL STAGE

TRYPANOSOMAL STAGE

EARLY STAGE

LATE STAGE

WINTERBOTTOM'S SIGN — ENLARGED LYMPH NODES

Fig. 16. Life cycle of *Trypanosoma gambiense* and *Trypanosoma rhodesiense*.

pains, and a rash. Delayed sensation to pain with deep hyperesthesia, Kerandel's sign, may be present. There is a slight microcytic anemia, moderate leukocytosis with an increase in the monocytes and lymphocytes, and an increased sedimentation rate. The superficial lymph nodes are enlarged. Winterbottom's sign consists of the enlargement of the postcervical group. The trypanosomes are present in the blood, lymph nodes, and bone marrow. The patient now becomes hyperactive.

Gradually the chronic phase of the disease ensues, with the development of characteristic central nervous system changes. There is a perivascular infiltration of endothelial, lymphoid, and plasma cells, leading to ischemic softening of tissues and petechial hemorrhages. A diffuse meningoencephalitis and meningomyelitis develops. The fever and headache now become pronounced. Evidence of nervous impairment becomes prominent with (1) lack of interest and disinclination to work; (2) avoidance of acquaintances; (3) morose and melancholic attitude alternating with exaltation; (4) mental retardation and lethargy; (5) speech low and tremulous; (6) tremors of tongue and limbs, intention tremors, even choreiform movements; (7) gait slow and shuffling; (8) altered reflexes. The spinal fluid shows increased protein and cells. The terminal sleeping stage now develops, and gradually the patient becomes more and more difficult to rouse; death ensues either from the disease or intercurrent infections such as malaria, dysentery, and pneumonia, aided by starvation. Prognosis is favorable if treatment is instituted before serious involvement of the nervous system occurs. Untreated infections may progress to a fatal termination or develop into a chronic or latent disease.

Diagnosis. Trypanosomiasis may be suspected when a patient from an endemic area has an acute infection with irregular fever and palpable lymph nodes, particularly in the postcervical triangle, or has developed a chronic disease with somnolence, personality changes, and neurologic symptoms. A definite laboratory diagnosis is made by finding the trypanosomes in the blood, lymph nodes, and bone marrow in the early disease and in the spinal fluid in the late disease, while a presumptive diagnosis is obtained by detecting changes in the cerebrospinal fluid and by complement-fixation and formol-gel tests.

Multiple examinations of thick blood films should be made, since the trypanosomes may be few or present irregularly after the early stages of the disease, and the examination of the centrifuged sediment of 10 to 20 ml of hemolyzed blood may be advantageous. The inoculation of laboratory rodents and even cultures of blood and tissues have been reported to be useful adjuncts to microscopic examination. At times trypanosomes may be found in the cerebrospinal fluid. A fluorescent antibody test is of value.

The protein content and the more sensitive cell count of the spinal fluid, indices of the stage of infection, are of therapeutic and prognostic value. For evaluating the results of treatment the disease may be divided according to the spinal fluid findings into three stages: (1) early, with normal spinal fluid of under three cells and protein concentration 25 mg/100 ml; (2) intermediate, with 3 to 10 cells and protein under 38 mg/100 ml; and (3) late, with more than 40 cells and protein over 38 mg/100 ml. The nonspecific formol-gel test and other flocculation tests which detect excess serum globulin in trypanosomiasis, leishmaniasis, and other diseases are useful as screening tests or when other diagnostic facilities are not available.

Treatment. The chemotherapy of African sleeping sickness is usually effective when it is begun early in the disease during the blood-lymphatic stage. After the central nervous system becomes involved, therapy is less successful. The available drugs are toxic to man, and some strains of trypanosomes become resistant to them. Suramin sodium is useful during early infection, and if it proves toxic to the patient pentamidine may be used in its place. For late infection with involvement of the central nervous system tryparsamide is used; as this drug is ineffective in *T. rhodesiense* infections and as *T. gambiense* infections are becoming resistant to it, Mel B (Arsobal), which appears to be effective against both early and late stages of both diseases, is replacing it. Nitrofurazone has recently been used against infections that failed to respond to tryparsamide or Mel B, but it must be used with care as it may cause peripheral neuritis and hemolytic anemia.

SURAMIN. Suramin (Antrypol, Bayer 205, Naphuride, Germanin, Moranyl,

Naganol, and Fourneau 309) is a carbamide compound. Used in early African trypanosomiasis and onchocerciasis. Administered intravenously in a 10 percent solution in freshly distilled water at maximal dose of 1 g every 4 to 7 days to a total of 10 g. Its toxicity is low, but it is a renal irritant, producing in some patients albuminuria, dermatitis, and gastrointestinal disturbances, or in supersensitive persons circulatory collapse. Contraindicated in renal disease.

TRYPARSAMIDE. Tryparsamide (Fourneau 270, Orsanine, Trypanarsyl meurice), a pentavalent arsenic derivative with an arsenic content of 25 percent, was one of the first effective drugs for African trypanosomiasis. Useful in late Gambesian trypanosomiasis; of little value in Rhodesian trypanosomiasis. Administered intravenously in a 20 percent freshly prepared aqueous solution at weekly intervals for 8 to 15 injections. The initial dose of 1 g is gradually increased to 3 g (not to exceed 0.04 g/kg). Rest period of 1 month between courses. Acute toxicity low, but drug may cause optic atrophy, jaundice, nephritis, abdominal colic, and dermatitis. Eye symptoms call for its immediate discontinuation. Contraindicated in ocular disease. Production of arsenic-fast strains is a disadvantage.

PENTAMIDINE. Pentamidine (Lomidine, 800 M and B) is an aromatic diamidine. Used in early African trypanosomiasis. Administration is preferably intramuscular, in 3.0 ml of distilled water, as a solution of pentamidine isethionate (75 percent base), but it may be given intravenously in 10 ml of distilled water. A course of 4 mg/kg may be given daily or on alternate days for 5 to 10 injections, and a second or further courses after 1 week. For prophylaxis 5 mg/kg may be given at intervals of 6 months for *T. gambiense* and of 2 months for *T. rhodesiense* in single or divided doses. Pentamidine is less toxic than the other aromatic diamidines, stilbamidine and propamidine. Transitory immediate reactions, which are largely due to fall in blood pressure and hypoglycemia, include rapid pulse, vertigo, faintness, salivation, nausea, vomiting, sweating, itching, and puffiness of eyelids. Contraindicated in renal disease.

MELARSOPROL. Mel B (Arsobal), an alkyl mercapto derivative of melaminylphenylarsenoxide, is a trivalent melarsen oxide combined with BAL (British antilewisite). Used in early and late African trypanosomiasis, especially in cases refractory to tryparsamide. Administered intravenously in a 5 percent solution in propylene glycol. The daily dose is 3.6 mg/kg for 4 consecutive days, then a rest of 7 days and a second series of four daily doses. In patients with severe meningo-encephalitic involvement, the first doses are given at intervals of several days. Toxicity of therapeutic dose is too great for field use. In excessive dosage the drug produces symptoms of arsenic toxicity, such as headache, fever, vomiting, and erythema, but it is nontoxic to the kidneys and optic nerve. No contraindications except arsenic sensitivity. Drug-fast strains may develop.

Prevention. Prevention includes the reduction of sources of infection in man, the protection of man from infection, and the control of riverine tsetse flies. Man may be protected by reducing exposure to tsetse flies and by chemoprophylaxis. Chemoprophylaxis and mass treatment have markedly reduced the incidence of Gambian trypanosomiasis in many localities. The use of Suramin at 3-month intervals has been replaced by pentamidine isethionate at 6-month intervals for Gambian and at 2-month intervals for Rhodesian trypanosomiasis. Successful prophylaxis involves wholesale inoculations, treatment of carriers, persistence of prophylaxis for 4 to 5 years in highly endemic areas, and speedy action to minimize drug resistance.

Exposure to the day-biting riverine species may be lessened by avoidance of streams and waterholes during the warm dry season; elimination of the flies at watercrossings; restriction of travel in fly-infested regions to nighttime; the use of headnets, leggings, and gloves; and the application of repellents. In some instances, mass removal of local populations from fly-infested areas has proved advantageous, and the spread of the disease may be reduced by border quarantine of infected migrants. The control of the riverine tsetse flies comprises the reduction of their habitats and breeding places, and their destruction by insecticides and other methods.

Trypanosoma rhodesiense

Disease.   Rhodesian trypanosomiasis, East African sleeping sickness.

Life Cycle.   See Fig. 16. Similar to *T. gambiense* except in the species of its insect vector. Antelopes, and possibly other wild game and domesticated cattle, are reservoir hosts. The principal insect vectors are the woodland tsetse flies (*Glossina morsitans, G. pallidipes,* and *G. swynnertoni*), but it is capable of developing in other species (Page 282). *T. rhodesiense* (Fig. 15.2) is morphologically indistinguishable from *T. gambiense.*

Epidemiology.   The incidence of Rhodesian trypanosomiasis is lower, and epidemics are less frequent than in the Gambian disease. The disease is endemic among the cattle-raising tribes of East Africa and tends to spread to new territory. It is present in Northeastern and Southern Rhodesia, Nyasaland, Mozambique, Tanganyika, and eastern Uganda. Its endemicity, as well as its geographic distribution, is determined by the woodland habitat of its principal vectors.

The study of reservoir hosts in wild game is complicated by many species being natural hosts of the pathogenic trypanosomes of domesticated animals. The existence of wild life reservoirs is indicated by finding infected tsetse flies in areas uninhabited by man for years and by the acquisition of infection by travelers in areas not traversed by man for periods exceeding the normal life of this fly. The vector flies feed chiefly upon ungulates and, infrequently, on man.

Pathogenicity.   Rhodesian trypanosomiasis runs a more rapid and fatal course than does the Gambian disease, often terminating within a year. The pathologic changes in the acute disease are similar to those of Gambian sleeping sickness, but the febrile paroxysms are more frequent and severe, the glandular enlargement less pronounced; edema, myocarditis, weakness, and emaciation are more prominent. Chronic lesions in the central nervous system are less frequently encountered, since death intervenes before marked cerebrospinal changes occur. Thus, while mental disturbances may develop, there are seldom tics, choreic movements, convulsions, or the typical sleeping sickness syndrome. Untreated cases tend to run a fatal course.

Diagnosis.   Similar to *T. gambiense.*

Treatment.   See under *Treatment* for *T. gambiense* above. The Rhodesian disease requires earlier and more intensive treatment than the Gambian. Suramin is only effective in the very early disease and should be administered within 3 weeks of the onset of symptoms to effect a cure. Pentamidine is less effective. Mel B does not replace Suramin in the early disease, but it is of value in patients with disease too advanced for Suramin. More information is needed as to its capabilities, particularly in regard to its synergistic action with Suramin. Tryparsamide may be used following Suramin in borderline neurologic involvement.

Prevention.   The prevention of Rhodesian tryponosomiasis involves medical, veterinary, entomologic, agricultural, and social problems arising from the redistribution of populations and the control of vectors. Its control requires constant supervision to detect new cases, to keep track of the old, and to regulate agriculture. The woodland tsetse flies are more difficult to eradicate and control than the riverine species (Page 282). The detection and treatment of infected persons is the same as for *T. gambiense*, but in spite of the scattered foci the few chronic cases make the task easier. Contact between man and tsetse flies may be broken by the removal of inhabitants from fly-infested areas to open country in close settlements and by discriminative clearing of bush in essential fly habitats and in the outer fringes of forests. Chemoprophylaxis, repellents, nets, and screens may give some protection to the individual.

Trypanosoma cruzi

Disease.   American trypanosomiasis, Chagas' disease.

Morphology.   See above. In the blood the trypanosomes appear either as long, thin flagellates about 20 μ in length or as short stumpy forms about 15 μ in length, with pointed posterior ends. In stained blood smears they have a U or S shape, a free flagellum about one-third of the body length, a granular cytoplasm, a deeply staining central nucleus, and a large kinetoplast (Fig. 15.3). In the tissues the round or oval aflagellate leishmanian forms in cells or in cysts are more common than the flagellated trypanosomes. Crithidial forms may also be present.

Life Cycle.   The vertebrate hosts are man and domesticated and wild animals. At least 28 species of reduviid bugs—*Panstrongylus, Rhodnius, Eutriatoma,* and *Triatoma*—have been found naturally infected with trypanosomes resembling *T. cruzi*, but the principal vectors are *T. infestans, T. sordida, P. megistus,* and *R. prolixus* (Page 265). Reduviid bugs may remain infected over 2 years or possibly for life.

Transmission to vertebrates is by the fecal contaminative method after cyclic reproduction for 8 to 20 days in the intestine of the reduviid bug. During the night the bug bites man, and since the bug frequently defecates at the time of biting, the bite wound is readily contaminated (Fig. 17). Infections are produced also in uncontaminated bites, evidently from the regurgitation of metacyclic trypanosomes. Infection may also be transmitted by the contamination of mucous membranes or abraded skin by infective feces, or by handling infected animals, although *T. cruzi* cannot penetrate unbroken skin. Blood transfusion may be a source of infection. Dogs and cats are the most important reservoir hosts.

Epidemiology.   Chagas' disease is prevalent throughout South America and most of Central America, where an estimated 7 million persons are infected.

Surveys using xenodiagnosis and complement fixation reveal an incidence of 12 to 17 percent in endemic areas. Its prevalence is highest in the rural districts and poorer classes living in thatched adobe huts, the walls of which offer excellent hiding places for the insect vectors. The clinical disease is more common in children than adults, and from two-thirds to four-fifths of the patients are under 21 years of age. In Brazil the disease is often severe with cardiac complications, while in Chile it is less severe and often asymptomatic. In North America it is present in southern Mexico, but only two autochthonous cases have been reported in the southwestern United States, where *T. cruzi* is widely distributed in reduviid bugs. One serum specimen, from a boy 8 years old, out of 1,909 serums from individuals in various

TRYPANOSOMA CRUZI

CHAGAS' DISEASE

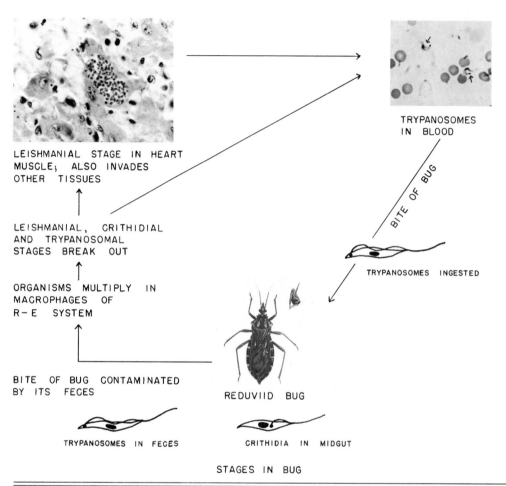

TRYPANOSOMES
IN BLOOD

LEISHMANIAL STAGE IN HEART
MUSCLE; ALSO INVADES
OTHER TISSUES

BITE OF BUG

TRYPANOSOMES INGESTED

LEISHMANIAL, CRITHIDIAL
AND TRYPANOSOMAL
STAGES BREAK OUT

ORGANISMS MULTIPLY IN
MACROPHAGES OF
R–E SYSTEM

BITE OF BUG CONTAMINATED
BY ITS FECES

REDUVIID BUG

TRYPANOSOMES IN FECES

CRITHIDIA IN MIDGUT

STAGES IN BUG

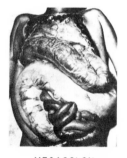

MEGACOLON

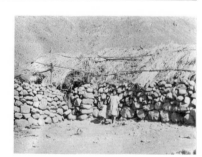

HOME OF MAN AND
BUG (TRIATOMA) IN CHILE

Fig. 17. Life cycle of *Trypanosoma cruzi.*

areas in Texas gave a significant serologic titer. It is possible that many infections go unnoticed due to the difficulty of diagnosis and to the fact that it is rarely considered in the differential diagnosis in the United States. Six out of 941 serums from Georgia residents gave positive reactions; two of the positively reacting serum specimens were from hospital patients suffering from "diffuse myocardial disease."

Nine species of triatomids and 14 species of mammals have been found infected with *T. cruzi* in the United States. One explanation for the absence of Chagas' disease in the United States is that the triatomids live under the bark of trees and animal burrows, as man's abode does not satisfy the bug's housing demands. It is also true that certain species of triatomids do not defecate as they feed, hence the absence of contaminative infection.

Pathology and Symptomatology. It is generally believed that the metacyclic trypanosomes, soon after their entrance into the mammalian host, are engulfed by the macrophages of the reticuloendothelial system, in which they multiply to erupt in 4 or 5 days, some entering the blood and others penetrating the cells of the various organs. Within the cells they assume the leishmanian form and continue to reproduce until the distended cells rupture, liberating leishmanian, trypanosomal, and crithidial forms, the first two apparently being capable of invading new cells. Different strains have predilection for certain tissues; most strains invade the fixed macrophages of the various tissues, while others prefer the cardiac and skeletal muscles.

The cells of the host react to invasion by vacuolation, hyperchromatosis, and hypertrophy. The basic pathologic process is essentially a parenchymatous degeneration of the affected tissues and an exudative inflammatory reaction, probably allergic, of the interstitial structures, followed later by proliferative changes. The course of the disease is represented first by the local lesion, the primary chagoma, at the site of the inoculation, and later by metastatic lesions throughout the body. The site of the infection is often on the head and on the eyelids.

After an incubation period of 1 to 2 weeks, there is an abrupt onset of daily fever, erythematous rash, and adenitis of the cervical, axillary, and iliac glands. Infection in the orbital region leads to unilateral conjunctivitis and edema of the eyelids, Romaña's sign. The liver and spleen may enlarge. Although any organ may be invaded, the most damaging lesions in man are in the heart and brain (Fig. 18), resulting in disability and even death. The heart enlarges and various arrhythmias develop leading to heart block. Autopsy reveals acute and chronic myocarditis. Healing may take place, and the resulting fibrosis give rise to chronic myocardial insufficiency.

A severe complication of the acute disease is diffuse meningoencephalitis with focal necrosis of the mesoglial cells, with neurologic signs, convulsions, and psychic manifestations.

Clinically, *T. cruzi* produces an acute or a chronic disease which may last 20 years or longer. It is serious and often fatal in young children, but is less severe and tends to become chronic in older children and adults. As a rule the chronic infection has no characteristic symptoms and many asymptomatic cases pass unrecognized. Megaesophagus and megacolon are not uncommon; this dilatation is due to a degeneration of autonomic nervous plexuses secondary to the toxins of *T. cruzi* (Fig. 17). The mortality rate is unknown because of the many unrecognized asymptomatic cases. The prognosis for children with the acute disease, especially the meningeal form, is unfavorable; and residual lesions may be present in

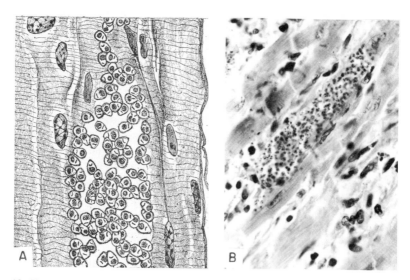

Fig. 18. *Trypanosoma cruzi* in tissues. A, section of striated muscle of infected guinea pig showing leishmanial forms. (× 1000) (Redrawn from Vianna, 1911); B, section of human heart with leishmanial forms and showing muscle destruction. (× 500)

survivors. Young adults with chronic heart infections rarely live beyond middle age.

Diagnosis.   The disease may be suspected when general and cardiac symptoms are present in patients of poor economic status in endemic regions. Laboratory diagnosis is made by finding the parasite in the blood or tissues, or by serologic methods. *T. cruzi* is present consistently in the blood only during the first 6 weeks of the disease, and it may be detected in thick blood smears. The histologic appearance of biopsied lymph nodes may be highly suggestive. *T. cruzi* may be confused with *T. rangeli* in the blood and *Leishmania braziliensis* in the tissues, but it may be differentiated by its large kintoplast. When the parasites are few, material from the blood, lymph nodes, bone marrow, and spleen may be cultured or injected into animals. The diagnostic method of choice, particularly in the chronic disease, is xenodiagnosis. Trypanosome-free reduviid bugs are allowed to feed on the blood of the suspected patient; the bugs are later examined for the metacyclic trypanosomes. This method is credited with 80 percent efficiency. Complement fixation (Machado-Guerreiro test) is performed with antigens of *T. cruzi*. It is valuable in revealing chronic cases and rarely gives positive reactions with other diseases; however, only about half of the patients with the acute disease give positive reactions. The hemagglutination and fluorescent antibody tests are also of value.

Treatment.   Treatment is unsatisfactory, since there is no drug that destroys the tissue-inhabiting organisms. Of the numerous types of compounds the eight aminoquinolines (Primaquine) appear to be most useful by eradicating the trypanosomes from the blood and thus preventing massive tissue invasion. A dose of 10 mg daily combined with 1 g of tetracycline, for 3 weeks or longer, given orally, appears to have some effect early in the infection. Nitrofurans and amphotericin B give promise of being of value against this infection. The chronic disease with intracellular invasion by the leishmanian stages, resists therapy; hence, only symptomatic therapy remains.

Prevention.   Preventive measures call for the destruction of the triatomid vectors and the protection of man from their bites. Since the replacement of insanitary houses with modern dwellings is economically impractical, the destruction of reduviid bugs in these houses by insecticides seems the best available method of combating the disease.

Other Species of South American Trypanosomes in Man

T. rangeli is found in South and Central America. A high percentage of children are infected in Venezuela. Except for the organism's small kinetoplast it may be mistaken for *T. cruzi*. It produces no symptoms in man or lower mammals. The natural reservoir hosts are dogs in urban areas, and monkeys, opossums, and anteaters in rural areas. The chief insect vector is *Rhodnius prolixus*. Transmission probably occurs through the proboscis.

PARASITIC LEISHMANIA OF MAN

The genus *Leishmania* includes flagellates that occur as leishmanias in vertebrate hosts and as leptomonads in invertebrate hosts and cultures.

Morphology. The typical leishmanian parasite in the vertebrate host is a small oval protozoon, 2 to 6 μ by 1 to 3 μ, with no flagellum or undulating membrane (Fig. 14 and 15.5, 6). Toward the posterior end is an oval vesicular nucleus which has a delicate membrane, submembranous chromatin, and a central karyosome. Anterior and tangential to the nucleus is a rod-shaped kinetoplast of variable size that contains the parabasal body, rhizoplast, and dot-like blepharoplast. Both nucleus and kinetoplast contain deoxyribonucleic acid. In the cytoplasm are mitochonodria, neutral red vacuoles, and basophilic and volutin granules containing ribonucleic acid. In cultures or in the invertebrate host, the parasites range from the leishmanian to the typical leptomonad form. The latter, equipped with a long delicate anterior flagellum, varies from a pyriform to a long, slender, spindle shape, 14 to 20 μ by 1.5 to 4 μ (Fig. 14).

The motile flagellate has a higher metabolism than the nonmotile leishmanian form, and utilizes carbohydrates, mainly dextrose, in its aerobic respiratory activities. In cultures, oxygen consumption and metabolic activities are dependent upon the dextrose in the medium. Food is absorbed from the tissues of the host. Reproduction occurs by longitudinal binary division in both leishmanian and flagellate forms, a new flagellum being formed by one daughter blepharoplast. The parasites die immediately at 45° C, but they survive for years when held at —70° C. Leishmanias may be cultivated in noncellular mediums (Page 328), tissue cultures, and chick embryo.

Life Cycle. The life cycle involves an alternate existence in a vertebrate and an insect host (Fig. 19). The natural reservoir hosts other than man include domesticated and wild mammals. The invertebrate hosts are sandflies, *Phlebotomus*. Only those species closely associated with man are important vectors of human leishmaniasis. After a blood meal the flagellates develop in the gut of the insect, in 8 to 20 days, to infective forms that migrate forward to the pharynx, buccal cavity, and mouth parts, where they may produce partial or complete blockage; they are dislodged by the efforts of the blocked sandflies to ingest blood. Transmission also may take place by contamination of the bite wound and by contact, but congenital transmission is of no practical importance. Infections have been produced in ex-

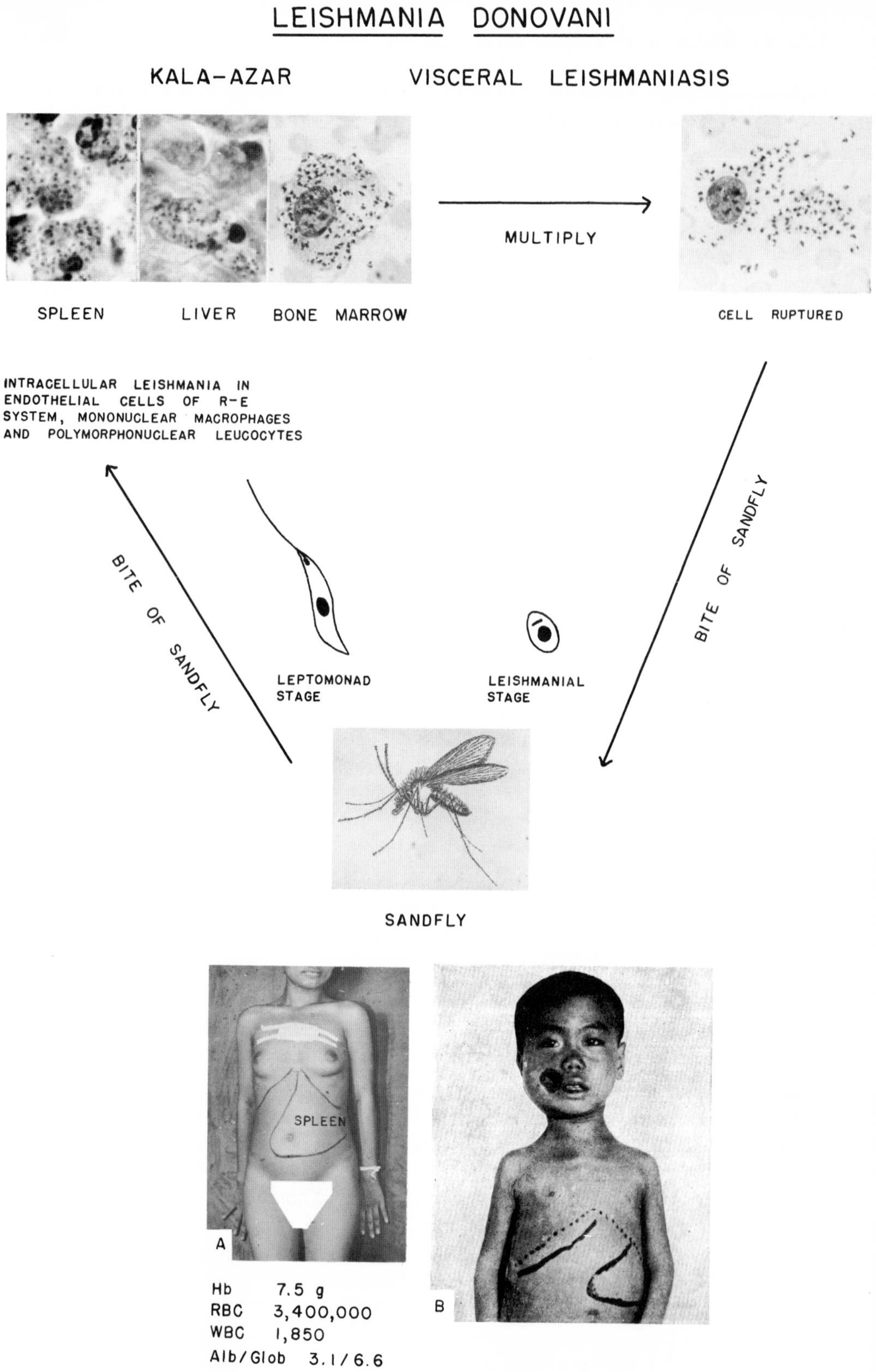

LEISHMANIA DONOVANI

KALA-AZAR   VISCERAL LEISHMANIASIS

SPLEEN   LIVER   BONE MARROW   CELL RUPTURED

MULTIPLY

INTRACELLULAR LEISHMANIA IN
ENDOTHELIAL CELLS OF R-E
SYSTEM, MONONUCLEAR MACROPHAGES
AND POLYMORPHONUCLEAR LEUCOCYTES

BITE OF SANDFLY   BITE OF SANDFLY

LEPTOMONAD   LEISHMANIAL
STAGE   STAGE

SANDFLY

Hb	7.5 g
RBC	3,400,000
WBC	1,850
Alb/Glob	3.1 / 6.6

Fig. 19. Life cycle of *Leishmania donovani*. A, diagnosed by sternal puncture; B, cancrum oris and enlargement of liver and spleen. (Photograph from Taiwan.)

perimental animals by parenteral injections, by contamination of the conjunctiva, and by oral administration. When the flagellates gain access to man, they lose their flagella, assume a leishmanian form, and multiply chiefly within the mononuclear and polymorphonuclear macrophages of the blood and cells of the reticuloendothelial system. When the cells rupture, the free parasites invade other cells or are phagocytosed.

Three species, similar in morphology but differing in cultural characteristics, clinical manifestations, geographic distribution, and species of vectors, are found in man: (1) *L. donovani* the etiologic agent of visceral leishmaniasis or kala-azar, (2) *L. tropica* of cutaneous leishmaniasis or oriental sore, and (3) *L. braziliensis* of mucocutaneous leishmaniasis. The three species are composed of a number of strains that differ in virulence, type of lesion, biologic characteristics, and adaptation to different vectors.

Immunity. Animals vary in natural resistance. Young animals are more susceptible than old, and individuals vary in susceptibility. Malnutrition and debility predispose to clinical attacks. Recovery from kala-azar and oriental sore gives a lasting immunity. Immunization with cultures or with material from human lesions or the spleens of infected animals has proved successful against oriental sore. Only about 5 percent of the persons thus vaccinated against *L. tropica* acquire oriental sore in endemic areas as compared with 63 to 93 percent of nonvaccinated persons. Reports on the effectiveness of immunization with killed organisms are conflicting. Agglutinins, precipitins, lysins, complement-fixing antibodies, and sensitizing antibodies may be produced in laboratory animals by the injection of living or dead organisms. Complement-fixing antibodies in kala-azar may be detected with antigens prepared from the flagellates or, strange to say, from acid-fast bacilli.

Leishmania donovani

Disease. Kala-azar or black disease, visceral leishmaniasis, dumdum fever, tropical splenomegaly.

In mammalian tissues *L. donovani* is a small, intracellular, nonflagellated oval body of uniform size, 4.2 by 2.8 μ (Fig. 15.5 and 20). In the gut of infected sandflies or in cultures, it assumes the leptomonad form (Fig. 15.7).

There are three main types of infection presumedly caused by separate strains: (1) the classic kala-azar of India that affects chiefly adults, does not occur in dogs, and has no known reservoir host; (2) the Mediterranean or infantile kala-azar that is prevalent in children throughout the Mediterranean countries, China, Middle Asia, and Central and South America, occurs frequently in dogs, and has wild reservoir hosts in jackals and possibly foxes in Middle Asia and wild dogs in South America; and (3) Sudanese kala-azar that affects adults, is somewhat resistant to antimony treatment, does not occur in dogs, and may have an unknown wild animal host. Strain variation has handicapped attempts to differentiate these types by the biologic characteristics of their organisms.

Life Cycle (Fig. 19). The important insect vectors are sandflies, *Phlebotomus*. In addition to man, the dog is the most important host.

Epidemiology. *L. donovani* is found in all continents except Australia: in Mediterranean Europe, in Asia (China, India, Middle Asia, and Southwest Asia), in North and East Africa, and in Central and South America.

Age, sex, and general resistance apparently affect susceptibility. In Mediterranean Europe, the infection is chiefly confined to children; in Middle Asia it is rare in those over 10 years; in China about one-third of the infections are in children under 10 years; and in Brazil about half of the cases occur in children under 6 years. Males acquire the disease more frequently than females. Its incidence is highest in rural areas and in squalid surroundings where conditions are favorable for sandflies.

Man is the chief source of infection and is the only known host in India and East Africa. In the other countries, where the infantile type predominates, dogs are another important source of infection, and in Middle Asia wild jackals and in South America dogs are also reservoir hosts. The disease is chiefly transmitted from man to man, or from dog to dog to man by various species of *Phlebotomus*. Also the possibility of mechanical transmission by insects, blood transfusion, and droplet infection must be considered. A well-documented infection in a female who had never been out of England established the transmission by sexual intercourse. Her husband had been infected and insufficiently treated in 1941; they married in 1953, and in 1955 the wife developed a vaginal lesion containing typical leishmania organisms. At this time lymph node biopsy of the husband revealed leishmania, which were cultured.

Pathology and Symptomatology.   A primary lesion at the site of infection is rarely observed, but minute papules have been described in infants. The phagocytosed parasites are present only in small numbers in the blood, but they are numerous in the reticuloendothelial cells of the spleen, liver, lymph nodes, bone marrow, intestinal mucosa, and other organs (Fig. 20), and there is marked hyperplasia of the reticular cells and increased vascularity of the tissues.

The incubation period is usually 1 to 4 months, but may be much longer. The initial fever, which lasts for 2 to 4 weeks, is usually intermittent with a daily rise to 102 to 104° F. Sometimes there is a pathognomonic double daily rise. Chills and sweating may be present, and the patient may present a malaria-like picture with which leishmaniasis is often confused. Diarrhea and dysentery are not uncommon and are related to heavy intestinal infection. Despite these symptoms the patient has a good appetite, and toxemia is absent. Later there is considerable weight loss and emaciation. The spleen gradually enlarges owing to the enormous increase of reticuloendothelial cells, many of which are heavily parasitized. Likewise, the liver may be enlarged owing to proliferation of the Küpffer cells which contain parasites.

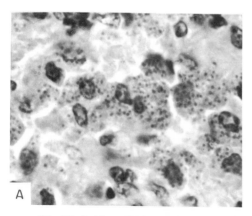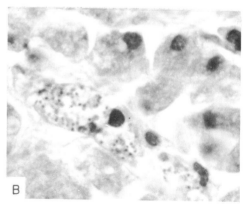

Fig. 20. *Leishmania donovani* in A, spleen (× 900); B, liver (× 950).

Serum glutamic oxalacetic transaminase is increased. Amyloid degeneration of renal glomeruli is found at autopsy.

A marked leukopenia with a relative monocytosis and lymphocytosis, anemia, and thrombocytopenia develop. The anemia is due to a reduced red cell life span and a mild degree of ineffective erythropoiesis. The plasma proteins undergo marked changes, with a reversal of the albumen: globulin ratio due largely to the elevation in the gamma globulins.

Skin changes develop as the disease continues and may consist of darkly pigmented erythematous, granulomatous areas with numerous parasites, or hypopigmented areas with few parasites.

General debility and leukopenia render the patient especially susceptible to secondary infections—e.g., cancrum oris, noma, pulmonary infections, and gastrointestinal complications. The untreated disease usually progresses to a fatal termination within 2 years, although fulminating infections may cause death within a few weeks, and chronic infections may persist for years. The clinical manifestations of the disease have been regarded as an expression of the breakdown in the parasite-host relationship due to an inadequate supply of gamma globulin for maintaining protective antibodies.

Diagnosis. In endemic areas, kala-azar may be suspected in a patient who has a persistent, irregular, remittent fever often with a double daily peak, leukopenia, and splenomegaly. Absolute diagnosis is made by finding the parasite in material from the blood and tissues by smear, culture, or inoculation of animals. In untreated patients the blood is usually examined first by smear or, preferably, by culture; if the result is negative, sternal, splenic, hepatic, or lymph node punctures are performed. Splenic puncture reveals the highest percentage of positive findings and is the method of choice in skilled hands, but sternal or hepatic puncture, although less certain, are safer procedures. When the parasites are relatively few, multiple cultures in N.N.N. medium of splenic or hepatic material give the most reliable results.

Diagnosis may be made by the complement-fixation and the fluorescent antibody tests. The formol-gel test or other nonspecific flocculation tests are useful for screening patients in clinics.

Treatment. Patients require bed rest during the acute disease, as well as a well-balanced high protein and vitamin diet, good nursing care, and auxiliary treatment with sulfonamides and antibiotics for secondary bacterial infections (such as bronchopnuemonia, diarrhea, and cancrum oris). Preliminary blood transfusions should be given to patients with severe anemia, edema, or bleeding from the mucous membranes. Systemic chemotherapy includes the antimonials and aromatic diamidines. The pentavalent antimonials are the standard chemotherapeutic agents. Sodium antimony gluconate, ethylstibamine, and the diamidines, pentamidine and stilbamidine, are effective. The aromatic diamidines may be used to advantage in antimony-resistant infections; antimony-sensitive, relapsing, or tuberculosis patients, and in the Mediterranean and Sudan areas. Stilbamidine, although the most toxic, is the most effective of the aromatic diamidines.

NEOSTIBOSAN. Neostibosan (ethylstibamine) is an organic pentavalent antimony derivative of phenyl stibonic acid with an antimony content of 41 to 44 percent. Administered intravenously in a freshly prepared 5 percent solution and intramuscularly in a 25 percent solution. For leishmaniasis daily intravenous doses, starting with 2 ml (0.1 g) increasing to a maximum of 6 ml (0.3 g), are given for 10 days to a total of 2.4 to 3.0 g. Toxic symptoms, probably allergic, such as nausea, vomiting, dyspnea, and urticaria may develop after irregular or repeated treatments. Contraindications are cardiac, pulmonary, or renal disease.

SOLUSTIBOSAN.   Solustibosan (sodium antimony gluconate) is a pentavalent antimony compound with an antimony content of 27 percent, prepared in a stable solution ready for injection. Results in visceral leishmaniasis are equal to those of neostibosan and urea stibamine. It is administered intravenously as a solution containing 20 mg antimony per milliliter, and intramuscularly as one of 100 mg or as an oil suspension of 54 mg per milliliter. The concentrated solutions are useful for treating children and for local injections for treatment of oriental sore. Intravenous injections of 12 to 18 ml are given daily for 10 days to a total of 2.4 to 3.6 g antimony, or 6 ml may be administered daily for 30 days. Intramuscular injections are made daily for 10 days to a total of 2 to 3 g for adults. The toxic symptoms are sharp rigor, temperature of 105° F, severe abdominal pains, vomiting, and diarrhea. Contraindicated in pulmonary or renal disease and in antimony-sensitive persons.

DIAMIDINES.   Stilbamidine (diamidinostilbene, 744 M and B) is the most effective, but the most toxic, of the aromatic diamidines. Used in visceral leishmaniasis, particularly in antimony-resistant cases. Administered intravenously in a freshly prepared 1 percent solution in distilled water. A course of treatment comprises 10 daily injections, starting at 0.025 g (2.5 ml) and increasing each day by 0.01 g, until a total of about 0.7 g has been given. In resistant cases the daily dose or the number of injections is increased so as to give a total of 1.0 to 1.3 g. The drug may also be administered on alternate days. Treatment should not be repeated within 4 weeks.

Its high toxicity precludes its use in outpatient clinics and field work. The immediate toxic reactions include fall in blood pressure, dyspnea, faintness, headache, sweating, formication, vomiting, and epigastric pains. The late symptoms in 3 to 4 months after treatment are systemic disorders resulting from degenerative lesions in the liver and kidneys and changes in the nervous system, particularly affecting the trigeminal nerve. Contraindicated in renal disease.

Pentamidine isethionate is useful in antimony-resistant infections; 2-4 mg/kg of body weight intramuscularly are given daily up to 15 doses. It is less toxic than stilbamidine.

Prevention.   The treatment of infected persons and the elimination of diseased dogs will reduce the sources of infection. Sandflies may be controlled by the destruction of their breeding grounds near human habitations and by the use of insecticides, particularly the residual spraying of houses with DDT (Page 278). Man may be protected by compactly built houses with fine mesh screening, and by repellents.

Leishmania tropica

Disease.   Oriental sore, Delhi ulcer, Aleppo, Delhi or Baghdad boil, cutaneous leishmaniasis.

The leishmanian (Fig. 15.6) and the leptomonad (Fig. 15.8) parasites are similar to those of *L. donovani*. In smears from the cutaneous lesions, leishmanias may be observed intracellularly in mononuclear and polymorphonuclear leukocytes and epithelial cells, or extracellularly when released by the rupture of these cells.

There are two nosologic types of oriental sore due to different strains: (1) the dry or urban type that runs a chronic course with late ulceration, and (2) the moist or rural type that has an acute course with early ulceration.

Life Cycle.   The reservoir hosts for the moist type are gerbils and other wild rodents. Experimental infections have been produced in mice, hamsters, rats, guinea pigs, dogs, and monkeys. The insect vectors are species of *Phlebotomus*.

Epidemiology.   Oriental sore is endemic in Asia Minor and in Middle and Southwest Asia, and to a lesser extent in North Africa, Mediterranean Europe, and South and Central America. The incidence of oriental sore is high in some endemic regions, such as the Dead Sea area of Jordan and the southern part of the Soviet Union bordering Asia Minor; at times the disease may even assume an epidemic form. Experimentally, infections have been transmitted cyclically by *P. papatasii* after feeding on cultures or lesions; and mechanically by the bite of the stable fly, *Stomoxys calcitrans,* and by the contamination of wounds with infective insect feces. The moist type is transmitted from gerbil to man, and man to man by sandflies in rural areas. The infection rate, which remains constant during the year in gerbils because of the optimal conditions in their burrows, explains the high incidence in man in isolated settlements during the seasons when sandflies attack man.

Pathology and Symptomatology.   In man the disease is limited to the cutaneous tissues and, occasionally, the mucous membranes. The difference between the moist and dry types is quantitative rather than qualitative. In the infected area there is hypertrophy of the corium and cellular infiltration of the dermal layers with epithelioid and lymphoid elements. The parasites are found both intra- and extra-cellularly, particularly in the histiocytes. The infiltrative stage is followed by a papular or nodular stage with dilated and anastomosing capillaries and, finally, by lysis of the tissues. Ulceration is produced by the penetration of the basement membrane by the parasites and the disintegration of the epidermis. The neighboring secondary lesions, which have a tuberculoid structure with few or no parasites, are generally regarded as allergic reactions.

The usual incubation period varies from several weeks to several months, but periods as long as 3 years have been recorded in experimental infections. The small initial papule continues to enlarge, acquires a glazed purplish appearance, and becomes covered with brown scales. By the third or fourth month, it becomes an indurated crusted ulcer that discharges a thin offensive pus. Single or multiple lesions may occur on the exposed body. At times the coalescence of ulcers and secondary bacterial invasion may result in extensive ulceration and even a generalized infection. Chills and fever may accompany the appearance of new sores. Uncomplicated sores heal in 2 to 10 months, but leave depigmented retracted scars, which are often disfiguring (Fig. 21).

Diagnosis.   The type and distribution of the lesions, and the presence of the parasites in the material from the indurated margin of the ulcer, establish the diagnosis. Cultures may be prepared if the microscopic examination is negative. Positive reactions to an intracutaneous test with an *L. tropica* antigen may be obtained as early as the second month and can persist for years. A positive reaction is characterized by a red area with a central papule that appears in 8 to 15 hours and reaches a maximum in 48 hours. Positive reactions have been obtained in 93 percent of persons with established sores, in 98 percent of those recovered from the infection, and in 7 to 13 percent of those with no history of infection.

Treatment (Oriental Sore.)   In endemic areas when the lesions are not on the face, it may be advisable to withhold treatment until sufficient time has elapsed

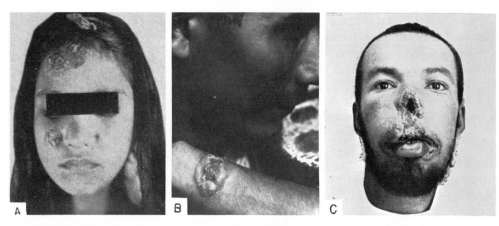

Fig. 21. Dermal and mucocutaneous leishmaniasis. A, lesions on forehead, right and left cheek. (Courtesy of Dr. H. K. Giffen, American Mission Hospital, Assiut, Egypt.) B, lesion on arm. (Courtesy of Army Medical Museum.) C, mucocutaneous form. (From Strong, Stitt's *Diagnosis, Prevention and Treatment of Tropical Diseases,* 7th ed., 1944. Courtesy of The Blakiston Co.)

for the patient to acquire immunity; but in nonendemic areas treatment may be instituted at once. If there are only a single or a few ulcers, local treatment is usually sufficient. Various types of local treatment have been used, including penicillin or bacitracin for bacterially infected ulcers, roentgen rays, electrocoagulation, carbon dioxide snow, and infiltration with Stibophen. The early lesions respond well to infiltrations of Quinacrine, 1 to 2 ml of a 10 percent solution given weekly for 1 to 5 weeks. The sores should be protected by dressings to prevent bacterial contamination and autoinoculation. For multiple lesions and advanced lesions, systemic treatment with Neostibosan (see under *Treatment* for *L. donovani* above) is advisable.

Prevention.   Protective covering of the ulcers reduces the chances of transmission by contact or insect vectors. The poisoning of rodents in their burrows has proved effective in reducing human infection in neighboring villages. The control of sandflies by the residual spraying of houses with DDT has markedly lowered the incidence of the disease in countries where the dry type of oriental sore is prevalent. Many may also be protected from sandflies by screens, nets, and repellents. Active immunization with living organisms provides effective protection, although immunity requires several months to develop.

Leishmania braziliensis

Disease.   American leishmaniasis, nasopharyngeal or mucocutaneous leishmaniasis, espundia, uta, chiclero ulcer, and forest yaws (Fig. 21C).

There are three nosologic types of the disease evidently due to different strains: (1) the Mexican or chicle ulcer type in which the lesions are chiefly confined to the ears and which runs a chronic course with few parasites, little ulceration, and no metastatic mucosal lesions; (2) the uta type in which the cutaneous lesions resemble those of oriental sore, with many parasites in the early lesions and few in the late, rarely extending or metastasizing to the mucous membranes; and (3) the espundia type in which there are frequently polypoid or ulcerative metastases or extensions to the mucocutaneous and cutaneous surfaces. The first two types are usually found above an altitude of 2,200 feet, and the third in warmer regions below that level.

Life Cycle. *L. braziliensis* undergoes cyclic development in species of sand-flies *Phlebotomus,* the chief vector apparently being *P. intermedius* (Page 277). Among the wild animals the agouti is suspected of being a reservoir host, and natural infections have been found in tapirs, cavies, civets, and capybaras. No reservoir hosts have been discovered in domesticated animals, although dogs are under suspicion.

Epidemiology. *L. braziliensis* is present from Yucatán, Mexico, throughout much of South America. The disease is rural rather than urban. It is most prevalent in adult males because of occupational exposure. In Brazil one-third of the espundia cases are in children. The prevalence and seasonal distribution of the disease is related to the density of sandflies, to their association with man, and to temperature and humidity. The parasite has been found in 0.23 percent of sand-flies in Brazil, chiefly in *P. intermedius*. The disease may be transmitted by direct contact, as well as by the bite of sandflies. The high incidence in forest workers suggests a reservoir source in wild animals, but none, except possibly the agouti, has been detected.

Pathology and Symptomatology. The pathology of the cutaneous lesion is similar to that of oriental sore. The initial lesion, probably at the site of the bite, starts as an impetiginous focus, a fissure on the lip, or a small papule, which becomes red, itchy and at times vesiculated during the primary phase of 1 to 4 weeks. Then a punched-out painless ulcer with a granular base, an undermined indurated margin, and a scanty purulent discharge persists for from 6 months to several years, although most lesions heal with a pliable depigmented scar in 12 to 15 months. The lesion extends by the formation of small peripheral nodules to a diameter of 3 cm in 2 to 3 months, and not infrequently is accompanied by regional adenitis. The parasites, mostly intracellular, are numerous in the early lesions, but are rare in the chronic; they are seldom found in mucous lesions of espundia.

In the Mexican type three-fifths of the lesions are on the ear. The incubational period is 2 to 6 weeks. The lesions on the ear run a long chronic course with little ulceration and few parasites; others undergo necrosis and mutilating cicatrization. The cutaneous lesions elsewhere on the body tend to heal spontaneously within a few weeks, leaving only small scars.

The lesions of the uta type are similar to those of the Mexican, except for less predilection for the ears. They rarely extend to the mucous membranes.

In the espundia type the incubational period is 2 to 3 months. The initial lesion is usually cutaneous, but at times it may be mucosal. About three-fourths of the patients with cutaneous lesions of over 1 year's duration show secondary lesions, chiefly of the nose. The secondary lesions are painful and may cause great deformity. The eroding ulcer often destroys the cartilage of the septum so that the tip of the nose is depressed to give a characteristic parrot beak or camel nose. In the mouth and pharynx there is thickening of the lips and the affected parts. The lesions are accompanied by fever, moderate hyperchromic anemia, malaise, and, if the larynx is affected, by loss of voice. The chief complaint is nasal obstruction. The organisms not infrequently are present on intact mucosa, and the metastatic lesions may arise after the healing of the primary cutaneous lesions.

Leishmaniasis tegumentaria diffusa reported from Venezuela and Ethiopia is an extraordinary variety of the disease in which the parasite spreads throughout the skin, giving rise to an almost incurable condition resembling lepromatous leprosy.

In the Mexican and uta types the prognosis is favorable; the lesions eventually heal spontaneously and respond readily to treatment. In the espundia type, prognosis is unfavorable when the mucous membranes are severely involved, but the early lesions tend to respond to treatment, and occasionally the cutaneous and even the secondary lesions may heal spontaneously.

Diagnosis. Clinically the disease requires differentiation from yaws and syphilis. *L. braziliensis* may be found by microscopic examination or culture of biopsied material and smears from the indurate margins of the ulcers and, at times, from the lymph nodes. The parasites are numerous in the early, and scarce in the late, lesions. The intracutaneous Montenegro test with whole or fractionated antigens of cultured *L. braziliensis* is considered the diagnostic method of choice in clinics and in surveys. The reaction of the delayed type becomes positive in 1 to 4 weeks after the appearance of the initial lesion and persists for life.

Treatment. In view of the destructive mucocutaneous lesions, intravenous therapy with ethylstibamine (Neostibosan, see under *Treatment* for *L. donovani* above) should be instituted as soon as the diagnosis is made. Sodium antimony tartrate and stibophen may be used in subsequent therapy. Amphotericin B also has therapeutic value. Antibiotics should be used if bacterial infection is present. Pyrimethamine and cycloguanil pamoate are of value in Central American dermal leishmaniasis.

Prevention. Preventive measures include protection against sandflies (Page 278) and avoidance of contact infection. Infected persons should be treated, and the lesions protected from sandflies. Protection of forest workers is a difficult problem. Active immunization may prove feasible in the future.

Toxoplasma gondii

Toxoplasma gondii was first found in the African rodent *Ctenodactylus gondi* in 1908; Janku in 1923 described toxoplasmic chorioretinitis; and in 1939 Wolf et al. isolated the parasite and established it as the cause of the congenital neonatal disease. Numerous species of *Toxoplasma* have been described, but it appears that there is only a single species capable of infecting a wide variety of hosts. It is a protozoan belonging to the sporozoa.

Morphology. This obligate, intracellular parasite is pyriform in shape and approximately 3 to 6 μ. This parasite has a cell membrane, a spheroid-to-oval nucleus with a central karyosome, and several organelles of unknown function (Fig. 22).

Life Cycle. *T. gondii* multiplies by binary fission within the host's cell. Endodyogeny, a process of internal budding, has also been described. The distended tissue cells rupture, and the parasites, progressing with a gliding movement, enter new cells. The host's cell may become greatly hypertrophied and distended with 50 to 3000 parasites contained in a cyst. *T. gondii* consumes oxygen, utilizes dextrose, evolves CO_2; its respiration is cyanide sensitive. It will grow in any mammalian or avian tissue culture.

Epidemiology. Toxoplasmosis is cosmopolitan, and antibody surveys indicate that from 20 to 80 percent of various populations are infected. Children have

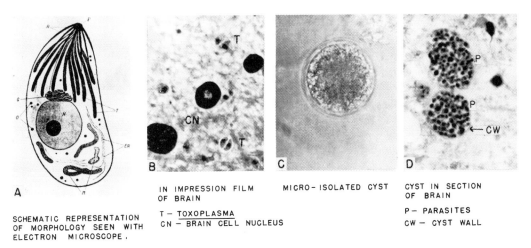

A SCHEMATIC REPRESENTATION OF MORPHOLOGY SEEN WITH ELECTRON MICROSCOPE.

B IN IMPRESSION FILM OF BRAIN

T – TOXOPLASMA
CN – BRAIN CELL NUCLEUS

C MICRO-ISOLATED CYST

D CYST IN SECTION OF BRAIN

P – PARASITES
CW – CYST WALL

ER – ENDOPLASMIC RETICULUM
G- GOLGI APPARATUS; M- MITOCHONDRIA; N- NUCLEUS; O- OSMIOPHILIC GRANULES
P- POLE RING; R- RADIAL RIBS; T- TOXONEMES

Fig. 22. *Toxoplasma gondii*. (A and C from Toxoplasmosis with Special Reference to Uveitis. Edited by A. E. Maumenee; The Williams and Wilkins Co., 1961. (A, courtesy of Ludvik; C, courtesy of R. Lainson; D, courtesy of H. C. Neu.)

the fewest positive tests. Although infection is common, disease is rare. Neonatal toxoplasmosis is credited with an incidence of 70 per 100,000. This congenital infection is acquired by transplacental transmission from mothers who have had an asymptomatic or unrecognized infection. *Toxoplasma* cysts have been found in beef, pork, lamb, poultry, rabbits, and dogs. Persons with trichinosis have a high *Toxoplasma* infection rate, suggesting pork as a source of infection; however, orthodox Jews and vegetarians have been reported to have high infection rates as do herbivorous domestic and wild animals. The prevalence rates in Hindu vegetarians and meat-eating Moslems in India were very similar. The presence of the organisms in the tissues, secretions, excretions, and dejecta presents numerous transmission possibilities; and laboratory animals have been infected by several routes of inoculation. Accidental human infections have occurred from lesions produced by contaminated needles. *Toxoplasma* has been transmitted by *Toxocara* eggs.

Pathology and Symptomatology. Ordinarily, *T. gondii* is a relatively benign, well-adapted parasite, and its disease-producing properties have been attributed to virulent strains or especially susceptible hosts.

CONGENITAL TOXOPLASMOSIS. The acute infection, considered to be due to the acquisition of the parasite by the mother shortly before delivery, is characterized by a severe febrile illness involving many organs. When transmission to the fetus takes place earlier in pregnancy, the acute infection has waned at the time of birth, and the infant may be afebrile. In this so-called subacute form, the cardinal tetrad—intracerebral calcification, chorioretinitis, hydrocephaly or microcephaly, and psychomotor disturbances and convulsions—may be noted at birth or shortly thereafter. Visceral and muscular lesions are also present.

There may be spasticity, opisthotonos, retraction of the head, stiff neck, and even paralysis. Anemia and leukocytosis with an absolute increase in monocytes and lymphocytes are present in about half of the patients. The spinal fluid shows increased pressure, xanthochromia, round-cell pleocytosis, a high protein content, and, occasionally, the organisms. The cerebral lesions may undergo calcification, appearing in roentgenographs as small round bodies, broad bands or scattered granules. Toxoplasmic cysts, which may persist for years without causing tissue reaction, may be present in apparently healthy tissues near the necrotic areas. Occasionally their rupture may give rise to edema, cellular infiltration, and necrosis, possibly an allergic reaction.

The chorioretinal lesions in infants are severe, extensive, and bilateral. There is an intense edema of the retina and various degrees of degeneration and necrotic inflammation with perivascular and general cellular infiltration. There may be an optic neuritis. Death may occur, or the infant may survive with a chronic infection or residual lesions. Mild forms of the disease in children or adults may be manifested by only retinochoroiditis with destruction of the macula.

ACQUIRED TOXOPLASMOSIS.   After infection and regional lymph node invasion, the parasite is blood-borne to many organs where intracellular multiplication takes place. Parasitemia persists for several weeks; and with the production of antibody, cysts form in various tissues; the patients are asymptomatic. There are three main clinical types of acquired postnatal toxoplasmosis: (1) The more common, mild lymphatic form resembling infectious mononucleosis. It is characterized by cervical and axillary lymphadenopathy, malaise, muscle pain, and irregular low fever. Slight anemia, low blood pressure, leukopenia, lymphocytosis, and slightly altered liver function may be present. (2) Acute, fulminating, disseminated infections, often with a skin rash, high fever, chills, and prostration. Meningencephalitis, hepatitis, pneumonitis, and myocarditis may be present. (3) Chronic toxoplasmosis with retinochoroiditis or posterior uveitis. This form of toxoplasmosis is difficult to diagnose, as the symptoms are vague and indefinite. Muscular weakness, weight loss, headache, and diarrhea may be present. It must be remembered that an estimated 65 percent of the retinochoroiditis and uveitis in the United States is NOT due to *Toxoplasma* infection. The existence of numerous persons with latent or cured toxoplasmosis and the few fatal cases in adults indicate the general mildness of the infection in man. Neonatal infections are fatal more often, produce subacute or chronic neurologic infections or residual lesions in children, or pass into a quiescent state. The future offspring of a symptomless mother who has previously given birth to an infected infant, very seldom if ever acquire the disease congenitally.

Diagnosis.   (See flow chart below.) The Sabin-Feldman dye test is the most useful serologic test. The test is based on the failure of living *Toxoplasma* organisms, in the presence of antibody and an accessory factor, to stain with methylene blue. Parasites not exposed to antibody stain readily. Because of the common occurrence of *Toxoplasma* antibodies in the general population, diagnosis by serologic means requires demonstration of a change from negative to positive, a rapidly ascending titer, or maintenance of a high titer.

The complement-fixation test becomes positive more slowly than the dye test. Because of this difference, its special usefulness is in the revelation of active infection when the dye test antibody levels are already high and stable. A negative complement-fixation test becoming positive or having an increase in titer, together with stable, high, dye test titers, are indicative of an active infection.

The hemagglutination test becomes positive later than the dye test, but in other respects correlates well with it.

SEROLOGIC DIAGNOSIS OF TOXOPLASMOSIS
FLOW CHART

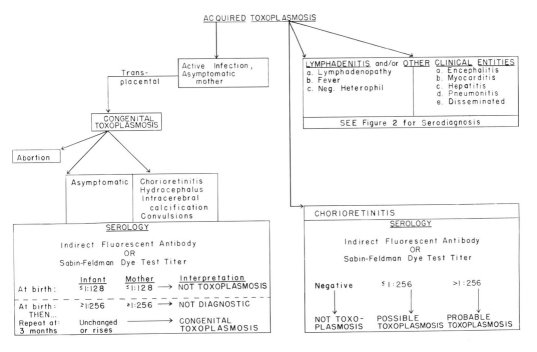

TEST

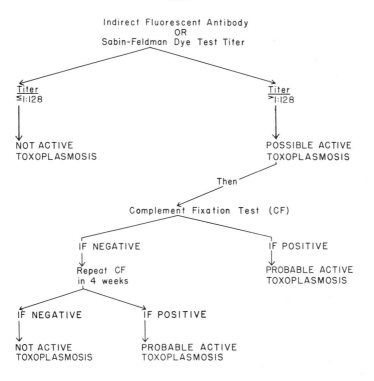

The *Toxoplasma* skin test reaction is of the delayed tuberculin type. As it becomes positive months after the onset of infection, a positive test early during an illness excludes acute toxoplasmosis.

Isolation of the parasite by the injection of the patient's blood, cerebrospinal fluid, lymph nodes, muscle, and other tissues into mice has yielded positive results during the acute phase of the disease. Biopsy material long after convalescence also may give positive results.

Treatment. All symptomatic infections should be treated with pyrimethamine (Daraprim) 1 mg/kg of body weight daily divided into two equal doses, after 2 or 3 days this dose may be reduced by half. Triple sulfonamides: 2 to 6 g daily for adults, and 100 to 150 mgs daily for infants and children. Therapy should be continued for a month. Both drugs act as inhibitors of nucleic acid synthesis— sulfadiazine competes with the para-aminobenzoic acid activity, and pyrimethamine is a folic acid antagonist.

Chronic ocular toxoplasmosis will usually respond to the above therapy. However, National Institutes of Health investigators have employed first-day loading doses of pyrimethamine as great as 200 mg. Relapses and failure to respond to therapy are considered to be at least partially due to hypersensitivity, and therefore corticosteroids are added to the standard therapy.

The usual sulfonamide toxic manifestations may be encountered, and these drugs stopped if they occur. High doses of pyrimethamine may cause thrombocytopenia, agranulocytosis, and anemia, which may be reversed by the administration of folinic acid (Leucovorin). Pregnant women should not be treated with pyrimethamine until the possibility of fetal damage is better understood.

Prognosis. Mothers who give birth to infants with congenital infection usually have normal children subsequently. The mortality and sequelae among the congenital group is high. Complete recovery from moderate, acute, acquired disease without sequelae is usual. Approximately half of the patients with retinochoroiditis respond well to therapy; however, relapses and treatment failure occur.

Prevention. No practical measures for the prevention of toxoplasmosis are known, but thorough cooking of all meats is suggested.

PATHOGENIC TISSUE PROTOZOA OF UNCERTAIN TAXONOMY

The taxonomic position in the Protozoa of the genera *Sarcocystis* and *Pneumocystis* of man and animals is uncertain. They do not fit well in the SPOROZOA, and their true nature remains in doubt.

Genus *Sarcocystis*

Species of the genus *Sarcocystis* are widely distributed parasites of birds, reptiles, and mammals. The parasite in man, designated as *S. lindemanni,* may represent one or more of the several species in mammals. Man is an incidental host.

Classification. Most parasitologists place the genus *Sarcocystis* under the SPOROZOA.

Life Cycle. In the striated muscles the parasites form long tubular masses of spores called Miescher's tubes. The size of the cylindrical bodies varies with the species and the stage of development; in cattle they sometimes reach 5 cm in length. The mature Miescher's tube has an outer membranous layer and an inner layer from which trabeculae pass into the interior to form various-sized noncommunicating chambers filled with sickle-shaped spores in varying stages of development. The mature spore, 10 to 15 μ in length, is surrounded by a thin membrane and contains a nucleated sporozoite and, at one end, an obliquely striated polar capsule. The spores, when liberated, are motile and travel with a slightly rotary, gliding movement.

The life cycle is not completely known. It was formerly believed that the parasite was transmitted directly by the ingestion of flesh containing Miescher's tubes. Transmission by feeding experiments in mice and guinea pigs, however, is not always successful, and infections in herbivorous animals are difficult to explain. It is now considered that the common method of infection is indirect. Carnivorous or omnivorous animals eliminate an infective stage of the parasite in their feces and urine, and actual infection is acquired by an animal through the ingestion of material contaminated by infective feces or urine.

Pathogenicity. Most species cause no material damage to their hosts except in heavy infections. Human infection is rare, and since it usually causes no particular damage or symptoms, is not readily discovered except at autopsy. One patient experienced painless swelling of the arms and legs for 9 months. The WBC was 15,000 with 40 percent eosinophils, the SGOT was normal, and the fluorescent antibody test positive for *Sarcocystis*. Some 22 cases of human infection, in which the parasite was found in the skeletal muscles or in the muscles of larynx, heart, and tongue, have been reported.

Pneumocystis carinii

Pneumocystis carinii, an extracellular parasite, is presently classed as a protozoan and is a cause of an interstitial plasma cell pneumonia.

Morphology and Life Cycle. The oval or round organisms are 1 to 2 μ in diameter and are nucleated. Usually eight of these daughter cells are found clumped together in a viscous capsule 6 to 9 μ in diameter (Fig. 23). Multiplication is by fission. The organisms are abundant in the pulmonary exudate, and, hence, transmission is probably by droplet to close contacts.

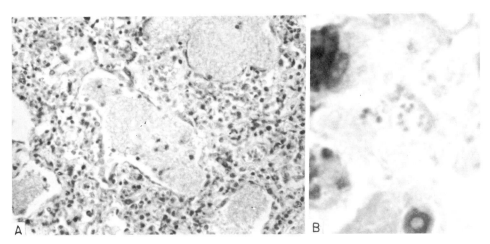

Fig. 23. *Pneumocystis carinii* in lungs. A, note "ground glass" appearance of exudate and interstitial plasma cells ($\times$ 250); B, organism showing 8 daughter cells ($\times$ 2000).

Epidemiology. *Pneumocystis* infection is cosmopolitan in man, rodents, dogs, and several domestic animals. In man, clinical infections are primarily found in infants and are uncommon in adults. This organism probably is of low virulence, and multiplies to damaging proportions in hosts of lowered resistance. Thus, it is most commonly found in enfeebled, premature, and malnourished infants, and in institutional epidemics; it produces a highly fatal pneumonia. When found clinically in older children and adults, this infection is usually associated with debilitating diseases such as leukemia, Hodgkin's disease, and other malignancies, which obscure it. Hypogammaglobulinemia may also dispose to infection.

Pathology and Symptomatology. The lungs of children with this disease are firm, and the cut surfaces are gray and airless. Microscopically, the most striking change is the thickened alveolar septums, infiltrated with plasma cells, leukocytes, and histiocytes; hence, the name interstitial plasma cell pneumonia. The alveolar epithelium is thickened and partly desquamated, and the alveoli are filled with fat-ladened cells, parasites, and exudate giving a foamy appearance. The alveolar exudate becomes organized and is replaced by fibrous tissue or resorbs completely (Fig. 23).

The disease begins, after an incubation period of 20 to 30 days, with anorexia, failure to thrive, and weight loss, followed shortly by a progressive dyspnea. Within 1 to 2 weeks after the onset of symptoms, respiratory distress ensues with 90 to 130 respirations per minute, cyanosis, and a nonproductive cough. X-ray films of the chest reveal a marked infiltration of the lung. Death is due to asphyxia caused by blockage of the alveoli and bronchioles by exudate.

Diagnosis. In epidemics the high respiratory rate and ground-glass appearance of the lungs on X-ray is useful for diagnosis. The organisms may be found in the sputum. A rising complement fixation titer is diagnostic. Diagnosis is confirmed at autopsy by the characteristic pulmonary pathology and the clusters of eight parasites.

Treatment. Numerous therapeutic agents have been tried with temporary enthusiasm. Presently, pentamidine isethionate (See Page 64 *Treatment* for *T. gambiense* above) intramuscularly, at a rate of 4 mg per kilogram per day for 14 days is reported to give excellent results. Stilbamidine and Neostibosan are also reported to be of value. Supportive measures such as oxygen, antibiotics, and good nutrition are important. Steroids should not be given.

MALARIA PARASITES OF MAN

Genus *Plasmodium*. The malarial parasites of man are species of the genus *Plasmodium* of the class SPOROZOA in which the asexual cycle (schizogony) takes place in the red blood cells of vertebrates and the sexual cycle (sporogony) in mosquitoes. The members of this genus, which cause malaria in mammals and birds, have closely similar morphology and life cycles.

Disease. Malaria, paludism, intermittent fever, chills and fever, Roman fever, Chagres fever, marsh fever, tropical fever, coastal fever, and ague. The term malaria is derived from two Italian words *mal* (bad) and *aria* (air). Hippocrates divided miasmic fevers into continuous, quotidian, tertian, and quartan types, the last three being attributed to malaria. Legend, or possibly history, suggest that in 1638 the Countess d'El Chinchon, wife of the Viceroy of Peru, was cured of malaria by the bark of quinine-producing trees, an incident that gave rise to the name cinchona for quinine.

Species. *Plasmodium malariae* was described in 1880 by Laveran; *P. vivax* was named in 1890 by Grassi and Feletti, *P. falciparum* in 1897 by Welch, and *P. ovale* in 1922 by Stephens. In 1898 Ross published a description of the sporogony of the avian species *P. relictum* in culicine mosquitoes; about the same time Grassi et al. reported a similar sexual cycle in *P. falciparum* in anopheline mosquitoes. Since 1917, studies of clinical malaria and chemotherapy have been conducted in syphilitic patients, as the fever produced by malaria is therapeutic in cerebral syphilis. Between 1948 and 1955, the exoerythrocytic cycles of the malarial parasites of man were demonstrated.

Morphology. The diagnostic morphology of the human plasmodia in the blood is shown in Figures 24 through 27. The cytoplasm is irregular in shape at different stages of development, and contains chromatin, pigment, and granules. The malarial pigment is a denatured protein complex, hemozoin or hematin, metabolized by the parasites at the expense of the erythrocyte. It is not present in exoerythrocytic parasites in the liver cells. The gametocytes can be differentiated from the old trophozoites by more compact cytoplasm, absence of chromatin division, and scattered peripheral pigment.

PLASMODIUM FALCIPARUM

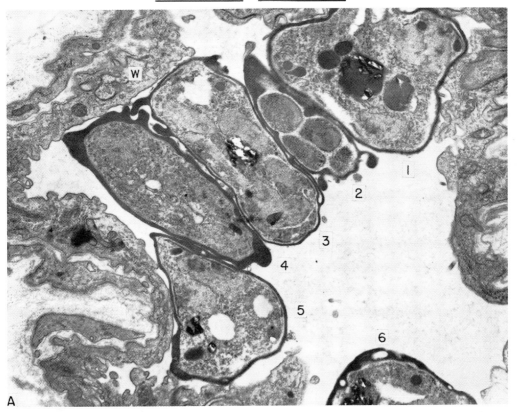

Fig. 24. A, Electron micrograph of schizonts in red blood cells in veins. Note distortion of red blood cells which are closely adhering to wall of vein. 1-6, infected red cells; W, wall of vein. (Courtesy of S. Luse and L. H. Miller.)

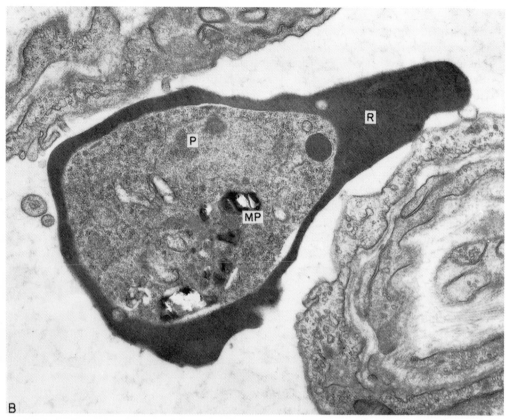

Fig. 24. B, Electron micrograph of schizont in red blood cell in vein. Note distortion of red cell. R, red cell; P, parasite; MP, malarial pigment. (Courtesy of S. Luse and L. H. Miller.)

Instances of human infection with species of questionable status or of primate origin have been reported. In malarial surveys mixed infections with two or more species have been encountered in 1 to 9 percent of infected persons, the incidence depending upon the local prevalence of the infecting species. Mixed infections with *P. vivax* and *P. falciparum* are the most common, followed by *P. falciparum* and *P. malariae,* and least frequent *P. vivax* and *P. malariae.* Infection with all three species is found very rarely.

The number of parasites observed in the peripheral blood varies with the species, *P. falciparum* being the most numerous, at times infecting 10 to 40 percent of the red blood cells (Table 5). Multiple invasion of the red blood cells is common with *P. falciparum,* rare with *P. vivax,* and very rare with *P. malariae.* The malarial parasites have a predilection for certain red blood cells. *P. vivax* and *P. ovale* have an affinity for the reticulocytes; *P. falciparum* is apparently indifferent to the age of the cells, and *P. malariae* seems to prefer the mature cells.

PLASMODIUM VIVAX (Fig. 25).   The erythrocytes invaded by *P. vivax* become pale, deficient in hemoglobin, and enlarged. Since *P. vivax* has an affinity for the large reticulocytes, the increase in size may be more apparent than real. The early trophozoite appears as a small hyaline disc with the nucleus on one side, giving a signet ring appearance. As the trophozoite grows it becomes an irregular finely pigmented organism that shows marked ameboidal activity. After 36 hours it fills over half of the enlarged red blood cell, its nucleus divides, and it becomes a schizont. It loses its activity, almost fills the distended cell, and contains accumulations of pigment in the cytoplasm. Approaching 48 hours the schizont reaches its maximal size, 8 to 10 μ, and undergoes segmentation. The pigment accumulates eccentrically, the divided nucleus with portions of cytoplasm forms 16 round or oval cells, 1.5 to 2.0 μ in diameter, the merozoites. The gametocytes are oval, nearly fill the erythrocyte—the microgametocyte with a pale pink diffuse nucleus and pale blue cytoplasm, the macrogametocyte with darker blue cytoplasm and a compact nucleus often located at the periphery of the parasite. Fine, round, uniform pink or reddish granules, Schüffner's dots, are often present in the stained cells infected with *P. vivax.*

PLASMODIUM MALARIAE (Fig. 26). *P. malariae* is smaller, less active, less abundant, and utilizes less hemoglobin than *P. vivax.* The stained ring form resembles that of *P. vivax,* but the cytoplasm is a deeper blue, and the parasite is smaller, less irregular, and more compact. The growing trophozoite acquires coarse granules of dark brown or black pigment and may assume a band shape across the cell. It contains threadlike masses of chromatin, occasionally a vacuole, and marginal accumulations of dark coarse pigment. At 72 hours the mature segmenting schizont, which almost fills the unenlarged red blood cell, resembles a daisy or rosette in having a central compact mass of greenish-black pigment surrounded by 8 to 10 oval merozoites, each with a red chromatin mass and blue cytoplasm. In cells infected with *P. malariae* fine pink granules, Ziemann's dots, occasionally may be demonstrated. The gametocytes are similar to those of *P. vivax,* but are smaller and contain less pigment.

PLASMODIUM FALCIPARUM (Fig. 27). *P. falciparum* differs from the other plasmodia of man in that, except in severe fatal infections, only the ring forms of the early trophozoites and the gametocytes are ordinarily seen in the peripheral blood. Schizogony takes place in the capillaries of the internal viscera including the heart, and very few of the schizonts are found in the peripheral blood (Figure 24). The infected red blood cells are of normal size. Multiple infection of the red blood cell is a common characteristic. The presence of the characteristic small ring forms, many with double chromatin dots, even without the gametocytes, is often sufficient to identify this species. Two chromation dots (Nuclei) are frequently found in *P. falciparum* ring forms, and occasionally in *P. vivax* and *P. malariae* rings. The oval or round schizonts, seldom found in the blood, resemble those of *P. vivax,* but do not fill the cell. The segmenting schizonts usually contain 16 to 24 small merozoites. The immature gametocytes gradually acquire an elliptical shape, stretching the corpuscular covering. When fully developed they have a characteristic banana shape, the so-called "crescent." In cells infected with *P. falciparum* there is sometimes a bluish basophilic stippling and cytoplasmic precipitates known as Maurer's dots that appear as irregular red spots, clefts, or bands in the cytoplasm.

PLASMODIUM OVALE. *P. ovale,* a rare parasite of man, is similar to *P. vivax* and *P. malariae* in several characteristics. The infected red blood cells are slightly enlarged, of oval shape, and contain at an early stage large Schüffner's dots. The irregular and fimbriated appearance of the red blood cells is of diagnostic importance. The pigment is scattered throughout the growing organism in fine greenish-brown granules with a distinctive pattern; it is centrally massed in the segmenting schizont, which nearly fills the infected cell. *P. ovale* resembles *P. malariae* in the growing trophozoite and early schizont stages, although they do not form distinct bands. Mature schizonts have massed pigment and usually eight merozoites. In thick blood films it is practically impossible to differentiate *P. ovale* from *P. malariae*, except when Schüffner's dots are present.

Physiology.   *P. falciparum* has the shortest life span in man and *P. malariae* the longest due to the variation in the length of their exoerythrocytic stage (Table 5). The metabolic requirements of avian and simian plasmodia have been studied in suspensions of parasites or in tissue cultures. Heavy metal catalysts of the cytochrome system, labile proteins, proteinases, and certain dehydrogenase systems play a part in the metabolism of the parasites. Oxygen is utilized by means of a heavy metal respiratory enzyme, possibly the iron porphyrin cytochrome oxidase. Dextrose is oxidized more rapidly by parasitized, than by normal, red blood cells; lactate is oxidized only by parasitized cells. *P. vivax* utilizes over three times more dextrose and lactate than *P. falciparum*.

Nourishment is obtained from the blood and tissues of the host. Hemoglobin is converted into hematin, which becomes the malarial pigment, and globulin. The protein of the erythrocyte is broken down and about half of the amino acids are synthesized by the plasmodia. In addition to carbohydrates, proteins, and fats, the plasmodia apparently require methionine, riboflavin, and *p*-aminobenzoic, pantothenic and ascorbic acids. Of these, the most necessary for growth is methionine, which markedly increases the severity of infection in monkeys.

Life Cycle.   The life of the plasmodia is passed in two hosts, a vertebrate and a mosquito (Fig. 28). The asexual cycle in the vertebrate host is known as schizogony, and the sporulating sexual cycle in the mosquito as sporogony.

SCHIZOGONY.   The infectious *sporozoite* from the salivary glands of an infected *Anopheles* mosquito is injected into the blood stream of man through the bite of the insect. This slender motile organism, within 30 minutes, enters a liver parenchymal cell, initiating the *exoerythrocytic* (EE) portion of the life cycle. It is called exoerythrocytic because it is not yet in the red blood cell. Within the liver cell, the developing parasite becomes a *cryptozoite*. Division of this cryptozoic schizont results in the production of 15,000 to 40,000 *cryptozoic merozoites* within the liver cell, in 6 to 9 days, depending upon the species of malaria. The weakened parasitized liver cell ruptures, freeing the merozoites. Most of these are phagocytosed, but some succeed in entering new liver cells to repeat the reproductive cycle. Since all of this occurs before red blood cells are infected, it is called the *pre-erythrocytic* portion of the *exoerythrocytic* cycle.

It appears that only one exoerythrocytic cycle is developed by *P. falciparum*, whereas the other species may continue this cycle for years—hence, relapses may occur after years have passed.

The *erythrocytic* cycle of the parasite begins when a cryptozoic merozoite invades a red blood cell. The parasite is first seen as a small chromatin mass surrounded by a little cytoplasm which assumes a ring shape, a *trophozoite*. As the trophozoite grows, the cytoplasm increases in size, becomes irregular, and begins to develop pigment. The trophozoite develops into the young *schizont*, eventually becomes a mature segmenting schizont which ultimately splits into merozoites. With the completion of segmentation, the red cell ruptures, and the merozoites, pigment, and cellular residue escape into the blood plasma where the parasites that escape phagocytosis enter other red blood cells to repeat the schizogonic cycle.

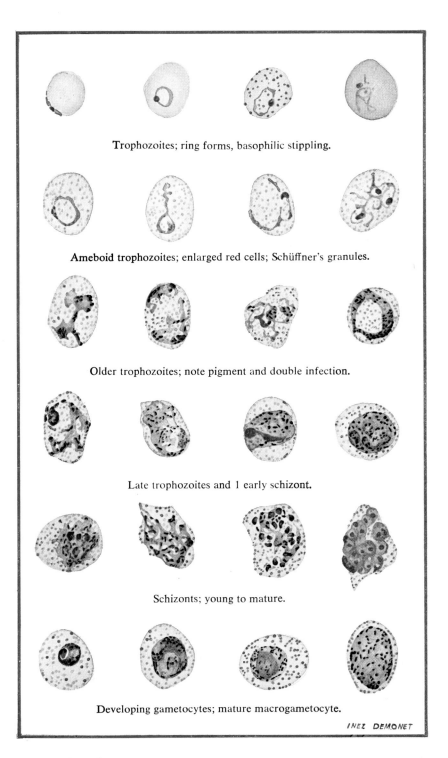

Trophozoites; ring forms, basophilic stippling.

Ameboid trophozoites; enlarged red cells; Schüffner's granules.

Older trophozoites; note pigment and double infection.

Late trophozoites and 1 early schizont.

Schizonts; young to mature.

Developing gametocytes; mature macrogametocyte.

INEZ DEMONET

Fig. 25. *Plasmodium vivax.*

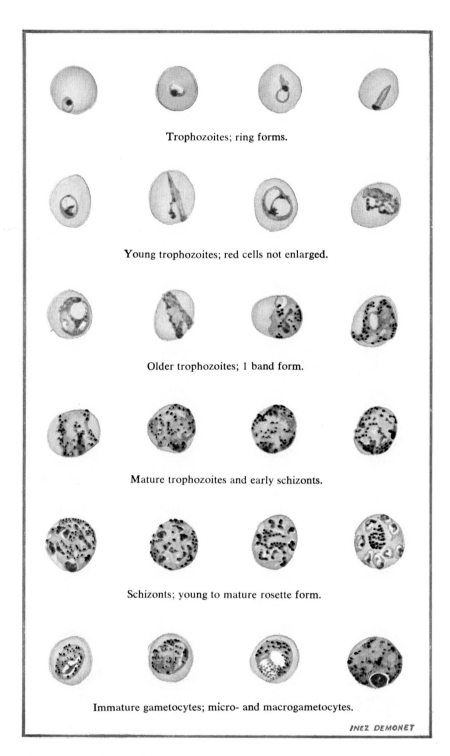

Trophozoites; ring forms.

Young trophozoites; red cells not enlarged.

Older trophozoites; 1 band form.

Mature trophozoites and early schizonts.

Schizonts; young to mature rosette form.

Immature gametocytes; micro- and macrogametocytes.

INEZ DEMONET

Fig. 26. *Plasmodium malariæ.*

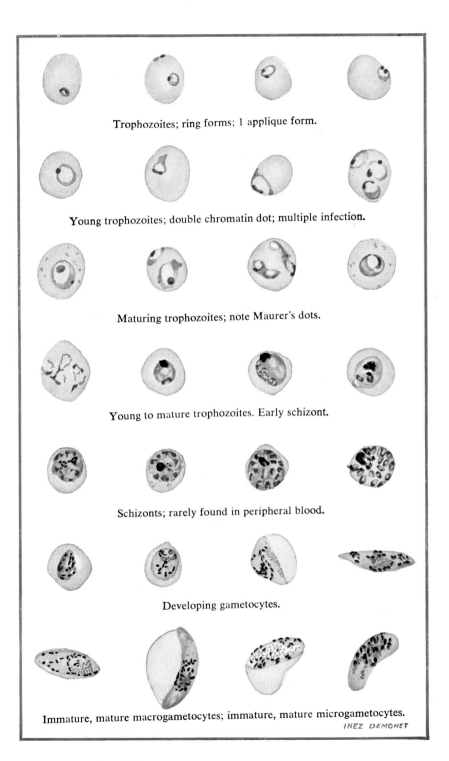

Trophozoites; ring forms; 1 applique form.

Young trophozoites; double chromatin dot; multiple infection.

Maturing trophozoites; note Maurer's dots.

Young to mature trophozoites. Early schizont.

Schizonts; rarely found in peripheral blood.

Developing gametocytes.

Immature, mature macrogametocytes; immature, mature microgametocytes.

INEZ DEMONET

Fig. 27. *Plasmodium falciparum.*

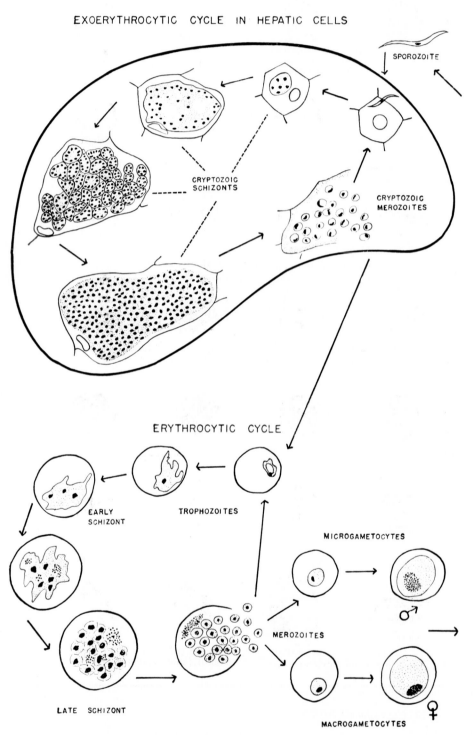

Fig. 28A. Malaria life cycle in man; asexual.

MALARIA

MOSQUITO

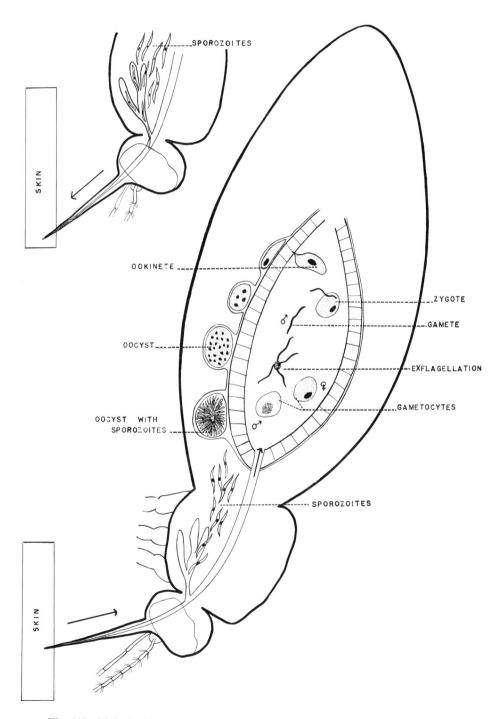

Fig. 28B. Malaria life cycle in mosquito; sexual.

Some of these merozoites which now invade erythrocytes, instead of developing into schizonts, become *gametocytes,* sexual stages.

SPOROGONY.   Sporogony proper takes places in the mosquito. The gametocytes ingested with the blood meal, unlike the schizonts, are not digested with the cellular elements. In the male *microgametocyte* the single chromatin dot divides into 6 to 8 nuclei which migrate to the periphery of the parasite (Fig. 29). There, several whiplike, actively motile filaments, the uninuclear *microgametes,* are thrust out and finally detached from the parent cell. This process is known as exflagellation. In the meantime, the female *macrogametocyte* has matured to a *macrogamete* consisting of a globular body of cytoplasm with a concentrated mass of chromatin. Fertilization is achieved by the entry of the microgamete into the macrogamete, forming a zygote. MacCallum, the noted pathologist, as a second year medical student was the first to observe this phenomenon. This is the key that opened to Ross, who was awarded a Nobel Prize, the riddle of the life cycle of malaria in the insect vector. MacCallum reported his findings at a scientific meeting of his august elders and, due to his apparent youth, succeeded in convincing them only with great difficulty, after due consideration, and against their better judgment.

In 12 to 24 hours after the mosquito's blood meal the *zygote* changes into a worm-like form, the *ookinete,* which penetrates the wall of the mosquito's gut and develops into a spherical *oocyst* between the epithelium and the basement membrane. Here it increases to several times its original size (Fig. 29). Within the oocyst thousands of sporozoites develop; with the rupture of the oocyst they are liberated into the body cavity and ultimately migrate to all the tissues of the mosquito, some penetrating the salivary glands. When the mosquito feeds on man the sporozoites gain access to the blood and tissues and enter upon their exoerythrocytic cycle. The sporogonic cycle in the mosquito takes 8 to 12 days.

Congenital infection with the three common species has been reported and is due to a breach in the placental barrier. The placenta acts as a barrier, since massive infection of the placenta may occur without infection of the child.

Malaria may be transmitted by blood transfusion from an infected donor or by a contaminated syringe. The majority of transfusion infections in temperate climates are due to *P. malariae* as this parasite may remain unnoticed in the donor for 30 or more years. In malarious areas any species of malaria may be transfused to a recipient. Severe *P. falciparum* outbreaks have resulted from the common-syringe technic among drug addicts. Transfusion malaria infections reproduce only the erythrocytic cycle, and therefore are usually easily eradicated.

Pathology.   The pathologic changes are primarily vascular—i.e., the destruction of erythrocytes and the blockage of the capillaries in the internal viscera—and

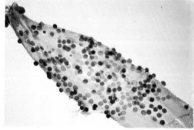 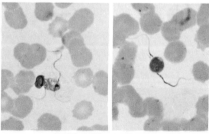

OOCYSTS ON STOMACH   EXFLAGELLATION OF
OF MOSQUITO   MICROGAMETOCYTE

Fig. 29. Stages of sexual life cycle of malaria in mosquito.

secondarily the anoxemic impairment of the tissues of the liver and other organs occurs. Each successive rupture of merozoites from the red blood cells stimulates a humoral and cellular reaction resulting in the phagocytosis of the parasites, infected cells, pigment, and cellular debris by the wandering histiocytes and the fixed macro-phages of the reticuloendothelial system, especially of the spleen—hence, its en-largement. The deposition of pigment which is formed by the malarial parasite during its erythrocytic development, results in a slate-gray or black color of the cerebral cortex, spleen, liver, kidneys, and other organs. The hematin, or possibly its nitrogenous complex hemozoin which is found in the parasite, in the infected cells, and free in the blood stream, is phagocytosed first by the leukocytes of the blood and later by the fixed and wandering macrophages of the reticuloendothelial systems. Its deposition by these cells in the various organs enhances the chronic in-flammatory reaction. The free hemoglobin that is not converted into hematin is rapidly changed into bilirubin, which is absorbed by the liver and secreted in the bile. The iron from the hemoglobin is not immediately utilized to form new hemo-globin and is deposited as hemosiderin in the parenchymatous cells of the liver and other organs. In primary vivax malaria the red blood cells may show only a 10 to 20 percent decrease, but in falciparum malaria greater destruction may take place. The marked anemia of malaria patients usually cannot be explained solely on the basis of the destruction of infected red blood cells, and it is possible that an auto-immune hemolysis contributes to the anemia. Tissue anoxia is brought about by the reduction in red blood cells, the multiple thromboses of the small blood ves-sels, and the decrease in circulating blood volume. The adhesiveness of the infected erythrocytes, and the physical and chemical changes in the blood plasma, cause the clumping and the adherence of the blood cells to the capillary endothelium. Serious circulatory disturbances, chiefly associated with falciparum infections, are produced through the blocking of the capillaries by clumped parasitized erythro-cytes and phagocytes, increased plasma viscosity, and slowing of the capillary cir-culation. During the febrile paroxysm there is a temporary increase in serum potassium, dextrose, cholesterol, and lecithin, and a decrease in phosphorus. The total plasma proteins, principally the serum albumin, are reduced during the acute and latent stages, while the euglobulin and the gamma globulin are often increased. The sedimentation rate is increased during the acute stages. A reticulocytosis fol-lows the regression of fever and the disappearance of the asexual parasites. In acute infection the spleen is dark brown, moderately enlarged, hemorrhagic, soft, and is susceptible to spontaneous or traumatic rupture. When an initial vivax infection is checked, the spleen tends to decrease in size.

In acute vivax infections the liver is soft, smooth, congested, dark brown, and slightly enlarged. In chronic infections it is enlarged and firm. There is hyperplasia of the endothelial cells of the interlobular veins and of the sinusoidal Küpffer cells, which later become hyperplastic and contain fine yellowish-brown pigment. Para-sitized erythrocytes and numerous macrophages loaded with parasites, red blood cells, and pigment are present in the interlobular veins and dilated sinusoids. The parenchymatous hepatic cells show cloudy swelling, nuclear abnormalities, numerous mitoses, fatty infiltration, decrease in biliary pigment, and reduced glycogen con-tent. There is little evidence of permanent damage, although the disposal of bili-rubin, hemosiderin, and, possibly, hematin places a heavy load on the liver. Hepatic dysfunction may be determined by flocculation reactions, which persist in chronic infections, and by early transitory changes in dye excretion. It is possible that

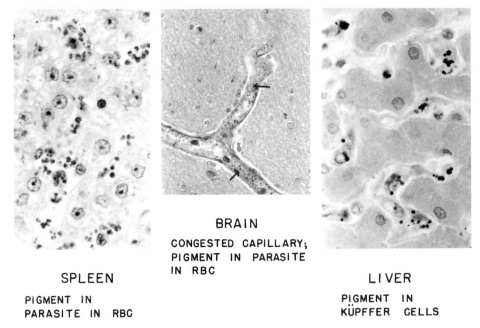

BRAIN

CONGESTED CAPILLARY;
PIGMENT IN PARASITE
IN RBC

SPLEEN

PIGMENT IN
PARASITE IN RBC

LIVER

PIGMENT IN
KÜPFFER CELLS

Fig. 30. Malaria parasites and pigment in organs.

altered dye excretion may result from decreased blood flow to the hepatic cells rather than from hepatic changes. A slight increase in the SGOT and SGPT has been reported in falciparum infections.

In fatal falciparum infections the brain is edematous, dark red, and markedly congested. Macroscopically, the cortex is dusky gray or brown, and petechial hemorrhages may be visible in the perivascular tissues. The cerebral capillaries are filled with numerous infected red cells, pigmented parasites, pigment, and phagocytes. The retarded circulation gives rise to an anoxic necrosis of the perivascular tissues (Fig. 30).

Lesions in the kidney, usually infrequent or slight, are predominantly those of an intracapillary glomerulonephritis associated with lipoid nephrosis.

Interstitial pneumonitis may occur in acute falciparum infections, and the heart may show petechial hemorrhages, partially blocked myocardial capillaries, and fatty degeneration and cloudy swelling of the cardiac muscles. Hemorrhages in the medulla and cortex of the adrenals, retinal hemorrhages, and concentration of plasmodia in the placenta resulting in abortions and recrudescense of the infection after delivery have been described in falciparum infections.

Symptomatology. The clinical manifestations of malaria are characterized by intermittent febrile paroxysms, secondary anemia, and splenic enlargement; it tends to progress from an acute to a chronic state. During the acute stage there are intermittent febrile episodes, and during the subsequent chronic stage periods of latency broken by a series of relapses, similar to the acute primary attack. The differential clinical characteristics of infections with the four malarial species which infect man are outlined in Table 5.

The incubation period varies from 9 to 40 days and represents the interval between the bite of the infecting mosquito and the onset of clinical symptoms. On the

Table 5. Clinical Differentiation of the Malarias

	Plasmodium vivax	*Plasmodium malariae*	*Plasmodium falciparum*	*Plasmodium ovale*
Name	Benign tertian	Quartan	Malignant tertian, subtertian, aestivoautumnal	Benign tertian
Pre-erythrocytic cycle (days)	8	12	6	9
Prepatent period (days)	11–13	15–16	9–10	14–15
Incubation period (days)	14 (12–17) or up to 6–12 months	28 (18–40) or for years	11 (9–14)	17 (16–18)
Erythrocytic cycle (hours)	45	72	48	49
Para-erythrocytic cycle	Present	Present	Not present	Present
Parasitemia (per cu mm) Average Maximum	20,000 50,000	6,000 20,000	100,000–500,000 2,000,000	9,000 30,000
Primary attack Severity Febrile paroxysm (hours) Duration (weeks)	Mild to severe 8–12 2–4	Mild 8–10 4–8	Severe 16–36 or longer 2	Mild 8–12 3
Relapses Tendency Period of recurrence	++ Long	+++ Very long	+ Short	++ Long
Duration of infection (years)	1.5–5.0 (14)	1–30	0.5–1.5	Probably same as *P. vivax*

other hand, the incubation period may be prolonged in vivax infections of 6 to 12 months or more, and in malariae and ovale infections for years. Thus, in the temperate zones a tertian infection acquired in the summer or autumn may not produce the acute disease until the following spring. Clinical malaria may develop many months after cessation of suppressive therapy. The primary attack of acute malaria comprises a series of paroxysms over a period of at least 2 and often more weeks, followed by a long latent period characterized by the relapses of chronic malaria. The febrile paroxysms are associated with progressive red blood cell destruction, debility, and splenic enlargement. The benign type is due usually to *P. vivax, P. malariae,* or *P. ovale.* The pernicious or malignant type is chiefly caused by *P. falciparum.*

During the prodromal period of a week or more, when the number of parasites are increasing in the blood through the early asexual cycles, there are no diagnostic clinical manifestations, although lassitude, lack of appetite, vague pains in the bones and joints, and a daily or irregular fever and chilliness may be present. In non-endemic areas, the first diagnosis is often INFLUENZA. The initial or primary attack is characterized by a series of intermittent febrile paroxysms recurring at varying intervals: 48 hours for *P. vivax* and *P. ovale,* 48 hours for *P. falciparum,* and 72 hours for *P. malariae.* The actual time in different vivax strains varies from 43.6

to 45.1 hours. The paroxysms begin with a cold stage or rigor of about an hour during which the patient has a shaking chill, although his temperature may be above normal. A hot stage of longer duration follows, in which the patient has a hot dry skin, flushed face, a temperature of 103 to 106° F, a full rapid pulse, headache, nausea, often vomiting, and convulsions in young children. Then the patient perspires profusely, the temperature falls, and the headache disappears, so that in a few hours he is exhausted but symptomless. The febrile paroxysm usually lasts 8 to 12 hours but is longer in falciparum infections (Table 5). The paroxysm has been variously attributed to hemolysis from the destruction of the red blood cells, to shock from the freed hemoglobin, or metabolic products. Virulence is often, but not always, correlated with the intensity of parasitemia.

Paroxysmal periodicity corresponds to the end of the schizogonic cycle, when the merozoites of the mature schizonts, together with their pigments and residual debris, erupt from the red blood cell into the blood stream—literally a foreign protein injection. The relationship of schizogonic cycle to paroxysmal periodicity is shown in Figure 31. In acute infections there is a moderate leukocytosis with granulocytosis, but with the fall in temperature a leukopenia with relative monocytosis and lymphocytosis develops. White cell counts from 3,000 to 45,000 have been reported. Early in the infection there may be a marked, transient thrombocytopenia. Only very few patients show malarial jaundice, and hemoglobinuria appears only when the plasma level of hemoglobin is above the renal threshold. There is an acute enlargement of the spleen in about one-fourth of patients with acute malaria. Pain in the left upper quadrant and epigastrium may be caused by stretching of the splenic capsule, a small ruptured infarct, or a subcapsular hemorrhage. Kidney function usually is not disturbed in patients with an ordinary case of malaria. Nephritis, however, with scanty urination, massive albuminuria, granular cylindrical casts, generalized edema, diminished blood proteins, moderate hypertension, and macroscopic or microscopic hematuria may be present and divert the diagnosis away from malaria. Albumin is present in the urine in about 2 percent of patients with acute malaria. Serious ocular lesions are seldom encountered in malarial infections, but in acute attacks the most frequent complications are headache and periocular pain, dendritic or herpetic keratitis with discomfort, photophobia and lacrymation, and in falciparum infections hemorrhage and allergic uveitis. Herpes labialis is not uncommon.

A pernicious form of malaria is observed in falciparum infections, and death in acute malaria is confined almost exclusively to this type of disease, which sometimes takes the form of coma, convulsions, and heart failure without high fever. Pernicious infection is characterized by capillary obstruction by the adhesive infected cells and cerebral involvement. The cerebral type assumes a comatose form with apathy, stupor, and coma, but it may be meningitic or encephalitic with delirium, psychotic disturbances, paralysis, and convulsive seizures (Fig. 30). Rapid collapse into coma is due to anoxia, cerebral edema, and increased cerebral pressure. In the septicemic infection, which may simulate a variety of diseases, there may be high fever, headache, delirium, symptoms of sunstroke, cyanosis, and hemorrhages in the internal organs. When both the circulatory and the nervous systems are involved, the disease may assume the fatal algid form with rapid loss of strength, cardiac weakness, circulatory collapse, and extensive intestinal hemorrhages.

In the natural course of malaria the acute symptoms subside, relapses become

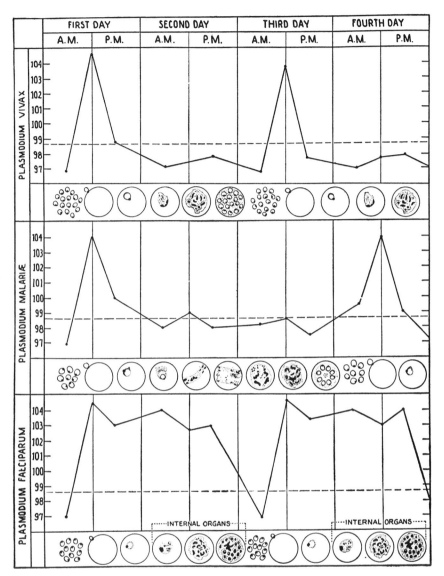

Fig. 31. Temperature curves in malaria showing relation to growth and schizogony of malarial parasites.

fewer, latency develops, and eventually most patients are freed of the infection through the development of acquired immunity. As a rule, falciparum infections disappear in less than 1 year, and vivax infections in about 1½ years, although a few may last as long as 5 years and even longer. Malariae infections persist much longer, and instances of relapses after 20 years and transfusion infections after 30 years have been reported. Chronic malaria is usually benign, but because of relapses, sequelae, and reinfections in endemic regions it may become a serious debilitating disease. Relapses are the most striking features of chronic malaria. In parasitic latency the parasites are present either as exoerythrocytic or as indetectable erythrocytic forms. All degrees of clinical manifestations may occur from symptomless carriers to patients with marked anemia, apathy, debility, and splenic enlargement. The standard liver function tests show some deviation from the normal in the majority of patients. Abnormal pregnancies are more common in malarial than in malaria-free women.

Blackwater fever is an acute hemolytic syndrome resulting from intravascular hemolysis. It is characterized by hemoglobinuria, fever, nausea, vomiting, jaundice, and sometimes by renal damage with oliguria and anuria. It appears to be closely associated with falciparum malaria, particularly in Africa. It is most prevalent in persons who have received treatment with quinine. The most striking pathologic feature is the intense hemolysis of the red blood cells, which are still susceptible to destruction when transferred into a normal individual. Likewise, the cells of a normal donor are hemolyzed in a blackwater fever patient. A number of unproved theories in explanation of this phenomenon have been postulated, including a glucose-6-phosphate dehydrogenase deficiency. Hemoglobinemia, bilirubinemia, and hemoglobinuria result from the inability of the liver to handle the excessive amounts of hemoglobin released by the destruction of the red blood cells. The fatality rate is 20 to 25 percent, and about half of the deaths are associated with renal failure. Recovery from untreated anuria is rare.

Diagnosis.   The definitive diagnosis of malaria is made in the laboratory by microscopic identification of the parasites in blood smears. The blood may be taken at any time in vivax, malariae, or ovale infections, as the various stages of the parasite are present in the peripheral blood throughout the cycle. Theoretically, in falciparum infections the blood is best taken just after the fever peak when the early rings are present and before the red blood cells with the later stages disappear into the capillaries of the internal organs to undergo schizogony. Although the late rings, trophozoites, and schizonts will be synchronized, a few laggard or precocious rings, out of step, "listening to another drummer," are found in the blood throughout the cycle. Gametocytes of all four species of malaria may be present in the blood continuously. Practically, the blood should be examined when the patient is first seen and at six-hour intervals thereafter until parasites are demonstrated. Parasites may be absent between attacks, after treatment, or during suppressive therapy. The blood should be examined on 3 to 4 successive days before malaria can be ruled out. A thin film (Page 326) should be examined for at least 15 minutes. The presence of pigment in the large mononuclears and polymorphonuclear neutrophils calls for a thorough search for parasites. The thick film (Page 326) in the hands of experienced workers is the most reliable method of detecting malarial parasites, especially if they are few in number. A 5-minute search should reveal the parasites. Both the thick and thin blood smears should be made on the same slide. When laboratory diagnosis is negative or not available, reliance must be placed on clinical signs and symptoms, and response to chemotherapy.

Treatment.   The treatment of malaria involves general and supportive measures and chemotherapy. During the acute attack the patient should have bed rest, cold sponging for the relief of fever, aspirin or sedatives for headache and general discomfort, and regulation of fluid intake and salt balance. The run-down, nonreactive, chronic patient with severe anemia and hypotension may require blood transfusions, liver extracts, iron, and a high vitamin and protein diet.

The chemotherapeutic agents may be classed as: (1) causal prophylactic drugs, for the destruction of the pre-erythrocytic parasites; (2) suppressive, for preventing the development of clinical symptoms; (3) therapeutic, for the treatment of the acute attack by destroying the asexual erythrocytic parasites; (4) radical cure for the destruction of the late exoerythrocytic forms; and (5) gametocytic and gametostatic.

Treatment of the acute attack calls for a powerful schizonticidal drug. Chloroquine and amodiaquine are the drugs of choice. In severe clinical malaria, parenteral administration of drugs, followed as soon as possible by oral administration, may be necessary to save life. Intravenous administration of quinine dihydrochloride has been the standard treatment for years in such cases. Chloroquine administered either intravenously or intramuscularly, or quinacrine intramuscularly, appear equally successful for comatose or patients who are vomiting.

Primaquine is the least toxic of the 8-aminoquinolines, which are the only drugs effective against the late exoerythrocytic and sexual forms, although chloroguanide and pyrimethamine so affect the gametocytes that they are unable to undergo sporogony in the mosquito. The combination of chloroquine, 300 mg, base with 45 mg primaquine once weekly for 8 weeks is successful in preventing relapses in vivax and malariae infections and producing radical cure. Primaquine is unnecessary in falciparum malaria, as there are probably no exoerythrocytic forms after the primary exoerythrocytic stage. Quinacrine should never be used with primaquine because of heightened toxicity.

In blackwater fever, the patient should be kept in bed, the fluid balance maintained, alkalosis prevented, edema avoided, and parenteral saline, plasma, or blood transfusions administered as required. Acute renal failure, due primarily to falciparum malaria, can be successfully treated with peritoneal dialysis. For the parasitemia, chloroquine, chloroguanide, or pyrimethamine may be given, but quinine, quinacrine, or primaquine should be avoided.

For malaria drug suppression chloroquine or amodiaquine are excellent and usually need be taken only weekly. Chloroguanide, which must be taken daily, and pyrimethamine weekly, are also used, but both may stimulate drug resistance. Quinine or quinacrine are recommended only when other drugs are not available.

Cycloguanil dihydrotriazine pamoate, (camolar) related to chloroguanide, a single injection of which (5 to 10 mg per kg of body weight) gives protection against malaria infection for 5 to 24 months, is an interesting new prophylactic. Four to 12 months' protection was obtained against mosquito-induced infections with strains of *P. falciparum* susceptible to proguanil and pyrimethamine, but strains resistant to antifolic drugs did not respond to the cycloguanil compound.

The addition of 25 mg weekly of DDS (diaminodiphenylsulfone) to chloroquine and primaquine shows promise in suppressing resistant falciparum infections.

The commonly used drugs are listed in respect to their action on the different phases of the plasmodia in Table 6.

Plasmodium falciparum strains resistant to chloroquine chemotherapy are found in several parts of the world; thus, the following therapy is suggested.

RECOMMENDED TREATMENT FOR RESISTANT MALARIA; SURGEON GENERAL, U. S. ARMY

1. In most cases of previously untreated falciparum malaria, the treatment consists of an initial dose of chloroquine phosphate, 1.0 g (600 mg of base), followed by 0.5 g (300 mg of base) 6 hours later, and then 0.5 g once daily for

Table 6. Chemotherapy of Malaria

Chemotherapeutic agent		Stage of plasmodium					
			Erythrocytic phase		Secondary		
Type	Drug	Primary tissue phase	Asexual forms	Sexual forms	Secondary tissue phase	Mosquito phase	Toxicity
Cinchona alkaloid	Quinine	—	+*	—	—	—	++
9-Amino-acridine	Quinacrine	—	++*	—	—	—	++
4-Amino-quinoline	Chloroquine	—	+++	—	—	—	+
	Amodiaquine	—	+++	—	—	—	+
8-Amino-quinoline	Primaquine	—†	—†	+	+	—	+++
Biguanide	Chloroguanide	+‡	++§	—	—	+	+
Pyrimidine	Pyrimethamine	+‡	++§	—	—	+	+

* Except for some strains of *P. falciparum.*
† Effective only in dangerously high doses.
‡ *P. falciparum* only.
§ Action too slow for treatment of acute attack.

the next 2 days, for a total dose of 2.5 g (1.5 g of base) in 3 days. If the patient is unable to take or retain oral chloroquine, give 250 mg of the hydrochloride, intramuscularly, and repeat in 6 hours, switching as soon as possible to the oral medication. This regimen should be employed initially for patients with any type of malaria who are not critically ill and for whom such therapy has already been administered.

2. In patients with *P. falciparum* malaria who (1) are gravely ill, (2) have not responded to the chloroquine treatment, (3) have a recrudescence despite a previous response to a course of chloroquine, the treatment of choice is quinine sulfate, 0.65 g every 8 hours for 7 to 10 days. Because of a tendency to develop postural hypotension, patients should be kept at bed rest during therapy. Urine output is measured, and if oliguria develops quinine should be temporarily discontinued. During oliguria, quinine blood levels may rise precipitously, and acute quinine toxicity may ensue.

3. Patients unable to retain quinine because of vomiting or coma, presumed due to falciparum malaria, the drug is given intravenously. This treatment carries a serious hazard and should be resorted to only when the patient's condition warrants the risk, and no other form of treatment is possible. Quinine is administered intravenously as the dihydrochloride, 600 mg in 600 ml of normal saline, by very slow intravenous drip with constant monitoring of the blood pressure and pulse to detect hypotension or arrhythmia. The same intravenous dose may be repeated at intervals of 8 hours if the patient's condition requires. Oral therapy, by stomach tube if necessary, should be utilized as soon as possible.

4. Patients who respond to quinine therapy but who later relapse should be retreated with quinine as above. The course of quinine may be maintained for 21 days at a dosage of 0.65g (10 grains) every 8 hours, as tolerated.

5. If asexual parasites persist during quinine therapy, regardless of the clinical response, the patient should receive a course of pyrimethamine (Daraprim), 50 mg

daily for 3 days, concurrently with sulfadiazine, 0.5 g every 6 hours for five days. Attention should be given to maintaining adequate hydration.

Quinacrine (Atabrine, Mepacrine) is an acridine derivative of methylene blue. It combines with the DNA of the malaria parasite and inactivates it. The suppressive dose by mouth is 0.1 g daily. Therapeutic dose; 0.2 g 4 times a day the first day, then 0.1 g 3 times a day for 6 days. Anorexia, nausea, diarrhea, headache, blurred vision, pruritis, yellow discoloration of the skin and mental symptoms may be encountered.

CHLOROQUINE. See Page 34 under *Treatment* for *E. histolytica*. In acute malaria it is administered orally as chloroquine diphosphate (62 percent chloroquine base) at an initial dose of 1.0 g followed 6 hours later by 0.5 g and 0.5 g on each of the next 2 days, making a total of 2.5 g (1.5 g base) in 3 days. For patients in coma or with persistent vomiting a rapid action chloroquine hydrochloride (89 percent base) is given intramuscularly at a dose of 250 mg of the hydrochloride followed in 6 hours by a second dose and then oral administration on the 3 succeeding days. Intravenous drip of 0.4 g of the base in 500 ml saline solution may be given over a 1 hour interval. The suppressive dose is 0.5 g of chloroquine diphosphate orally each week. It may be necessary to give this amount twice weekly.

Treatment and Suppression of Malaria in Children:
Dosage of chloroquine (base) for treatment of malaria

Age (yr.)	Initial dose (mg)	Dose, 6 hr. later (mg)	Daily dose for next 4 days (mg)
1	150	150	75
2–5	300	150	75
6–10	300	150	150
11–15	450–600	150	150

For children exposed to malaria in endemic areas, chloroquine will effectively suppress symptoms. The drug should be taken once a week, on Sunday, which is a day usually remembered, as follows. Dosage as chloroquine base: infants, 37 mg; children 1 to 4 years of age, 75 mg; children 5 to 8 years of age, 150 mg; children over 8 years of age, 300 mg.

AMODIAQUINE. Amodiaquine (Camoquin Cam-aqi, Miaquin, Flavoquine) is a 4-aminoquinoline drug. Santoquine (santochin) is a similar drug produced in Germany. It is used in acute malaria, but is slightly less active than chloroquine. Administered orally as dihydrochloride dihydrate (78 percent base) in a single dose of 0.6 g (base) or followed by 0.4 g for 2 days or more. Suppressive dose is 0.4 g weekly. The slight and rare toxic symptoms include lack of energy, inability to sleep at night, uneasiness in epigastrium, and loss of appetite.

PYRIMETHAMINE. Pyrimethamine (Daraprim, Malocide) is a diaminopyrimidine compound. It is a good malarial suppressive drug, but it acts too slowly for an efficient therapeutic agent, and it may produce drug-resistant strains. Administered orally at 25 mg per week for suppression, or 50 mg daily on 2 successive days for treatment of malaria. Toxicity is low, occasional gastrointestinal upsets.

CHLOROGUANIDE. Chloroguanide (Paludrine, Chloroquane, proguanil) is a biguanide that is used for the clinical treatment and suppression of malaria. It renders gametocytes incapable of developing in the mosquito and is a causal prophylactic for *P. falciparum*. It does not prevent relapses with *P. vivax*. Tablets contain 0.1 g of chloroguanide hydrochloride (87 percent base). An effective dosage appears to be 0.3 g daily for 5 or 10 days, or a single dose of 0.3 g followed by suppressive weekly doses of 0.1 to 0.3 g. About one-tenth of patients receiving from 0.1 to 0.6 g per day for 5 days show weakness, drowsiness, vomiting, diarrhea, pains in the back, and urticaria.

PRIMAQUINE.   Primaquine is the least toxic and the most effective of the 8-aminoquinolines. It is active against the sexual forms and the secondary exoerythrocytic phase of the parasite. It is administered orally as primaquine phosphate (57 percent base) at a daily dosage of 15 mg (base) in two divided doses for 14 days. Its administration with quinine notably reduces the high relapse rate in vivax malaria. Below a daily dosage of 30 mg (base) the only toxic effects are moderate abdominal cramps, mild anemia, and slight stimulation of leukocyte formation. An acute hemolytic anemia may occur, especially in the non-Caucasian races who may be deficient in glucose-6-phosphate dehydrogenase. The patient may show gastric irritation, cyanosis from methemoglobinemia, and leukopenia from depression of leukocyte formation. It is contraindicated in renal and hemolytic diseases.

QUININE.   Quinine, the chief alkaloid of the bark of the cinchona tree, for many years was the principal drug for the treatment of malaria. At present it is only used in combination with primaquine for relapsing malaria, for intravenous administration in severe acute malaria, and chloroquine-resistant falciparum infections. It is administered orally as the slightly soluble sulfate (83 percent anhydrous quinine) or intravenously as the soluble dihydrochloride (82 percent). The therapeutic dose is 2 g of quinine sulfate daily in three divided doses for 14 days, and for malaria suppression 0.65 g daily. Mild toxic manifestations are present in about half of the persons receiving 2 g per day, and in about 1 percent the side effects require discontinuation of treatment. Symptoms of cinchonism are tinnitus, slight deafness, dizziness, sense of constriction in the head, cardiac irregularity, gastric discomfort, and visual disturbances. Contraindicated in hemoglobinuria, renal disease, pregnancy, and optic neuritis. Since malaria parasites seldom become resistant to quinine, this drug assumes greater importance as malaria becomes resistant to the several synthetic therapeutic agents.

Epidemiology.   Human malaria was acquired from our simian ancestors. Cross infections between modern human and simian tertian and quartan plasmodia have been produced in the laboratory and have occurred naturally in the field. Man, however, is the only important reservoir of human malaria. The most important parasitic disease of man, it has a world-wide distribution in the tropics and subtropics, and also in areas in the temperate zone. It is not present in Hawaii, many southeastern Pacific Islands, and New Zealand as anopheline mosquitoes are absent from these areas. Over a billion persons live in malarious areas, and it is estimated that 100 million persons are infected and that 1 million die of it each year (Fig. 32). Surveys designed to determine the prevalence and intensity of the disease and the factors governing its local spread include: (1) collection of statistics of past and present morbidity and mortality, (2) spleen index, (3) parasite index, (4) mosquito density and infection rate, and (5) environmental features affecting transmission.

Splenic enlargement is a useful index of the prevalence of malaria. The largest spleens are found in vivax and the smallest in malariae infections; the highest incidence is in the younger age groups. The spleen index represents the percentage

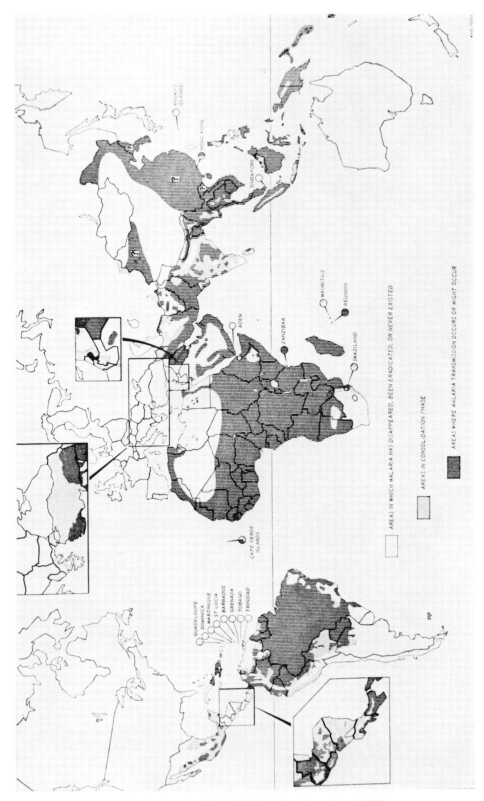

Fig 32. World malaria situation in 1966. (*WHO Techn. Rep. Ser.*, 1967.)

of children of 2 to 9 years of age with enlarged spleens. The adult spleen index is useful in estimating the immune status of a community. Since the spleen decreases rapidly in size after the cessation of an attack, the index should be taken at the height of the malarial season.

The parasite index of a community is the percentage of children from 2 to 9 years of age with detectable plasmodia in a single thick blood smear. Children, especially the very young in hyperendemic areas, show a higher parasitic index than adults. The infant parasitic index represents the infections acquired within a year.

The presence and intenstiy of infection in female *Anopheles* mosquitoes may be determined by the dissection of the stomach for oocysts and of the salivary glands for sporozoites. The bloodsucking habits in relation to man (anthropophilic) and animals (zoophilic) may be determined by precipitin tests on their blood meals. The percentage of infected mosquitoes, usually 0 to 10 percent in endemic areas, varies with the species and strain of the parasite, the susceptibility of the mosquito species, and its proximity to and attraction to man. Mosquitoes retain infectious sporozoites for some time but not necessarily for life. The number of sporozoites declines with repeated feedings, practically all being discharged after 20 blood meals.

The epidemiology of malaria is influenced by climate, topography, and the socioeconomic status of a country. A temperature between 16 and 34° C and a relative humidity over 60 percent are suitable for the transmission of malaria by favoring the breeding of mosquitoes and the cyclic development of the parasite. Agricultural practices may account for its decline in some localities and may favor its spread in others. Improved economics including better housing, nutrition, more antimalarial drugs, and reduction in mosquito breeding areas contributes greatly to malaria reduction.

Malaria is a self-limiting disease unless repeated infections occur. Prognosis is usually favorable in acute vivax and malariae malaria, grave in falciparum infections.

Immunity.   Knowledge of systemic immunity of man has been derived from studies on human plasmodia in syphilitic patients and volunteers. Natural immunity is probably associated with an ability to mobilize the reticuloendothelial system against the invading organism and to develop rapidly an additional acquired immunity.

Acquired active immunity is dependent upon present or past infection and the antigen stimulus of the parasite or its products. In hyperendemic areas natives are protected as infants by passive immunity from their mothers during the first 3 months, acquire an active infection during the first 3 years, and then develop an acquired immunity for life. In some East African tribes in hyperendemic regions all the infants are infected during the first year of life with minimal clinical symptoms and high parasitemia, while an immunity from repeated attacks enables adults to show mild or no signs of the disease in the presence of parasitemia.

Some persons are able to remain free of malaria in endemic areas, unless subjected to massive infective doses, while others acquire mild to severe infections. Negroes are subject to milder infections and respond more readily than whites to chemotherapy. Experimental massive sporozoite- and trophozoite-induced infections with American, Pacific, and Mediterranean strains of *P. vivax* have resulted in 96 percent of infections in whites and only 23 percent in Negroes.

There is an association of the sickle cell anemia trait and resistance to malaria. Sicklers over one year of age show fewer detectable infections, a lower parasitemia, and a milder disease than nonsicklers. The phenomenon may be connected with the metabolism of the abnormal hemoglobin or the nonparasitization of sickle cells. Patients whose red blood cells are deficient in glucose-6-phosphate dehydrogenase have lower malarial infection rates and lower parasite density rates than normal individuals.

Systemic immunity is a complex process involving the destruction of the parasite and tolerance to its activities. Both humoral and cellular defense mechanisms are involved, but the latter appears to be the more potent type. Agglutinins, precipitins, complement-fixing antibodies, and protective antibodies have been demonstrated in the serums of infected and immunized animals and man. The fall in parasite density occurs progressively and concomitantly with the rise in the antibody titer as determined by the fluorescent antibody technic. Cellular immunity depends primarily upon an increase in the number of macrophages through the mobilization of the cells of the reticuloendothelial system and an accelerated rate of phagocytosis. As immunity develops there is hyperplasia of the reticuloendothelial system and heightened activity of the phagocytic cells, which dispose of parasites, parasitized cells, pigment, and cellular debris. In mammals, immunity suppresses the blood infection but is unable to destroy the exoerythrocytic parasites. In human malaria the removal of the spleen in infected infants heightens the parasitemia.

The multiplicity of antigenic strains gives little hope for practical immunization. Thus, immunity against the Puerto Rican vivax does not protect against the Florida McCoy vivax strain. Immunity against one species of malaria does not protect against the others.

About one-fourth of malarial patients give falsely positive reactions with the Wassermann and Kahn tests for syphilis owing to changes in the serum globulin. These reactions are transitory and tend to disappear after the clinical attack.

Prevention. Prevention of malaria comprises: (1) reduction of gametocyte carriers, the source of infection; (2) mosquito control; and (3) protection of susceptible persons against mosquitoes. There is ample evidence that districts and even countries can be made malaria-free by mosquito control measures, although the cost may be beyond the resources of some countries. A marked reduction or eradication of malaria has been effected in the Americas, particularly in the United States, Barbados, Antigua, Martinique, Puerto Rico, Jamaica, Brazil, Argentina, Venezuela, Ecuador; in Italy, Greece, India, Indonesia, and Taiwan.

Measures for the control of malarial mosquitoes include: (1) eradication of breeding places, (2) destruction of larvae, and (3) reduction of adult mosquitoes (Page 275). Residual insecticides have proved particularly efficient in reducing the number of malarial mosquitoes which, after frequenting human habitations, survive long enough to transmit malaria. This does not imply mosquito eradication, but rather the elimination of anophelines which have invaded houses and fed on man and therefore are infected (Fig. 33).

The nonimmune person may be protected from malaria by reducing exposure to mosquitoes and by suppressive chemotherapy. Man may be protected from mosquitoes by screened houses, mosquito nets over beds, and repellents (Page 275). Chemotherapy alone will rarely eliminate malaria except in a few favorable localities, since it is impossible to discover and treat every infected person. At present there is no safe prophylactic drug capable of destroying the pre-erythrocytic plas-

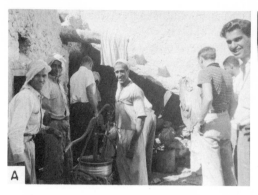
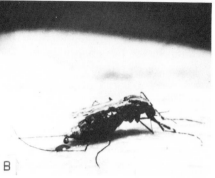

Fig. 33. Malaria control. A, DDT spray team in a village in Saudi Arabia; B, greedy *Anopheles* female overeating. She will fly, we hope, to a DDT'd wall in the house. (Courtesy Dr. J. B. Poole.)

modia of all species. Clinical prophylaxis is achieved by suppressive drugs that prevent the multiplication of the asexual erythrocytic parasites (see under *Treatment* above). The addition of chloroquine to table salt has proven effective in several areas.

As blood transfusions may be a source of malaria infection, the Red Cross recommends that blood donors must not have had an attack of malaria or an antimalarial drug in the past 2 years. Blood for use as plasma may be used from donors who have not had malaria or an antimalarial drug in the past 6 months. When in need of blood, and there is a question about the donor's malaria history, a course of therapeutic chloroquine is recommended. A fluorescent antibody test using antigen from malaria-infected red blood cells is useful in detecting malarial infections among prospective donors.

5

Nematodes

HELMINTHS

The term vermes designates wormlike animals of three phyla:
> Annelida, segmented worms
> Nemathelminthes, roundworms
> > Nematoda
> Platyhelminthes, flatworms
> > Cestoda—tapeworms
> > Trematoda—flukes

Annelida

The ectoparasitic leeches comprise the parasitic members of the phylum. The species of medical importance are either aquatic or terrestrial. They have variously sized, muscular, often pigmented, oval bodies with a tough cuticle, suckers at both ends, hard jaws, and a muscular pharynx.

The aquatic leeches, usually species of *Limnatis,* are injurious to man. The larger suck the blood of bathers; the smaller, taken in drinking water, infest the upper respiratory or digestive passages. At times they invade the vagina, urethra, and eyes of bathers.

The terrestrial leeches, especially species of *Haemadipsa* found in the Far East, live in damp tropical forests, where they attach themselves to travelers, even crawling inside clothing and boots. The painless and often unnoticed wound caused by the bite bleeds readily because of an anticoagulative secretion, hirudin, and heals slowly. Leeches may be removed, after loosening their hold, by applying a local anesthetic, a strong salt solution, or a lighted match. Travelers may be protected by impregnating their clothing with a repellent such as dimethyl phthalate.

Nemathelminthes—Nematoda

The nematoda include numerous free-living and parasitic species. The free-living forms are widely distributed in water and soil. The parasitic species live in plants, mollusks, annelids, arthropods, and vertebrates. It is estimated that over 80,000 species are parasites of vertebrates. The species parasitic in man range in length from 2.0 mm (*Strongyloides stercoralis*) to over a meter (*Dracunculus medinensis*). The sexes are usually separate. The male, which is smaller than the

99

female, commonly has a curved posterior end and, in some species, copulatory spicules and a bursa.

Morphology (Fig. 34).   The adult nematode is an elongate cylindrical worm, primarily bilaterally symmetrical. The anterior end may be equipped with hooks, teeth, plates, setae, and papillae for purposes of abrasion, attachment, and sensory response. The supporting body wall consists of: (1) an outer, hyaline, noncellular cuticle; (2) a subcuticular epithelium; and (3) a layer of muscle cells. The cuticle has various surface markings and spines, bosses, or sensory papillae. The thin, syncytial, subcuticular layer is thickened into four longitudinal cords—dorsal, ventral, and two lateral—which project into the body cavity and separate the somatic muscle cells into four groups. These cords carry longitudinal nerves and often lateral excretory canals. The body wall surrounds a cavity, within which lie the digestive, reproductive, and parts of the nervous and excretory systems. This cavity is lined by delicate connective tissue and a single layer of muscle cells.

The alimentary tract is a simple tube extending from the mouth to the anus, which opens on the ventral surface a short distance from the posterior extremity (Fig. 34). The mouth is usually surrounded by lips or papillae and, in some species, is equipped with teeth or plates. It leads into a tubular or funnel-shaped buccal cavity, which in some species is expanded for sucking purposes. The esophagus, lined with an extension of the buccal cuticle, has a striated muscular wall, a triradiate lumen, and associated esophageal glands. It usually terminates in a bulbar extension equipped with strong valves. Its size and shape are useful for species identification. The intestine or midgut is a flattened tube with a wide lumen which follows a straight course from the esophagus to the rectum. Its wall consists of a single layer of columnar cells. In the female the intestine leads into a short rectum lined with cuticle. In the male it joins with the genital duct to form the common cloaca, which opens through the anus. Around the anal orifice are papillae, the number and pattern of which aid in the identification of species.

There is no circulatory system. The fluid of the body cavity contains hemoglobin, glucose, proteins, salts, and vitamins, and fulfills the functions of blood. The nervous system consists of a ring or commissure of connected ganglia surrounding the esophagus (Fig. 34). From this commissure six nerve trunks pass forward to the head and circumoral region, and six nerve trunks, connected by commissures, extend posteriorly. Sensory organs are situated in the labial, cervical, anal, and genital regions.

The male reproductive organs are situated in the posterior third of the body as a single coiled or convoluted tube, the various parts of which are differentiated as testis, vas deferens, seminal vesicle, and ejaculatory duct (Fig. 34). The ameboid spermatozoa traverse the vas deferens to the dilated seminal vesicle and pass through the muscular ejaculatory duct into the cloaca. The accessory copulatory apparatus consists of one or two ensheathed spicules and, at times, a gubernaculum. In some species wing-like appendages or a copulatory bursa serve to attach the male to the female.

The female reproductive system (Fig. 34) may be either a single or a bifurcated tube, differentiated into ovary, oviduct, seminal receptacle, uterus, ovejector, and vagina. The ovum passes from the ovary into the oviduct where it is fertilized. The true shell, a secretory product of the egg, begins to form immediately after sperm penetration, the vitelline membrane separating from the inner layer of the shell. In the uterus the protein coat is added as a secretion of the uterine wall. There is

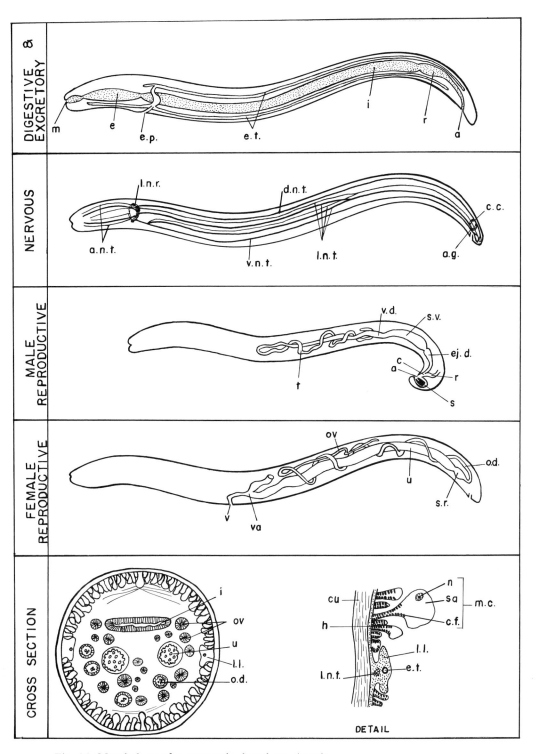

Fig. 34. Morphology of a nematode, based on *Ascaris*.

a, anus; a.g., anal ganglion; a.n.t., anterior nerve trunks; c, cloaca; cu, cuticle; c.c., circumcloacal commissure (male); c.f., contractile fibers; d.n.t., dorsal nerve trunk; e, esophagus; e.p., excretory pore; e.t., excretory tubules; ej.d., ejaculatory duct; h, hypodermis; i, intestine; l.l., lateral line; l.n.r., circumesophageal ring; l.n.t., lateral nerve trunks; m, mouth; m.c., muscle cells; n, nucleus; ov., ovary; o.d., oviduct; r, rectum; s, spicules, sa., sarcoplasm; s.r., seminal receptable; s.v., seminal vesicle; t, testis; u, uterus; v, vulva; va., vagina; v.d., vas deferens; v.n.t., ventral nerve trunk.

considerable variation in relative thickness of these layers. The daily output of a gravid female ranges from 20 to 200,000 eggs.

The excretory system consists of two lateral canals that lie in the lateral longitudinal cords. Near the anterior end of the body the lateral canals join in a bridge from which the terminal duct leads to a ventral pore in the region of the esophagus. Variations from this pattern, even to absence of the system, occur in some adult nematodes. Nematodes possess only longitudinal muscles, which produce their typical sinuous movements.

Adult worms react to touch, heat, cold, and probably to chemical stimulus. The penetration of the skin by hookworm larvae has been ascribed to thigmotropism.

Intestinal nematodes maintain their positions by oral attachment to the mucosa (*Ancylostoma*), by anchorage with their attenuated ends (*Trichuris*), by penetration of the tissues (*Strongyloides*), and by retention in the folds of the mucosa and pressure against it (*Ascaris*).

The methods of obtaining food may be classed as: (1) sucking with ingestion of blood (*Ancylostoma*), (2) ingestion of lysed tissues by embedded worms (*Trichuris*), (3) feeding on the intestinal contents (*Ascaris*), and (4) ingestion of nourishment from the body fluids (filarial worms). The metabolic processes of parasitic nematodes are essentially anaerobic, since the intestinal tract ordinarily contains little or no free oxygen. Aerobic metabolism may also take place, since they are not obligatory anaerobes. Carbohydrates are readily utilized and the glycogen content of the worms is high. A major portion of the total energy requirement of the female worm is expended in production of a large number of ova.

Existence within the host necessitates the development of protective mechanisms. Intestinal parasites resist the action of the digestive juices, and tissue invaders that of the body fluids. Protection against digestive action is afforded by the cuticle and by the elaboration of antienzymes. The free-living larval forms are capable of withstanding a wide range of environmental conditions. Desiccation, excessive moisture, and extremes of temperature retard growth and may even kill the larvae. The growth of both the larval and adult worms follows the typical logistic curve of animal growth.

The life span of nematodes varies: The female *Trichinella spiralis* is passed from the intestine in 4 to 5 weeks; *Enterobius vermicularis* has a life span of 1 to 2 months; *Ascaris lumbricoides* may live for about 1½ years; and hookworms have been observed to persist for at least 14 years.

Life Cycle. Parasitic nematodes pass through simple or complex life cycles both within and without the definitive host. Multiplication during the larval stages, so prevalent in trematodes, rarely occurs. In some genera (*Strongyloides*) it takes place during the free-living phase by the development of sexually mature free-living individuals that produce one or more generations. These larvae either resume their parasitic existence or again develop into mature free-living worms that produce further generations.

Most nematodes have only one host—the definitive—the larvae passing from host to host directly or after a free-living existence.

Transmission to a new host depends upon the ingestion of the mature infectious egg or larva, or the penetration of the skin or mucous membranes by the larva. Some species have an intermediate host in which the larva passes through a cyclic development. The intermediate host, usually an arthropod, ingests the parasite, which passes from the intestinal tract into the tissues. The same animal is both the definitive and intermediate host of *Trichinella spiralis*. The location of the adult parasite in the host, to a large extent, governs the escape of the eggs and the character of the life cycle. When the habitat of the parasites is in the intestinal tract, the eggs or larvae leave the host via the feces. When its habitat is elsewhere in the body, there are other avenues of escape: urine, sputum, skin, blood, lymph, or tissue fluids. During larval development, nematodes pass through several molts or ecdyses both inside and outside the host. Invasion of the host takes place through the intestinal tract or by the penetration of the skin or mucous membranes. In many instances the infective larvae within the egg shells are ingested in food. Nematodes, with few exceptions do not multiply in man, thus differing from many other pathogenic organisms.

Pathogenicity. The effect of parasitic nematodes upon the host depends upon the species, the intensity of the infection, and the location of the parasite. Simultaneous infection with several species of intestinal nematodes is common in tropical and subtropical countries. Injury may be produced by both adult and larval parasites. Intestinal parasites produce less local and systemic effect than tissue parasites. The local reactions from intestinal parasites result from irritation, invasion of the intestinal wall, and occasionally penetration to extraneous sites. The intestinal mucosa is damaged by biting and bloodsucking, by lytic ferments secreted by the parasite, and by mechanical irritation. The general reactions are produced by loss of blood, absorption of toxins, nervous reflexes, and protein sensitization. The larvae of certain species produce local and general reactions during their invasion, migration, and development in the host. The degree of local reaction and associated general reaction depends upon the sensitivity of the host to the protein products of the parasite. The circuitous routes of migration of the larvae in the host result in damage to organs not affected by the adult parasite. The local reactions in the liver, lungs, and other organs at times may destroy or encapsulate the larvae. In unnatural hosts, the larvae may pass through their invasive stages with injury to the host, but never become established as adult parasites.

Resistance to nematode infection depends upon the pre-existing or acquired incompatibility of the host to the parasite and upon the tolerance of its effects. Immunity is acquired through the invasion of the tissues by the parasite and its larvae or through the absorption of its products. Evidence of present or past infection may be shown by the presence of specific antibodies against the parasite or its products and cutaneous supersensitivity. Immunity is both humoral and cellular. The antigen-antibody combinations localize the irritating excretions and secretions of the worm, immobilize it, inhibit its physiologic activities, retard its development, and sometimes destroy it. The immobilized worms are surrounded by inflammatory reactions. Eosinophils, which appear late in the immune reaction, are probably associated with the detoxication of foreign proteins and form a barrier to absorption.

Nematodes differ in host specificity. Certain animals exhibit a definite resistance to infection. Adult *Ascaris lumbricoides* develops almost exclusively in man, although its larval cycle may take place in other animals. Innate resistance may differ in human races; for instance, Negroes are partially immune to hookworm infection. Old animals are usually more resistant than young, and good nutrition protects the host.

The acquisition of immunity by infection presumes an injury to the host sufficient to evoke a reaction. Nematodes that do not invade the tissues or secrete absorbable products produce slight if any immunity. Immunity acquired by natural infection may completely or partially protect against reinfection; may limit the size, egg-laying capabilities, and length of existence of the parasites; and may reduce the number of invading larvae. Constant reinfection tends to enchance immunity. Little success has attended attempts to immunize animals against nematodes by the parenteral injections of antigenic extracts of adult or larval worms. On the other hand, larvae attenuated by irradiation stimulate an immunity.

Antiserums containing various antibodies may be produced by infection or by the injection of the whole nematode or its antigenic fractions. The protective antibodies appear to be directed chiefly against the metabolic products of the worms. Both anti-adult and antilarval antibodies have been described. The presence of these antibodies and tissue sensitization is of practical importance in diagnostic serologic and skin tests.

6

Intestinal Nematodes of Man

Trichinella spiralis

Disease.   Trichinosis, trichiniasis, trichinelliasis.

Morphology (Fig. 35).   The infrequently seen adult is a small worm, the male measuring 1.50 mm by 0.04 mm, and the female 3.50 mm by 0.06 mm. It is characterized by: (1) a slender anterior end with a small orbicular nonpapillated mouth, (2) a posterior end bluntly rounded in the female and ventrally curved with two lobular caudal appendages in the male, (3) a single ovary with vulva in the anterior fifth of the female, and (4) a long narrow digestive tract. The larva has a spearlike burrowing tip at its tapering anterior end. It measures 80 to 120 μ by 5.6 μ at birth and grows but little until it has entered a muscle fiber, where it attains a size of 900 to 1,300 μ by 35 to 40 μ. The mature encysted larva has a digestive tract similar to that of the adult, and although the reproductive organs are not fully developed, it is often possible to differentiate the sexes.

Life Cycle.   The same animal acts as final and intermediate host, harboring the adult parasite temporarily and the larva for a longer period. In order to complete the life cycle, flesh containing the encysted larvae must be ingested by another host (Fig. 36). The larval parasite is found chiefly in man, hogs, rats, bears, foxes, walruses, dogs, and cats, but any carnivorous or omnivorous animal may be infected. Adult birds may temporarily harbor the adult parasite, but the larvae do not encyst in the muscles. Poikilothermal animals do not harbor the parasite.

When infective larvae are ingested by man, they pass to the upper small intestine where the capsules are dissolved and the larvae released in a few hours by the action of the digestive juices. The liberated larvae immediately invade the intestinal mucosa. The sexes may be differentiated in 18 to 24 hours. After fertilization the males are dislodged from the mucosa and carried out of the intestine, although sometimes they remain for several days. The female increases in size and, in about 48 hours, burrows deeply into the mucosa of the intestinal villi—from the duodenum to the cecum and even in the large intestine in heavy infections. At about the fifth day the viviparous female worm begins to deposit larvae into the mucosa and, sometimes, directly into the lymphatics and the mesenteric lymph nodes, from which they reach the thoracic duct and enter the blood stream. After passing through the hepatic and pulmonary filters, the larvae are carried to all parts of the body. They burrow into the muscle fibers by means of a spear-shaped apparatus at the anterior end. They are capable of encysting and developing only in striated muscle, particularly the tendinous portion. In other tissues, such as the myocardium

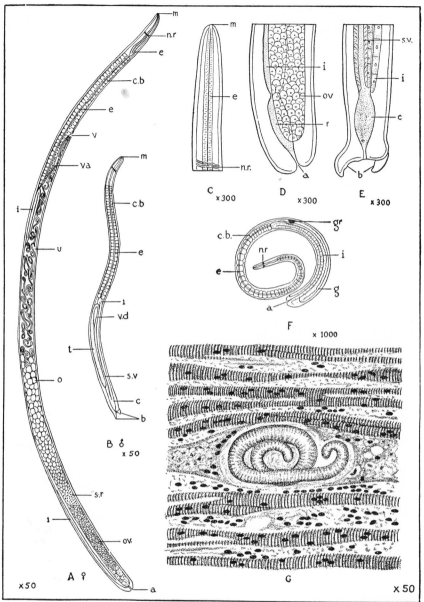

Fig. 35. Schematic representation of *Trichinella spiralis*. A, adult female; B, adult male; C, anterior end of worm; D, posterior end of female; E, posterior end of male; F, young larval worm; G, early encysted larva in muscle.

a, anus; b, bursa; c, cloaca; c.b., cell bodies; e, esophagus; g, gonads (anlage); gr, granules; i, intestine; m, mouth; n.r., nerve ring; o, ova; ov., ovary; r, rectum; s.r., seminal receptacle; s.v., seminal vesicle; t, testis; u, uterus containing larvae; v, vulva; va, vagina; v.d., vas deferens (C adapted from Leuckart, 1868).

and brain, they soon disintegrate and are absorbed. Among the muscles most heavily parasitized are the diaphragmatic, masseteric, intercostal, laryngeal, lingual, extraocular, nuchal, pectoral, deltoid, gluteus, biceps, and gastrocnemius. The larvae are mostly liberated within 4 to 16 weeks, but production continues with lessened intensity as long as the female worms remain in the intestine. Live female adults containing larvae were found in the intestine of a man who died on the fifty-fourth

TRICHINELLA SPIRALIS

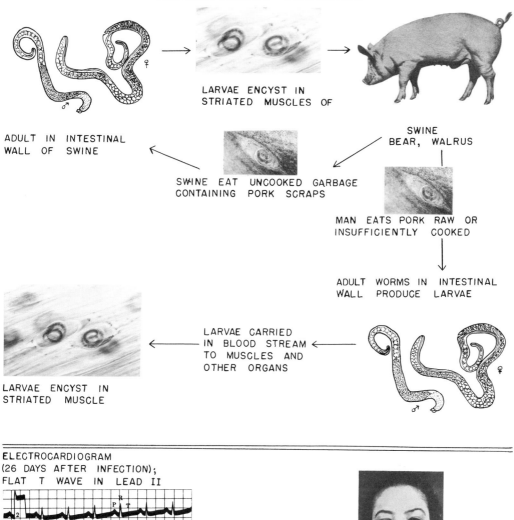

LARVAE ENCYST IN
STRIATED MUSCLES OF

SWINE
BEAR, WALRUS

ADULT IN INTESTINAL
WALL OF SWINE

SWINE EAT UNCOOKED GARBAGE
CONTAINING PORK SCRAPS

MAN EATS PORK RAW OR
INSUFFICIENTLY COOKED

ADULT WORMS IN INTESTINAL
WALL PRODUCE LARVAE

LARVAE CARRIED
IN BLOOD STREAM
TO MUSCLES AND
OTHER ORGANS

LARVAE ENCYST IN
STRIATED MUSCLE

ELECTROCARDIOGRAM
(26 DAYS AFTER INFECTION);
FLAT T WAVE IN LEAD II

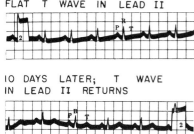

10 DAYS LATER; T WAVE
IN LEAD II RETURNS

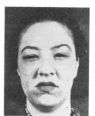

PERIORBITAL EDEMA

FEVER CHART IN MODERATELY SEVERE CLINICAL TRICHINIASIS

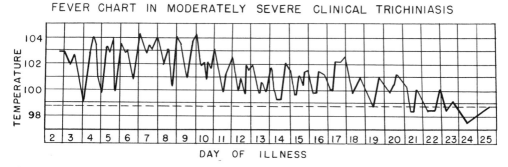

Fig. 36. Life cycle of *Trichinella spiralis*.

day of infection; his diaphragm contained 2,677 larvae per gram of muscle. A female worm produces approximately 1,500 larvae. Occasionally, larvae may be liberated into the intestinal lumen.

The larva grows rapidly in the long axis of the muscle, begins to coil on the seventeenth day and attains its maximal size about the twentieth day. Encapsulation begins about the twenty-first day; the larva is enclosed in a blunt, ellipsoidal, lemon-shaped capsule of muscle fiber origin, 0.40 by 0.25 mm, which is composed of an inner mantle of basophilic degenerative muscle plus epithelioid cells and fibroblasts and an outer hyaline covering derived from the sarcolemma. The permanent capsule is completed in about 3 months. The mesenchymal cells at the poles of the cyst become infiltrated with fat and are transformed into fat globules in about 6 weeks.

Calcification, which may begin as early as 6 months or within 2 years, ordinarily starts at the poles and proceeds toward the center. Usually the capsule calcifies first, but at times there may be a primary impregnation of the larva. Calcification is usually completed within 18 months. The newly formed cysts are invisible to the naked eye, but when calcified they appear as fine opaque granules. The calcified cysts are seldom if ever revealed by the roentgen rays. The adult female dies after passing her larvae and then is digested or passed out of the intestine.

Epidemiology. In 1947 Stoll estimated that there were 27.8 million infected persons in the world, of which three-quarters were in the United States. Its incidence is cosmopolitan, except in Asia, the islands of the Pacific, Puerto Rico, and Australia. The incidence of trichinosis in man may be determined by detecting encysted larvae in cadavers and by intracutaneous tests. Recent autopsy surveys have revealed an incidence of 4.5 percent in the United States. There are an estimated 100,000 new infections, largely subclinical, annually in the United States, of which only a few hundred are reported. The incidence is high in the northeastern states where there is a heavy consumption of garbage-fed hogs, and low in the southern and midwestern states where the hogs are grain-fed. In the United States, there has been a striking reduction in prevalence, mortality, and severity of *Trichinella* infection in man and swine during the past 25 years. The incidence of infection in the 60 million hogs in the United States is 1.5 percent. In garbage-fed hogs the incidence is 11.5 percent, and the number of larvae is 100 to 274 per gram of muscle, whereas in grain-fed hogs it is 0.6 percent and the larvae less than 5 per gram. In nature the enzootic disease is maintained by cannibalistic rats.

Trichinosis reaches its peak during the winter months when there is the greatest consumption of pork. Its incidence is less in the tropics and subtropics, chiefly owing to low consumption of pork products. Poor people in many countries cannot afford meat; an occasional bit of fish is their only protein. Religious bans on eating pork explain the absence of the disease among Hindus, Jews, and Moslems. Seventh-Day Adventists and other vegetarians are not exposed to infection. Catholics may be protected against it on Friday. Chinese, who consume large quantities of pork, are protected by their culinary custom of cooking it thoroughly.

Hogs become infected chiefly from eating uncooked meat scraps in refuse from slaughter houses, markets, and garbage from restaurants, hotels, and private homes; occasionally they may eat infected rats. Rats acquire the infection by eating garbage and discarded offal from slaughter houses and by cannibalism. Man may also acquire the infection by the ingestion of ground beef, as hamburger or steak tartar which is diluted with its cheaper competitor, pork. Beef, ground in a machine in which infected pork has been ground is a possible source of infection. Instances of human infection from bear and walrus meat have been reported. As bears leave their sylvan retreats and join man in picnic areas and suburbia, banqueting on his raw garbage, they will become even a greater threat to the nimrod.

Pathology. Except for the early intestinal lesions caused by the adult worms, the pathology of trichinosis is concerned with the presence of the larvae in the striated muscles and vital organs and with the reaction of the host to their activities, metabolic products, and, possibly, toxic secretions. The characteristic pathologic picture is found in the striated muscles that contain the encysted larvae. The muscle fibers, in 3 to 4 days after the invasion of the larva, increase in size, become edematous, develop a spindle shape, lose their cross striations, and undergo basophilic degeneration. The nuclei increase in number and size, stain intensely, and migrate toward the interior of the muscle cell. There is an acute interstitial inflammation about the parasitized muscle fiber, which reaches its peak in 5 to 6 weeks, with edematous swelling and cellular infiltration of polymorphonuclear neutrophils, eosinophils, lymphocytes, and, at times, foreign body giant cells. Later the inflammation and edema disappear, but the adjacent muscle fibers undergo hydropic degeneration and hyaline necrosis.

Symptomatology (Table 7). Because of the involvement of many organs the protean symptoms of trichinosis resemble those of many other diseases. The variability and severity of the clinical symptoms depend upon the number of worms, the size and age of the patient, the tissues invaded, and the general resistance of the patient. A distinction should be made between zoologic and clinical infection. Only a small percentage of infected persons have sufficient parasites to produce clinical trichinosis. The number of invading larvae in the muscles required to produce symptoms or cause death in man can only be approximated, since individuals vary in resistance: A 7-year-old boy who died during the fifth week of infection had the following number of larvae per gram of muscle: tongue 5,190, gluteus 5,025, masseter 4,560, and diaphragm 2,095. Seven patients who recovered had larval counts ranging from 1,240 to 2,800 per gram of muscle.

The predominating symptoms depend upon the organs affected. In typical clinical trichinosis the leading symptoms in order of prevalence are: eosinophilia; edema, chiefly orbital; muscular pain and tenderness, including joint pain, headache, fever, respiratory manifestations, and general weakness. Myocardial and central nervous system involvement also produce signs and symptoms. Trichinosis is the only helminthic infection that runs a consistent fever during its course. The fever may persist for several weeks and resemble that of typhoid fever. A rising eosinophilia associated with fever, edema of the face, myalgia, and recent gastrointestinal disturbances provide strong presumptive evidence of trichinosis, especially if there is a history of eating pork.

The disease is commonly divided into three clinical phases corresponding to the periods of: (1) intestinal invasion by adult worms, (2) migration of the larvae, and (3) encystment and repair. In the first there may be diarrhea; in the second and third, muscle pain and discomfort; and in the third, weakness and cachexia. The incubational period for the early intestinal symptoms is only 1 to 2 days, but for the migrating larvae in the tissues it is 7 to 28 days. Most of the symptoms appear in the second stage. Prognosis, although unfavorable in severe infections, is ordinarily good. If the patient survives the acute illness, he usually will recover slowly and show no residual ill effects, although muscle pain may persist for 6 months. In overwhelming infections death may take place in 2 to 3 weeks, but more often it occurs in 4 to 8 weeks from exhaustion, pneumonia, pulmonary embolism, cerebral involvement, or cardiac failure. Weakness, stiffness, rheumatic pain, loss of dexterity, and hemiplegia, persisting for years after recovery from the acute attack, are rare sequellae.

The presence of adult and larval trichinae produces an immunity that may be demonstrated by the production of antibodies, by passive protection tests, and by resistance to reinfection. In experimental animals, reinfection produces a nonspecific allergic inflammation which, in turn, directly effects expulsion of adult worms from the intestine due presumably to the creation of an unsuitable biochemical environment.

Diagnosis.   The definitive diagnosis often depends upon the several laboratory or biologic tests that are available. None of them are 100 percent accurate, and they should not negate a positive clinical diagnosis. Early in the infection, the skin test and complement-fixation and precipitin tests are usually negative. A negative test, followed by a positive test or rising titer is of great diagnostic significance.

Intradermal test, using an antigen prepared from *Trichinella* larvae diluted 1:10,000, gives an immediate reaction (within 30 minutes) in from 11 to 93 percent of infected individuals. A positive test is characterized by a blanched, ele-

Table 7. Trichinosis Symptomatology and Clinical Differential Diagnosis

Site of parasites	Signs and symptoms	Simulating disease
Young adults migrating into mucosa of small intestine	Nausea Vomiting Diarrhea Headache	Food poisoning Intestinal influenza Appendicitis
24–72 hours	Abdominal Pain	
Larvae in blood stream and striated muscles	Edema, periorbital * Conjunctivitis * Photophobia * Fever-chills-sweating *	— Conjunctivitis Measles Rheumatism
10–21 days	Muscle pain & spasm * Headache Eosinophilia * Dyspnea Dysphagia Sore throat Skin eruptions Pleurisy Bronchitis Cough, hemoptysis Hypostatic pnuemonia Diarrhea or constipation Abdominal pain	Arthritis Intercostal neuritis Periarteritis nodosa Dermatomyositis Laryngitis Influenza Scarlet fever Pleurisy (bacterial) Pneumonia (bacterial) Typhoid fever — — —
Larvae in myocardium	Precordial pain Tachycardia	— —
10–21 days	Dicrotic pulse Hypotension ECG changes Edema of extremities Venous & arterial thrombosis	Myocarditis Endocarditis — — — —
Larvae in brain and meninges	Headache, supraorbital Vertigo, tinnitis, Deafness	— Frontal sinusitis Meningitis
14–28 days	Mental apathy Delirium, stupor, coma Reflexes absent	Encephalitis Poliomyelitis —

* Very common.

vated wheal of 5 mm or more in diameter, surrounded by an area of erythema. The test may become positive as early as the eleventh day of infection, usually becomes positive by the seventeenth day, but may not develop until the third or fourth week. A delayed skin reaction appearing within 12 to 24 hours of the injection of the antigen may be elicited in approximately 10 percent of infected individuals on the second to sixth day of infection. This test may remain positive for several years. Falsely positive (7 percent) and falsely negative (10 to 15 percent) results have been reported.

The *complement-fixation* test usually does not become positive until the fourth week of the infection. It may remain positive for 1 to 2 years after the acute infection.

The *precipitin test* is reliable and becomes positive during the third or fourth week of infection. Serums of persons who recently have taken quinine or certain other drugs give a positive reaction, and falsely positive reactions have been encountered in patients with Hodgkin's disease, lymphosarcoma, acute leukemia, and infectious mononucleosis.

A *bentonite flocculation test* for the diagnosis of trichinosis is as sensitive as the complement-fixation test, and it too may remain positive for several years. The Hyland *latex test* gives results comparable to the bentonite flocculation test, and the reagent is commercially available.

Search for the adult worms in the feces and the larvae in the spinal fluid and other transudates and exudates is impractical, since they are seldom found even with concentration technics.

Eosinophilia is a most constant finding and diagnostic aid in trichinosis, and when it rises over a period of days, it is most suggestive. Eosinophilia of 40 to 80 percent is not unusual, and an accompanying leukocytosis is not uncommon. The eosinophilia may be greatly decreased or disappear at the appearance of a secondary bacterial infection or near the termination of an overwhelming fatal *Trichinella* infection. The eosinophilia usually appears in the second week, reaches its maximum during the third or fourth week of infection, and then gradually declines, returning to normal limits within 6 months. Old and subclinical infections may be accompanied by a slight degree of eosinophilia which remains stationary rather than increasing day by day.

The *erythrocyte sedimentation rate* is often elevated.

MUSCLE BIOPSY. Demonstration of living larvae in a fragment of the patient's muscle confirms the diagnosis. The invading larvae do not begin to coil until the seventeenth day of infection, thereby making detection easy, and, as only one biopsy is welcomed by the patient, it is suggested that it be done during the third or fourth week of infection. A small piece of muscle is removed by biopsy from the deltoid, biceps, gastrocnemius, or pectoralis major, usually near the tendinous attachments. A portion of the removed muscle may be sliced into thin strips which are compressed between two microscope slides or a "trichinoscope" and examined under the low power of a compound or a dissecting microscope. Old calcified cysts and calcified larvae must be properly evaluated, as they represent previous unsuspected infections and are not related to the current infection. Some of the muscle may be sectioned and stained and a search made for larvae, a technic which is more time-consuming and less sensitive than the compression technic. Muscle which has been examined by the compression method may also be digested in a pepsin hydrochloric acid medium, thereby freeing the larvae from their capsules; they may be found in the sediment.

Treatment.   Patients with trichinosis should be confined to bed and given adequate fluids, and a smooth, high-caloric, high-vitamin diet. Headache and muscle pain may be relieved by salicylates, although the latter may require codeine or morphine. Sedatives are useful, especially the barbiturates. Constipation may be relieved by enemas or a mild cathartic. Fluids should be restricted if an acute myocarditis results in congestive heart failure.

Steroids give symptomatic relief in trichinosis. Oral prednisone, 10 to 15 mg every 6 hours is recommended. Hormonal therapy does not affect the adult worms' fecundity or the number of larvae that successfully invade and encyst in the muscles. Recent studies suggest thiabendazole (25 mg orally per kilogram of body weight, twice daily for 5 to 7 days) is of value in trichinosis (see below under *Treatment for Strongyloides stercoralis*).

Prevention.   The ultimate eradication of trichinosis in man is dependent upon its elimination in hogs. Its prevalence in these animals can be greatly reduced by sterilizing garbage containing raw meat scraps. Until this goal is achieved, the prevention of human trichinosis is dependent upon the processing and refrigeration of pork products, the possible treatment of pork by irradiation, and the education of housewives in regard to the thorough cooking of pork. Federal inspection, which covers about 70 percent of the pork products in the United States, is macroscopic and therefore unreliable. The microscopic examination of pork, once used for exported pork in the United States from 1891 to 1906, was abandoned because of its unreliability under American conditions of automation. It is used in European and South American countries where volume and tempo are slower. The detection of trichinous hogs by serologic and intracutaneous tests has not been successful. Pork products may be processed by salting, smoking, and heating at a temperature not lower than 58.3° C (137° F). The slow-freezing process, now recommended by federal regulations, requires the holding of pork 6 to 27 inches thick for 30 days at —15° C or 12 days at —28.9° C. The more promising rapid-freezing process kills the larvae at —17.8° C in 48 to 72 hours and at —35° C in 2 hours. The freezing of all pork appears impractical under present conditions. Slow freezing would require the equivalent of all the freezing capacity in the country; rapid freezing would necessitate new installations, and the product would have to be handled in the frozen state until in the hands of the consumer. Storage in the deep-freeze units at —15° to —17.8° C in the home should prove effective.

Irradiation with cobalt-60 rays appears to be a promising method of treating pork. Irradiation at 18,000 rep will destroy or sterilize the encysted larvae, produces no ill effects in the consumer even at 40,000 rep, does not cause any change in flavor, and does not produce radio-resistant strains, although a few larvae may survive to maturity. Wholesale irradiation, however, presents practical difficulties.

The general public should be informed, through educational campaigns, of the danger of trichinosis, its method of transmission, and the necessity of thoroughly cooking pork, until its attractive pink color turns to a drab grey.

Trichuris trichiura

Disease.   Trichuriasis, trichocephaliasis, whipworm infection.

Life Cycle.   Man is the principal host of *Trichuris trichiura,* but it has also been reported in monkeys and hogs. Closely allied species are found in sheep, cattle, dogs, cats, rabbits, rats, and mice.

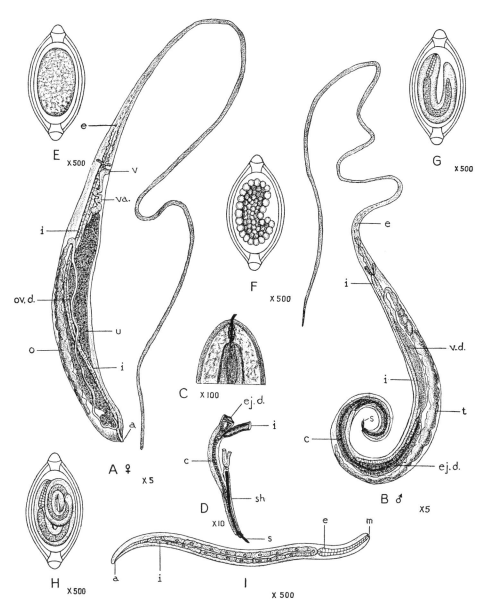

Fig. 37. *Trichuris trichiura.* A, female; B, male; C, anterior end showing spear; D, cloaca and copulatory organs of male; E, unicellular stage of egg; F, multicellular stage of egg; G, early larva in egg shell; H, mature larva in egg shell; I, newly hatched larva. (A-I adapted from Leuckart, 1876, except C, drawn from photograph by Li, 1933.)

a, anus; c, cloaca; e, esophagus; ej.d., ejaculatory duct; i, intestine; m, mouth; o, ovary; ov.d., oviduct; s, spicule; sh, sheath of spicule; t, testis; u, uterus; v, vulva; va., vagina; v.d., vas deferens.

The morphologic characteristics of *Trichuris trichiura* are (Fig. 37), (1) an attenuated whip-like anterior three-fifths traversed by a narrow esophagus resembling a string of beads; (2) a more robust posterior two-fifths containing the intestine and a single set of reproductive organs; (3) similarity in length of male,

TRICHURIS   TRICHIURA

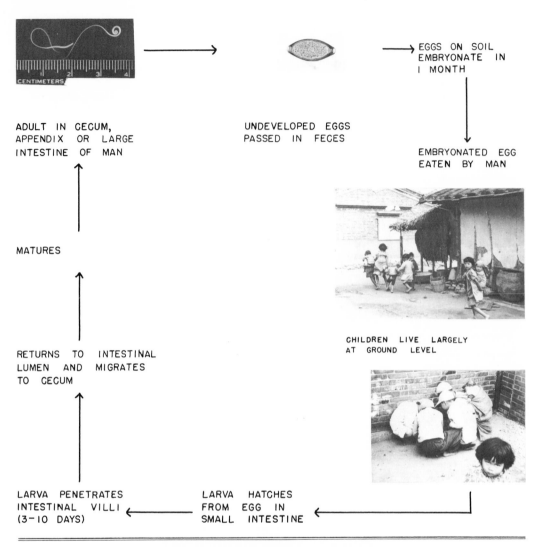

ADULT IN CECUM,
APPENDIX OR LARGE
INTESTINE OF MAN

UNDEVELOPED EGGS
PASSED IN FECES

EGGS ON SOIL
EMBRYONATE IN
I MONTH

EMBRYONATED EGG
EATEN BY MAN

MATURES

RETURNS TO INTESTINAL
LUMEN AND MIGRATES
TO CECUM

CHILDREN LIVE LARGELY
AT GROUND LEVEL

LARVA PENETRATES
INTESTINAL VILLI
(3-10 DAYS)

LARVA HATCHES
FROM EGG IN
SMALL INTESTINE

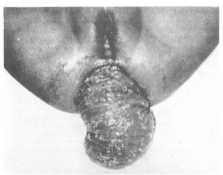

VERY HEAVY TRICHURIS INFECTION
WITH WORMS ON PROLAPSED RECTUM

Fig. 38. Life cycle of *Trichuris trichiura*.

30 to 45 mm, and female, 35 to 50 mm; and (4) the bluntly rounded posterior end of the female and the coiled posterior extremity of the male with its single spicule and retractile sheath. The number of eggs produced per day by a female has been variously estimated at 3,000–10,000. The eggs 50 to 54 μ by 23 μ, are lemon-shaped with plug-like translucent polar prominences. They have a yellowish outer, and a transparent inner, shell. The fertilized eggs are unsegmented at oviposition. Embryonic development takes place outside the host. An unhatched, infective, first-stage larva is produced in 3 to 4 weeks in a favorable environment—i.e., warm, moist, shaded soil. The eggs are less resistant to desiccation, heat, and cold than those of *Ascaris lumbricoides*.

Infection is direct; no intermediate host is required (Fig. 38). When the embryonated egg is ingested by man, the activated larva escapes from the weakened egg shell in the upper small intestine and penetrates an intestinal villus, where it remains 3 to 10 days near the crypts of Lieberkühn. Upon reaching adolescence, it gradually passes downward to the cecum. A spearlike projection at its anterior extremity enables the worm to penetrate into and embed its whip-like anterior portion in the intestinal mucosa of the host, whence it derives its nourishment. Its secretions possibly may liquefy the adjacent mucosal cells. The developmental period from the ingested egg to ovipositing adult covers about 30 to 90 days. Its life span probably covers many years.

Epidemiology.   The incidence of whipworm infection is high, but its intensity is usually light. It is estimated that 500 million persons throughout the world are infected, the incidence ranging as high as 80 percent in certain tropical countries. In the United States whipworm infection is found in the warm, moist South. Its distribution is coextensive with that of *Ascaris lumbricoides*. The highest incidence is found in the regions of heavy rainfail, subtropical climate, and highly polluted soil.

Children are more frequently infected than adults. The heaviest infections are in young children, who live largely at ground level, habitually contaminate the soil, and pick up infection from polluted dooryards. Infection results from the ingestion of embryonated eggs via hands, food, or drink that have been contaminated directly by infested soil or indirectly by playthings, domestic animals, or dust.

Pathology and Symptomatology.   *Trichuris* lives primarily in the cecum of man, but is also found in the appendix and lower ileum. In heavily parasitized individuals, the worms are distributed throughout the colon and rectum, and they may be seen on the prolapsed rectal mucosa that results from straining at the frequent stools (Fig. 38 and 39).

Although *Trichuris* is widespread and its incidence is high in many areas, the intensity of the infection is usually low. Light infections usually do not give rise to recognizable clinical manifestations, and the presence of the parasite is discovered only on routine stool examination. Some of the patients are given a tentative diagnosis of some form of appendicitis, the chronic type predominating.

Patients with very heavy chronic *Trichuris* infections present a characteristic clinical picture consisting of (1) severe anemia, (2) frequent small blood-streaked diarrheal stools, (3) abdominal pain and tenderness, (4) nausea and vomiting, (5) weight loss, and (6) occasional rectal prolapse with worms embedded in the mucosa. Headache and slight fever may occur. Extreme cachexia is sometimes seen with a fatal termination. Getz reported four infections with fatal terminations in Panamanian children who harbored from 400 to 4,100 worms.

The anemia that accompanies *Trichuris* infections may be marked, and hemo-

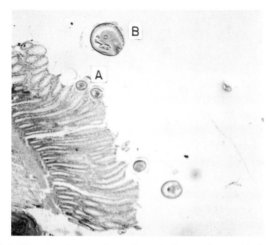

Fig. 39. Large intestine showing sections through A, esophagus, B, body of *Trichuris*.

globin levels as low as 3 gm per 100 ml have been reported. The worms apparently suck the blood of their host, and hemorrhage may occur at the site of their attachment. Approximately 0.005 ml of blood is lost per day per each *Trichuris*. Not infrequently, the *Trichuris* infection is accompanied by hookworm or *E. histolytica* infections, making it impossible to determine the exact role of *Trichuris* in the anemia and symptomatology. Studies indicate that children with light and moderate infections have hemoglobin values essentially identical to those of noninfected children. The white blood cell count may be increased, although the differential count may be essentially the same for parasitized and nonparasitized groups, and a relative lymphocytosis is usually present. Although eosinophilia is encountered occasionally in uncomplicated *Trichuris* infections, it is presumably the recently acquired infections that give this response, as chronic infections may be accompanied by a normal eosinophil count. *Trichuris* may attach to the appendiceal mucosa and provide an entrance for pathogenic bacteria and subsequent acute or subacute inflammatory processes.

Diagnosis.   Clinical trichuriasis cannot be differentiated from infections with other intestinal nematodes, although eosinophilia is present more consistently. Diagnosis is made by finding the characteristic lemon-shaped eggs in the feces. Light infections may necessitate the use of concentration methods (Page 324). Egg counts, although unreliable, have been used for determining the intensity of infection and for assaying the results of treatment.

Treatment.   Oral tetarachlorethylene (Page 127), thiabendazole (See Page 120), and hexylresorcinol (See Page 128) are only moderately effective against *Trichuris;* however, hexylresorcinol enemas are quite effective and of value in heavy infections. A new drug, stilbazium iodide (Monopar) shows considerable effect against *Trichuris*. Poorly nourished, debilitated, or anemic patients should receive a high-protein diet, vitamins, and iron. Dichlorovos is effective against Trichuris but not approved by the Federal government.

Prevention.   Infection in highly endemic areas may be prevented by: (1) treatment of infected individuals, (2) sanitary disposal of human feces, (3) washing of hands before meals, (4) instruction of children in sanitation and personal hygiene, and (5) thorough washing and scalding of uncooked vegetables, especially important in countries using nightsoil for fertilizer.

Strongyloides stercoralis

Disease.   Strongyloidiasis, Cochin-China diarrhea.

Life Cycle.   Man is the principal host of *Strongyloides stercoralis*. The parasitic female (Fig. 40), 2.20 by 0.04 mm, is a small, colorless, semitransparent filariform nematode with a finely striated cuticle. It has a short buccal cavity and a long, slender, cylindrical esophagus. The paired uteri contain a single file of thin-shelled, transparent, segmented eggs. The free-living female, smaller than the parasitic one, resembles a typical free-living rhabditoid nematode and has paired reproductive organs. The free-living male is smaller than the female and has a curved tail. The eggs of the parasitic form, 54 by 32 μ, are deposited in the intestinal mucosa; they hatch into rhabditiform larvae which penetrate the glandular epithelium and pass into the lumen of the intestine and out in the feces. The eggs are seldom found in the stool except after violent purgation. This parasite has three types of life cycle.

I. DIRECT CYCLE, LIKE HOOKWORM.   After a short feeding period of 2 to 3 days in the soil, the rhabditiform larva (Fig. 41), 225 by 16 μ, molts into a long, slender, nonfeeding, infective, filariform larva about 700 μ in length. The infective filariform larvae penetrate the skin of man, enter the venous circulation, and pass through the right heart to the lungs, where they penetrate into the alveoli. From the lungs the adolescent parasites ascend to the glottis, are swallowed, and reach the upper part of the small intestine, where they develop into adults. Occasionally some larvae pass through the pulmonary barrier into the arterial circulation and reach various organs of the body. During their migration in the host the larvae pass through two molts to become adolescent worms. Mature oviposting females are produced in about 28 days after the initial infection.

II. INDIRECT CYCLE.   In the indirect cycle the rhabditiform larvae develop into sexually mature free-living males and females in the soil. After fertilization the free-living female produces eggs that develop into rhabditiform larvae. These may become infective filariform larvae within a few days and enter new hosts, or they may repeat the free-living generations. The indirect method appears to be associated with the optimal environmental conditions for a free-living existence in tropical countries, while the direct method is more frequently followed in the less favorable, colder regions. Strains may show chiefly one or the other type of development or a mixture of both types.

III. AUTOINFECTION.   At times the larvae may develop into the filariform stage in the intestine and, by penetrating the intestinal mucosa or the perianal skin, establish a developmental cycle within the host. Autoinfection explains persistent strongyloidiasis, as long as 36 years, in patients living in nonendemic areas.

Epidemiology.   The distribution of *Strongyloides* infection runs parallel to that of hookworm, but its prevalence is lower in the temperate zones. It is especially prevalent in tropical and subtropical areas, where warmth, moisture, and lack of sanitation favor its free living cycle. In the United States it occurs in the rural South. Man alone is responsible for the perpetuation of strongyloidiasis.

Pathology and Symptomatology.   The parasitic females penetrate the mucosa of the intestinal villi, where they burrow in serpentine channels in the mucosa, depositing eggs and securing nourishment. The worms are most frequently found

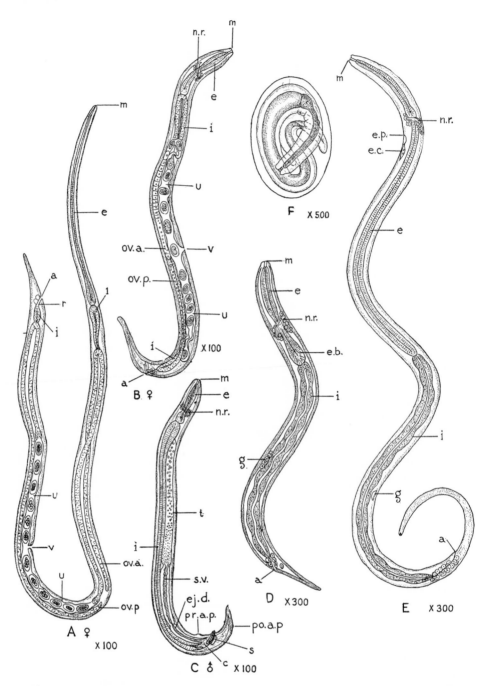

Fig. 40. *Strongyloides stercoralis.* A, parasitic female; B, free-living female; C, free-living male; D, rhabditiform larva; E, filariform larva; F, egg containing mature larva of *S. simiae.* (A-E redrawn or adapted from Looss, 1911; F adapted from Kreis, 1932.)

a, anus; c, cloaca; e, esophagus; e.b., esophageal bulb; e.c., excretory cell; ej.d., ejaculatory duct; e.p., excretory pore; g, genital rudiment; i, intestine; m, mouth; n.r., nerve ring; ov.a., anterior ovary; ov.p., posterior ovary; po.a.p., postanal papilla; pr.a.p., preanal papilla; r, rectum; s, spicules; s.v., seminal vesicle; t, testis; u, uterus; v, vulva.

STRONGYLOIDES STERCORALIS

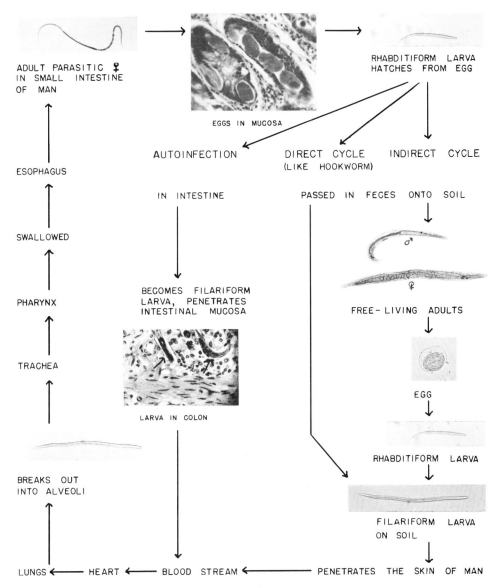

Fig. 41. Life cycle of *Strongyloides stercoralis*.

in the duodenum and upper jejunum, but in heavy infections the pylorus, both the small and large intestine, and the proximal biliary and pancreatic passages may be involved.

Many *Strongyloides* infections are light and go unnoticed by their human host as they produce no symptoms. Moderate infections with the parasitic females embedded primarily in the duodenal region may cause a burning, dull or sharp, non-radiating midepigastric pain. Pressure to this area may elicit pain and tenderness. Nausea and vomiting may be present; diarrhea and constipation alternate. Longstanding and heavy infections result in anemia, weight loss, and chronic dysentery accompanied by a low-grade fever. The latter suggests secondary bacterial invasion of the intestinal lesions. In heavy infections, all of the signs and symptoms are more marked, and death may ensue. One of our patients with overwhelming strongyloidiasis had a fatal *Escherichia coli* infection which was probably carried to her blood stream by the numerous filariform larvae migrating from her intestine. At autopsy, parasitic female worms were found embedded in the mucosa, all the way from her stomach to the lower colon. There was a moderately chronic inflammation of her gastrointestinal tract. In her lungs there was extensive recent hemorrhage and scattered foci of acute lobular pneumonia; filariform larvae were found in the lungs, liver, gallbladder, pancreas, adrenals, thyroid and parathyroid glands, lymph glands, and gastrointestinal tract.

There is often a moderate leukocytosis and eosinophilia, although in many infections the eosinophil count is normal. Intestinal strongyloidiasis differs from hookworm infection in that the parasite causes an immediate inflammatory irritation of the intestine, whereas in hookworm disease marked symptoms do not occur until anemia has developed. Prognosis is favorable except in severe cases involving autoinfection. The chemotherapeutic eradication of the worms, however, is relatively easy.

Diagnosis. Clinical diagnosis is uncertain, since strongyloidiasis presents no distinctive clinical picture. The sequence of an atypical bronchitis or pneumonitis followed in a few weeks by a mucous or watery diarrhea, epigastric pain, and eosinophilia is suggestive.

Laboratory diagnosis includes the examination of the feces and duodenal contents by direct or concentration methods. The presence of characteristic rhabditiform larvae in fresh feces is diagnostic; in heavy infections they may be found in simple film preparations. The duodenal fluid of suspected subjects should be examined if the feces are negative, as the duodenal fluid gives slightly higher positive findings. The rhabditiform larvae of *Strongyloides* differ morphologically from those of hookworms, which are rarely found in fresh feces (Fig. 44), while the embryonated *Strongyloides* eggs, slightly smaller than those of hookworms, can only be obtained by a drastic purge or by duodenal intubation. Cultivation of the feces for 48 hours will produce filariform larvae and free-living adult *Strongyloides*, but only rhabditiform hookworm larvae.

Treatment. Thiabendazole (Mintezol) is the drug of choice; 25 mg/kg body weight, twice daily for 2 or 3 days. No special diet or purgation are required. Side effects consisting of anorexia, nausea, vomiting, and dizziness are not uncommon. Less frequent are diarrhea, epigastric distress, pruritis, drowsiness, and headache. The following have rarely been associated with the administration of thiabendazole: bradycardia, hypotension, collapse, conjunctival injection, fever, chills, rash, angioneurotic edema, leukopenia, crystalluria, and transitory rise in the SGOT.

Pyrvinium pamoate (Povan) 50 mg of the base three times a day for 8 days is recommended for persons over 80 pounds weight and 50 mg of the base two times a day for 8 days for persons less than 80 pounds. This drug is given after meals.

Prevention. The prevention of strongyloidiasis is similar to that of hookworm disease. The disease may be self-perpetuating for years because of autoinfection. Autoinfection may be reduced by cleanliness of the anal area, avoidance of constipation, and by treatment. Prevention essentially depends upon the sanitary disposal of human wastes and protection of the skin from contact with contaminated soil. Detection and treatment of subclinical carriers does not appear to be practical.

Hookworms of Man

Disease.   Ancylostomiasis, uncinariasis, necatoriasis, hookworm infection.

Species.   The species in man include: (1) *Necator americanus;* (2) *Ancylostoma duodenale;* and, rarely (3) *Ancylostoma braziliense;* (4) *Ancylostoma caninum;* and (5) *Ancylostoma malayanum.*

History.   Hookworm infection probably existed among the ancient Egyptians; the disease was described in Italy, Arabia, and Brazil long before *Ancylostoma duodenale,* the Old World hookworm, was discovered by Dubini in 1838. In 1877, following an epidemic among the laborers at the St. Gotthard tunnel in Switzerland, the metamorphosis of the free-living rhabditiform larva into the infectious filariform larva and the etiopathology, symptomatology, diagnosis, and therapy of hookworm infection were established. During 1905 to 1911 Looss described infection through the skin and the migratory route of the larvae through the body. Although hookworm disease was recognized in the United States as early as 1845, it was not until 1902 that Stiles described the New World hookworm, *Necator americanus,* which was brought to the United States from West Africa with the importation of slaves.

Morphology.   Adult hookworms are small, cylindrical, fusiform, grayish white nematodes (Fig. 42). The females (9 to 13 by 0.35 to 0.6 mm) are larger than the males (5 to 11 by 0.3 to 0.45 mm). *A duodenale* is larger than *N. americanus.* The worm has a relatively thick cuticle. There are single male and paired female reproductive organs. The posterior end of the male has a broad, translucent, membranous, caudal bursa with rib-like rays, which is used for attachment to the female during copulation.

The chief morphologic differences in the species are in the shape, buccal capsule, and male bursa. The vulva is located anterior to the middle of the body in *Necator* and posterior in *Ancylostoma,* and the caudal spine in the female is absent in *Necator.* In the buccal capsule *N. americanus* has a ventral pair and a less conspicuous dorsal pair of semilunar cutting plates, a concave dorsal median tooth, and a deep pair of triangular subventral lancets. *A. duodenale* has two ventral pairs of teeth, *A. braziliense* two ventral pairs, and *A. caninum* three ventral pairs.

The egg (Fig. 43) has bluntly rounded ends and a single thin transparent hyaline shell. It is unsegmented at oviposition and in two to eight cell stages of division in fresh feces. The eggs of the several species are almost indistinguishable, differing only slightly in size: *N. americanus* 64 to 76 by 36 to 40 μ. and *A. duodenale* 56 to 60 by 36 to 40 μ.

The hookworms attach themselves to the mucosa of the small intestine by their buccal capsules. The favorite site is the upper small intestine, but in heavy infections the worms may be present as far as the lower ileum. They suck the host's blood and mucosal substances by the tractile pull of the contracting and expanding esophagus (Fig. 43). An anticoagulating secretion facilitates blood sucking. Since the blood passes rapidly through the worm, it is possible that only simple diffusible substances are consumed. As much as 0.026 to 0.200 ml of blood may be withdrawn by a worm in 24 hours. Approximately 50 percent of the red blood cells

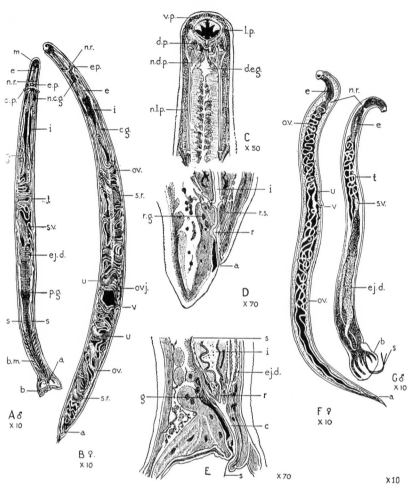

Fig. 42. Important hookworms of man. A, adult male *Ancylostoma duodenale* from ventral side; B, young adult female *A. duodenale* from right side; C, anterior end of *A. duodenale* from dorsal side; D, longitudinal section through posterior end of female *A. duodenale*, somewhat diagrammatic; E, longitudinal section through posterior end of male *A. duodenale*, not quite median; F, female *Necator americanus*; G, male *N. americanus*.

a, anus; b, bursa; b.m., bursal muscles; c, cloaca; c.g., cervical gland; c.p., cervical papilla; d.e.g., dorsal esophageal gland; d.p., dorsal papilla; e, esophagus; e.p., excretory pore; ej.d., ejaculatory duct; g, gubernaculum; i, intestine; l.p., lateral papilla; m, mouth; n.c.g., nucleus of cephalic gland; n.d.p., nerve of dorsal papilla; n.l.p., nerve of lateral papilla; n.r., nerve ring; ov., ovary; ovj., ovejector; p.g., prostatic glands; r, rectum; r.g., rectal ganglion; r.s., rectal sphincter; s, spicules; s.r., seminal receptable; s.v., seminal vesicle; t, testis; u, uterus; v, vulva; v.p., ventral papilla. (A-E redrawn from Looss, 1905; F and G redrawn after Placencia from Manson-Bahr, 1936.)

are hemolyzed during passage through the worm's intestine. *A. duodenale* infections may persist for 6 to 8 years and longer. The majority of *N. americanus* disappear within 2 years, others live 4 to 5 years. An experimental infection in an American scientist persisted for 14 years. The maximum daily egg output by a mature female has been estimated at 20,000 for *A. duodenale* and 10,000 for *N. americanus*. Egg production is constant; thus, the number of female worms may be

HOOKWORMS

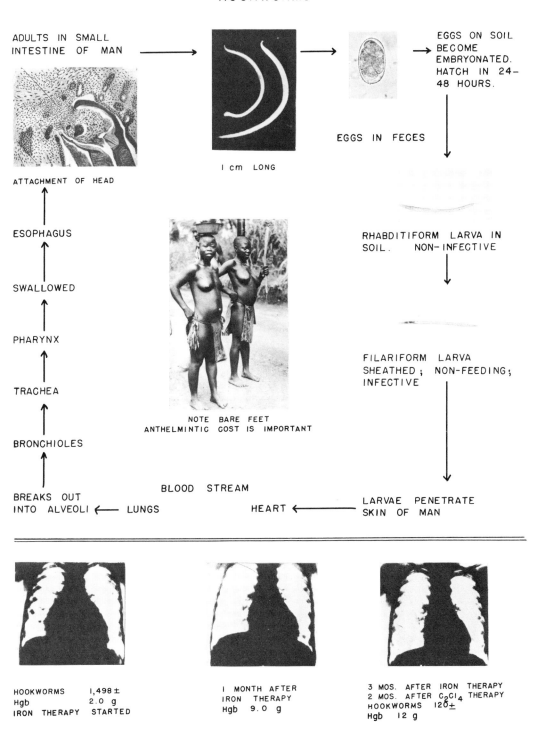

ADULTS IN SMALL
INTESTINE OF MAN

1 cm LONG

ATTACHMENT OF HEAD

EGGS ON SOIL
BECOME
EMBRYONATED.
HATCH IN 24–
48 HOURS.

EGGS IN FECES

ESOPHAGUS

SWALLOWED

PHARYNX

TRACHEA

RHABDITIFORM LARVA IN
SOIL.   NON–INFECTIVE

NOTE BARE FEET
ANTHELMINTIC COST IS IMPORTANT

FILARIFORM LARVA
SHEATHED ; NON–FEEDING ;
INFECTIVE

BRONCHIOLES

BLOOD STREAM

BREAKS OUT
INTO ALVEOLI ← LUNGS   HEART ←   LARVAE PENETRATE
SKIN OF MAN

HOOKWORMS   1,498 ±
Hgb   2.0 g
IRON THERAPY STARTED

1 MONTH AFTER
IRON THERAPY
Hgb 9.0 g

3 MOS. AFTER IRON THERAPY
2 MOS. AFTER C₂Cl₄ THERAPY
HOOKWORMS 120 ±
Hgb 12 g

CARDIAC ENLARGEMENT CAUSED BY ANEMIA

Fig. 43. Life cycle of hookworms of man.

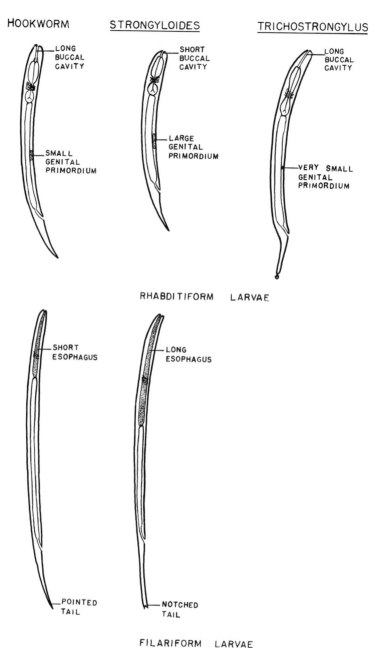

Fig. 44. Differentiation of nematode larvae from stool.

calculated from the egg count, and there are usually an equal number of males.

   Life Cycle (Fig. 43).   The life cycles of the several species of hookworm are similar. Man is almost the exclusive host of *A. duodenale* and *N. americanus,* although these species have been reported occasionally in primates and other mammals. The adults of *A. braziliense,* a parasite of wild and domestic felines and canines in the tropics, are infrequently found in man. *A. caninum,* the common hookworm of dogs and cats, is an extremely rare intestinal parasite of man.

The eggs, passed in the feces, mature rapidly and produce the rhabditiform larvae in 1 to 2 days under favorable conditions and an optimal temperature of 23° to 33° C. Eggs of *A. duodenale* die in a few hours at 45° C and in 7 days at 0° C.

The rhabditiform larvae (Fig. 44) of *A. duodenale* and *N. americanus* are somewhat larger, more attenuated posteriorly, and have a longer buccal capsule than the larvae of *Strongyloides stercoralis.* The newly hatched larvae, 275 by 16 μ, feed actively upon organic debris and grow rapidly to a size of 500 to 700 μ in 5 days. Then they molt for a second time to become slender, nonfeeding, infective filariform larvae (Fig. 44), which differ from the filariform larvae of *Strongyloides stercoralis* in the absence of notched clefts in the pointed tail and a shorter esophagus. The active filariform larvae, which frequent the upper half inch of soil and project from the surface, have a strong thigmotaxis that facilitates access to the skin of a new host. Hookworm larvae remain within a few inches of where they are deposited unless carried by floods or animals to other locations.

In heavily infested soil under tropical conditions, practically all the larvae are extremely active, rapidly consume their stored food, and die within 6 weeks; however, constant reinfestation maintains the supply in endemic areas. Although they require little moisture, drying is destructive. They survive best in shaded localities such as light sandy or alluvial soils or loam covered by vegetation, where they are protected from drying or excessive wetness. At 0° C larvae survive less than 2 weeks, at −11° C less than 24 hours, and at 45° C less than 1 hour.

The filariform larvae gain access to the host through hair follicles, pores, or even the unbroken skin. Damp clinging soil facilitates infection. The usual site of infection is the dorsum of the foot or between the toes; miners and farmers may acquire the infection on the hands, chiefly in the interdigital spaces; and fishermen have been infected by sitting on infested stream banks. The larvae enter the lymphatics or venules and are carried in the blood through the heart to the lungs, where because of their size they are unable to pass the capillary barrier and therefore break out of the capillaries into the alveoli. They ascend the bronchi and trachea, are finally swallowed, and pass down to the intestines. This larval blood and pulmonary migration takes about 1 week. During this period the larvae undergo a third molt and acquire a temporary buccal capsule, which enables the adolescent worm to feed. After a fourth molt at about the thirteenth day, they acquire adult characteristics, and mature egg-laying females are produced in 5 to 6 weeks after infection. Rarely, infection may occur by mouth, the larvae being taken into the body through drinking water or contaminated food.

Epidemiology. The present distribution has been brought about by the migration of people and extends in the tropical and subtropical zones between 45° N and 30° S latitude, except for the presence of *A. duodenale* in the northern mining districts of Europe. *N. americanus* is the prevailing species in the Western Hemisphere, in Central and South Africa, southern Asia, Indonesia, Australia, and the islands of the Pacific. *A. duodenale* is the dominant species in the Mediterranean region, northern Asia, and the west coast of South America. It is also found in smaller numbers in areas where *N. americanus* predominates.

It is estimated that throughout the world the hookworms, harbored by 700 million persons, cause a daily blood loss of 7 million liters, the total blood of more than a million people—a Washington, Taipei, or Bangkok.

The following factors favor hookworm maintenance and dispersal:

1. Infected individuals who defecate on the soil in areas frequented by others— fecal concentration in secluded areas near the house; return to this restricted area by members of the family leads to family infection. The one-room school without sanitary facilities is an excellent source of infection.

2. A sandy or loam soil which is a favorable culture medium for hookworm larvae. Clay soil, which packs tightly, is unsuitable for the larvae.

3. A warm climate which favors the development of the eggs and larvae and promiscuous defecation. Cold, snowy climes force man into shelter, hence the widespread use of the privy in such areas.

4. Moisture, 30 to 50 inches of rain, especially during the warm season of the year when egg and larval development are possible.

5. A poor, ignorant population who do not wear shoes. The population of half of the world do not wear shoes, cannot afford them, nor do they need them.

These conditions are found throughout the tropics, subtropics, and parts of the temperate zone. In Egypt, where little effort at concealment is made, defecation is widespread in the unshaded streets, yards, and fields, and the arid winds and sun destroy much of the potential infection. Hence, though hookworm is widespread, the infections are light, and hookworm disease is rare. In China, where mulberry trees are grown for the leaves to maintain silkworms, human nightsoil is used to fertilize the trees. In this sandy, moist, shady environment as many as 10,000 hookworm infective larvae were recovered from a soil sample. Picking of the mulberry leaves falls to the lot of women and, as would be expected, they are heavily infected. Cultivation of coffee, sweet potatoes and bananas offer similar opportunities for infection.

The Negro is less susceptible to *N. americanus* than whites, when they live under the same unsanitary conditions. The reasons for this are not clear. Since this parasite appeared early in Africa there may have been some natural selection. Possibly the thicker skin of the Negro offers more resistance to the larva's penetration. Nutrition may play some part, since Negroes appear to be better nourished than their poor-white neighbors. It has been demonstrated that dogs fed a protein- and vitamin-deficient diet fail to develop the degree of immunity to repeated hookworm infection that is acquired by their well-nourished litter mates.

Pathology and Symptomatology. When the larvae penetrate the skin they produce maculopapules and localized erythema. Itching is often severe, and as it is related to contact with the soil, especially on dewy mornings when the moisture permits the larvae to be at the surface, it is known as "ground itch" or "dew itch." If considerable numbers of larvae migrate through the lungs at one time or in sensitized individuals, a bronchitis or pneumonitis may result.

Hookworm disease is essentially a chronic infection, and the infected individual often shows no acute symptoms. Symptoms attributable to the adult worm usually do not develop until the onset of anemia. Infections with *A. duodenale* are more severe and produce symptoms with fewer worms than infections with *N. americanus,* as the former consumes more blood. Light infections produce no recognized symptoms, but elimination of the worms sometimes increases the vigor of children. The most prominent characteristic in moderate or heavy chronic hookworm infection is a progressive, secondary, microcytic, hypochromic anemia of the nutritional deficiency type. Clinical and experimental evidence indicates that the anemia is primarily due to the continuous loss of blood. The pathology and symptomatology are proportional to the number of worms and the nutritional intake of the patient. In adults an infection with 50 worms is subclinical, one with 50 to 125 worms is borderline, and one with 500 is serious. A combination of iron deficiency and hookworm infection appears necessary for the establishment of anemia, since it may be offset by the administration of iron. Malnutrition not only may produce anemia, but also may weaken the natural protective mechanism of the host so that an excessive number of worms may become established. Depending on the degree of anemia, which may be as low as 2.0 g of hemoglobin per 100 ml of blood, the patient experiences dyspnea on exertion, weakness, and dizziness.

The appetite may be enormous or poor and associated with pica. Nausea, vomiting, diarrhea, or constipation may be present. The heart shows hypertrophy, a hemic murmur is present, and the pulse is rapid. There is edema of varying degrees, and albumin is present in the urine. Heavily infected children may be physically, mentally, and sexually retarded. Early in the infection eosinophilia and leukocytosis are marked; as the infection becomes chronic the eosinophilia and leukocytosis both decrease, but the anemia persists. The stools may contain gross blood, and occult blood is readily found.

Diagnosis.   The clinical picture, though characteristic, is not sufficiently pathognomonic to permit differentiation from the nutritional deficiency anemias and edemas or from other helminthic infections. Final diagnosis depends upon finding the eggs in the feces. It is practically impossible to distinguish the eggs of *A. duodenale* from those of *N. americanus*. Hookworm eggs may be confused with the root parasite eggs of *Meloidogyne* (*Heterodera*) or those of *Trichostrongylus,* which are larger, more elongated, narrow at one end, and have a larger number of blastomeres (Fig. 141).

Eggs are found in direct fecal films, but in light infections concentration methods (Page 324) may be required. The direct coverglass mount is of value only where there are over 1,200 eggs per gram of feces; cases with less than 400 are often missed. The zinc sulfate centrifugal flotation and the acid-sodium-sulfate-triton-ether concentration methods increase the number of positive findings several fold. The collection of larvae from eggs hatched on strips of filter paper with one end immersed in water is reported to give a high percentage of positive findings. Egg-counting methods, such as the Stoll dilution eggcount (Page 325), that indicate the intensity of the infection are useful in surveys, and before and after therapy. It is important to distinguish the rhabditiform larvae of hookworm from those of *Strongyloides* and *Trichostrongylus* all of which may be found in stool specimens that are several days old (Fig. 44). In fresh stools the eggs of hookworm and *Trichostrongylus* will be found in the early stages of cleavage, and *Strongyloides* as rhabditiform larvae. It must be remembered that the patient may harbor more than one species of parasite.

Treatment.   Tetrachlorethylene is the drug of choice for the treatment of *Necator* as it is safe, effective, cheap, and a liquid. It has been given to millions of anemic patients without serious side effects, although transient vertigo, abdominal cramps and vomiting may occur. A single dose will remove 90 percent of the *Necator* and 65 percent of the *Ancylostoma;* bephenium hydroxynaphthoate (Alcopara) is especially effective against *Ancylostoma* as well as *Ascaris;* hence, it is useful in mixed infections. This drug is less effective against *Necator,* yet when repeated on several consecutive days it removes a high percentage of them.

Treatment of light infections in endemic areas, where reinfection is certain and rapid, is of questionable value. However, treatment of all individuals who will not again be exposed to infection is recommended, as a very light infection of 10 hookworms could remove as much as 3,500 ml of blood from their host in 5 years. An adequately high protein and vitamin diet, and iron therapy for the hypochromic anemia, will materially improve the health of the patient.

Tetrachlorethylene is a chlorinated aliphatic hydrocarbon. It is administered in gelatin capsules on an empty stomach in the morning at a dosage of 5 ml for adults and at 0.06 ml per pound of weight to children. Treatment may be repeated in 2 weeks if eggs are still found in the patient's stool.

Bephenium hydroxynaphthoate (Alcopara) is supplied in packets containing 5.0 g, equivalent to 2.5 g of bephenium ion. The usual adult dosage is one packet, 5.0 g of Alcopara granules twice in 1 day, total 10 gms. Children under 50 pounds in weight are given half the above amount. The drug is somewhat bitter and should be administered in milk, chocolate milk, orange juice, or a carbonated beverage. Food should be withheld for 2 hours after giving the drug, and no purgatives should be used. No serious side effects have been reported. It has been safely administered to seriously ill patients with hemoglobin level below 50 percent. A small percentage of patients may experience nausea and/or vomiting, which may be accompanied by diarrhea. In seriously debilitated patients, the possibility of electrolyte imbalance should be taken into consideration and corrective measures applied before giving the drug. Safety for use in pregnancy has not been established. In hypertensive patients the drug should be used with caution, because if the drug were appreciably absorbed, it might produce a brief marked fall in blood pressure.

Thiabendazole is effective against hookworm (See Page 120).

Hexylresorcinol (Crystoids anthelmintic) is moderately effective against hookworm, very effective against *Ascaris,* and of some value in trichuriasis. The adult dose is 1.0 g. The dose for children is 0.1 g for each year of age up to 10. The advantages of this drug are that it is nontoxic and that it will remove *Ascaris* as well as hookworm. The crystals will burn the mouth if the capsules are chewed, and the drug combines with protein and is soluble in fat, so that food must be avoided for 12 hours before and 4 hours after treatment.

Prevention.   Hookworm infection may be reduced or even eliminated in a community by: (1) the sanitary disposal of fecal wastes, (2) the protection of susceptible individuals, and (3) the treatment of infected individuals.

From a practical standpoint it is most important to treat persons showing clinical evidence of the disease. Mass treatment is advisable when the incidence is over 50 percent, the average worm burden over 150, and facilities for examining all of the population are not available. Unless mass treatment includes the entire population, is repeated at intervals, and is accompanied by improvements in sanitation, its effect is temporary.

Sanitation is the chief method of control. In rural communities, where sewerage systems are impracticable, promiscuous defecation may be curtailed by the construction of pit privies. Education of the public as to the method of transmission of hookworm infection and the proper use of privies is as essential as their installation. Attempts to enforce sanitary regulations are less effective than sanitary instruction

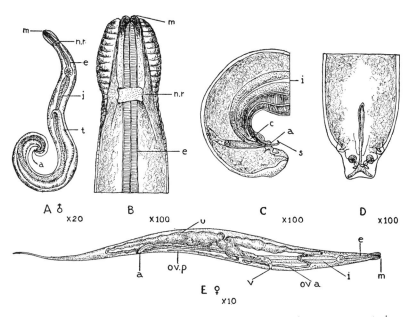

Fig. 45. *Enterobius vermicularis.* A, male; B, anterior end of worm; c, posterior end of male, lateral view; D, posterior end of male, ventral view; E, female.

a, anus; c, cloaca; e, esophagus; i, intestine; m, mouth; n.r., nerve ring; ov.a., anterior ovary; ov.p., posterior ovary; s, spicule; t, testis; u, uterus; v, vulva. (Redrawn from Leuckart, 1876.)

in the home, publicity campaigns, and training in the schools. The use of night soil as fertilizer in certain countries presents an economic and sanitary problem that may be solved by storage or by chemical disinfection of feces.

The protection of the susceptible individual in an endemic locality is largely an economic and educational problem. It involves the prevention of malnutrition by an adequate diet. The wearing of shoes, especially by children, is important but economically impossible in the tropics, and to the children unacceptable.

Enterobius vermicularis

Disease.   Enterobiasis, oxyuriasis, pinworm, seatworm.

Morphology (Fig. 45).   The small adult female worm (8 to 13 mm by 0.4 mm) has a cuticular alar expansion at the anterior end, a prominent esophageal bulb, a long pointed tail, and rigid body. The uteri of the gravid female are distended with eggs. The male, 2 to 5 mm in length with a curved tail and a single spicule, is seldom seen.

Life Cycle (Fig. 46).   Man is the only known host of *E. vermicularis.* The usual habitat of the mature pinworm is the cecum and the adjacent portions of the large and small intestines. Presumably it feeds on the intestinal contents, although it may consume cellular material. Immature females and males occasionally may be found in the rectum and lower part of the colon. At times the worms may travel upward to the stomach, esophagus, and nose. The gravid females, containing about 11,000 eggs, migrate at night to the perianal and perineal regions where the eggs are expelled in masses by contractions of the uterus and vagina under the stimulus of a lower temperature and aerobic environment. The eggs mature and are in-

ENTEROBIUS VERMICULARIS

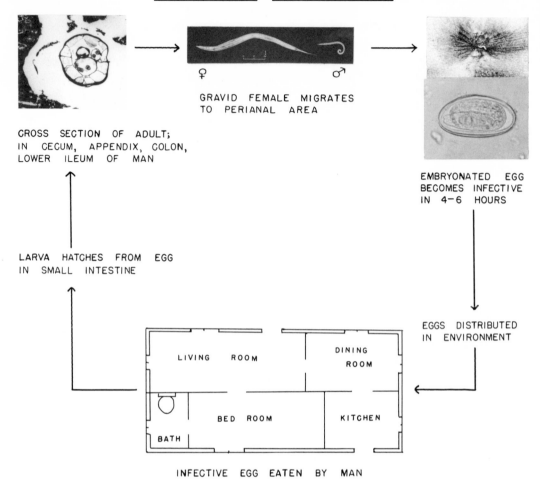

CROSS SECTION OF ADULT;
IN CECUM, APPENDIX, COLON,
LOWER ILEUM OF MAN

GRAVID FEMALE MIGRATES
TO PERIANAL AREA

EMBRYONATED EGG
BECOMES INFECTIVE
IN 4—6 HOURS

LARVA HATCHES FROM EGG
IN SMALL INTESTINE

EGGS DISTRIBUTED
IN ENVIRONMENT

LIVING ROOM   DINING ROOM

BED ROOM   KITCHEN

BATH

INFECTIVE EGG EATEN BY MAN

SCOTCH TAPE DIAGNOSIS

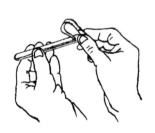

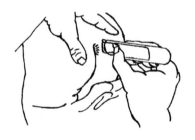

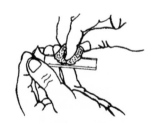

LOOP TAPE OVER END
OF SLIDE TO EXPOSE
GUMMED SURFACE

TOUCH GUMMED SURFACE
SEVERAL TIMES TO
PERIANAL REGION

SMOOTH TAPE
ON SLIDE

Fig. 46. Life cycle of *Enterobius vermicularis*.

fectious several hours after passage. Eggs are infrequently laid in the intestine; hence, stool examination is of little value.

Upon ingestion of the egg, the embryonic first-stage larvae hatch in the duodenum. The liberated rhabditiform larvae molt twice before reaching adolescence in the jejunum and upper ileum. Copulation probably takes place in the cecum. The duration of the cycle from the ingestion of the egg to the perianal migration of the gravid female may be as short as 2 to 4 weeks, but often is longer. The infection is self-limited and, in the absence of reinfection, ceases without treatment.

Epidemiology. Pinworm has the widest geographic distribution of any helminth, and its success is due to a close association with man and his environment. Stoll estimated that there are 208.8 million infected persons in the world, and 18 million in Canada and the United States. Surveys have revealed infection rates of from 3 to 80 percent in various groups. An Eskimo village gave a 66 percent infection rate, in tropical Brazil 60 percent, and in Washington, D.C. 12 to 41 percent. Although this parasite is more prevalent in the lower economic groups, mental institutions, and orphanages, it is not uncommon in the well-to-do and even in the seats of the mighty. Children are more commonly infected than adults, and the incidence in whites is considerably higher than in Negroes.

Infection of the same or another person may be effected by: (1) the important hand-to-mouth transmission from scratching the perianal areas or from handling contaminated fomites, (2) inhalation of airborne eggs in dust, and (3) retroinfection through the anus. Eggs hatch in the perianal region and the larvae migrate back into the large intestine. Heavy infections are effected by the transference of eggs from the perianal region to the hands and thence to the mouth directly or through contaminated food. In households with several pinworm-infected members, 92 percent of 241 dust samples collected from floors, baseboards, tables, chairs, davenports, dressers, shelves, picture frames, window sills, toilet seats, wash basins, bath tubs, bed sheets, and mattresses contained *Enterobius* eggs. The largest number of eggs was found in bedrooms. This study demonstrates how the infection is spread through families or groups living in the same environment. Pinworm eggs have been isolated from the dust of school rooms and the school's cafeteria, which could be the source of a new family infection. Fortunately most of these eggs are dead, as it has been shown that at usual room temperature (20 to 24.5° C) and a relative humidity of 30 to 54 percent less than 10 percent of eggs survived for 2 days. At summer temperature 36° to 37° C, and a relative humidity of 38 to 41 percent less than 10 percent of the eggs survived for 3 hours. These data explain why reinfection is not universal in a potentially infected environment. Dogs and cats do not harbor *Enterobius*, yet the eggs from their master's environment may be carried on their fur and serve as a source of infection.

Pathology and Symptomatology. *E. vermicularis* is relatively innocuous and rarely produces serious lesions. The clinical symptoms are due largely to the perianal, perineal, and vaginal irritation caused by the migrations of the gravid female worm, and less frequently to the intestinal activities of the parasite. In the former, the local pruritus and discomfort produce a chain of secondary reflex symptoms that tend to debilitate the patient—due to disturbed sleep.

Various observers have ascribed a number of signs and symptoms to the presence of pinworm—e.g., poor appetite, weight loss, hyperactivity, enuresis, insomnia, irritability, grinding of the teeth, abdominal pain, nausea, and vomiting— but it is often difficult to prove the causal relationship of pinworm. The gravid females may migrate into and become imbedded in the vagina, the fallopian tubes, into the peritoneal cavity, and even into the urinary bladder. They are frequently found in the appendix, but probably seldom are the cause of appendicitis.

Slight eosinophilia has been reported, but it is unusual. As this parasite has no tissue migrating stage and does not attach to the intestine, blood changes would not be expected.

The conscientious housewife's mental distress, guilt complex, and desire to conceal the infection from her friends is perhaps the most important trauma of this persistent, pruritic, parasite.

Diagnosis. Pinworm infection is suspected in children who show nocturnal perianal itching, insomnia, and nervous restlessness. Diagnosis is made by finding the adult worms or eggs. Often the first evidence of infection is the discovery of the adult worms on the feces after enemas or in the perianal region. Eggs are seldom found in the feces—in only about 5 percent of infected persons. They are best obtained by swabbing the perianal region. Graham's Scotch adhesive tape swab (Fig. 46) gives the highest percentage of positive results and the greatest number of eggs. In this method, a strip of sticky Scotch tape is applied to the perianal region, removed, and then spread on a slide for examination. The preparation is cleared by placing a drop of toluol between the slide and tape. A drop of iodine in xylol, which gives a stained background for the eggs as well as clearing, is preferred by some workers. Repeated examinations on consecutive days are necessary because of the irregular migrations of the gravid female worms. A single swabbing reveals only about 50 percent of the infections, three swabbings about 90 percent, and examinations on 7 consecutive days are necessary before the patient is considered free from infection. The swab for eggs is preferably made in the morning before bathing or defecation. In about one-third of infected children, eggs may be obtained from beneath the fingernails. The eggs are identified by their asymmetrical shape and well-developed embryo.

Treatment. The treatment of a person harboring pinworm is frequently unsatisfactory if other infected members of the household are untreated and remain as sources of infection. It is recommended, therefore, if it is not feasible to make several Scotch tape examinations and treat only those found to be infected, that all members of the household be treated simultaneously.

Piperazine (Antepar) is highly effective against pinworm when taken before breakfast and followed by a glass of water, which carries the drug to the cecum and colon, the habitat of the worms. Therapy is continued for 7 consecutive days employing the following daily dosage:

Patient's weight (lb)	Piperazine citrate syrup (ml)	Equivalent piperazine hexahydrate (g)
Up to 15	2.5	0.25
16–30	5.0	0.50
31–60	10.0	1.00
Over 60	20.0	2.00

Both tablets and a syrup are available. Overdosage with, or sensitivity to, piperazine may result in nausea, vomiting, dizziness, difficulty in focusing vision, and urticaria.

Pyrvinium pamoate (Povan) is effective in enterobiasis. Both tablets and a liquid preparation are available. The dose is 5 mg of the base per kilogram of body weight. Pyrvinium pamoate colors the stool bright red, and the suspension, if spilled, will stain. Nausea and vomiting may occur. As the cure rate from a single dose is approximately 90 percent, a second dose 1 week after the first treatment is recommended.

Thiabendazole (Mintezol) 25 mg/kg twice daily for 1 day to be repeated in 7 days is highly effective (see under *Treatment* for *Strongyloides stercoralis,* above). See Page 120.

Stilbazium iodide (Monopar) is highly effective and requires only a single dose, but it is still in the experimental stage.

Prevention. Personal cleanliness is essential; the fingernails should be cut short, the hands thoroughly washed after using the toilet and before meals, and the anal region washed on rising. A salve or ointment applied to the perianal area will help prevent the dispersal of eggs. Infected children should wear tight-fitting cotton pants to prevent contact of hands with perianal region and the contamination of the bed clothing. As the bathtub may be a source of infection, the use of a shower bath is suggested. In order to protect others the infected person should sleep alone, and his underwear, night clothes, and bed sheets should be carefully handled and laundered. Food should be protected from dust and from the hands of infected individuals. The difficulty of preventing dustborne and retroinfections may account for the frequent failure of strict hygienic measures.

Ascaris lumbricoides

Disease. Ascariasis, ascaris infection, roundworm infection.

Morphology. (Fig. 47). The white or pink worm is identified by: (1) large size, males 10 to 31 cm and females 22 to 35 cm; (2) smooth finely striated cuticle; (3) conical anterior and posterior extremities; (4) ventrally curved papillated posterior extremity of male with two spicules; (5) terminal mouth with three oval lips with sensory papillae; and (6) paired reproductive organs in posterior two-thirds of female, and a single long tortuous tubule in male.

The eggs (Fig. 47) measure 45 to 70 by 35 to 50 μ. There is an outer, coarsely mammillated, albuminous covering which serves as an auxiliary barrier to permeability, but may be absent. The egg proper has a thick, transparent, hyaline shell with a relatively thick outer layer that acts as a supporting structure, and a delicate vitelline, lipoidal, inner membrane that is highly impermeable. At oviposition the shell contains an ovoid mass of unsegmented protoplasm densely impregnated with lecithin granules. The typical infertile eggs (Fig. 141), 88 to 94 by 39 to 44 μ, are longer and narrower than fertile eggs, have a thinner shell with an irregular coating of albumen, and are completely filled with an amorphous mass of protoplasm, with refractile granules. Bizarre-shaped eggs without albuminous coating or with abnormally extensive and irregular coating are also found. The infertile eggs are difficult to identify and may be missed by the unwary and untutored. They are found not only in the absence of males but in about two-fifths of all infections, since repeated copulations are necessary for the continuous production of fertile eggs.

Life Cycle (Fig. 47). The adult worms normally live in the lumen of the small intestine. They obtain their nourishment from the semidigested food of the host and possibly from the cells of the intestinal mucosa. Male or female worms are found alone in very lightly infected persons. A female worm has a productive capacity of 26 million eggs, and an average daily output of 200,000. The eggs are unsegmented when they leave the host in the feces. Under favorable environmental conditions in the soil, infective second-stage embryos, after the first molt, are formed within the eggshell in about 3 weeks. The optimal temperature for development is about 25° C, ranging from 21° to 30° C. Lower temperatures retard development but favor survival. At 37° C they develop only to the eight-cell stage. Since eggs require oxygen, their development in putrefactive material is retarded.

ASCARIS LUMBRICOIDES

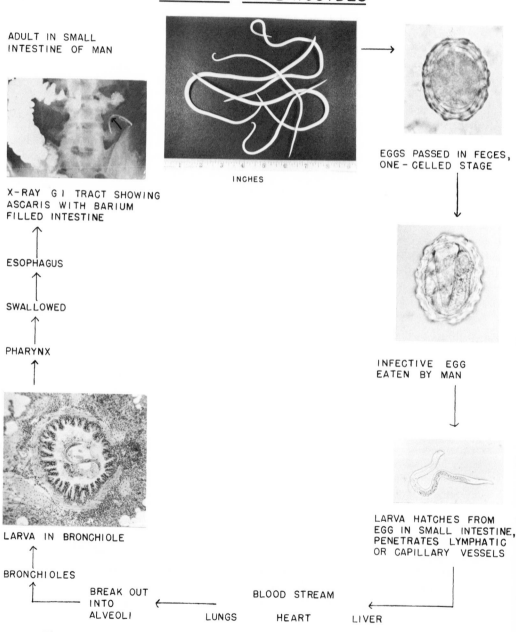

ADULT IN SMALL
INTESTINE OF MAN

INCHES

EGGS PASSED IN FECES,
ONE - CELLED STAGE

X-RAY G I TRACT SHOWING
ASCARIS WITH BARIUM
FILLED INTESTINE

ESOPHAGUS

SWALLOWED

PHARYNX

INFECTIVE EGG
EATEN BY MAN

LARVA IN BRONCHIOLE

LARVA HATCHES FROM
EGG IN SMALL INTESTINE,
PENETRATES LYMPHATIC
OR CAPILLARY VESSELS

BRONCHIOLES

BREAK OUT   BLOOD STREAM
INTO
ALVEOLI   LUNGS   HEART   LIVER

Fig. 47. Life cycle of *Ascaris lumbricoides.*

The infective egg, when ingested by man, hatches in the upper small intestine, freeing its rhabditiform larva (200 to 300 by 14 μ in size), which penetrates the intestinal wall to reach the venules or lymphatics. In the portal circulation they pass to the liver, thence to the heart and lungs. The larvae may reach the lungs 1 to 7 days after infection. As they are 0.02 mm in diameter and the pulmonary capillaries only 0.01 mm in diameter, they break out of the capillaries into the alveoli. Occasionally some reach the left heart by the pulmonary veins and are distributed as emboli to various organs of the body. In the lungs the larvae undergo their second and third molts. They migrate or are carried by the bronchioles to the bronchi, ascend the trachea to the glottis, and pass down the esophagus to the small intestine. During the pulmonary cycle the larvae increase fivefold, to 1.5 mm in length. On arrival in the intestine they undergo a fourth molt. Ovipositing females develop about 2 months after infection, and they live from 12 to 18 months.

Epidemiology. *A. lumbricoides* is a prominent parasite in both temperate and tropical zones, but it is more common in warm countries and is most prevalent where sanitation is poor. In ancient times when man was distinguished from other animals only by his upright position rather than by food or sanitary habits, the vast majority of men probably harbored this parasite. Over the centuries, as man's habits and sanitation gradually changed from those of a quadruped to those of "modern man," this ubiquitous parasite has partially lost its hold on him, although approximately 900 million of the earth's population harbor *Ascaris*. Some one million people in the United States, especially inhabitants of the mountainous and hilly areas of the South, are hosts of this persistent parasite. In many countries the incidence may reach 80 percent.

Ascariasis occurs at all ages, but it is most prevalent in the 5- to 9-year-old group of preschool and young school children, who are more frequently exposed to contaminated soil than adults. The incidence is approximately the same for both sexes. The incidence in Negroes is over three times that in whites, and the intensity of the infection is greater. The poorer urban and the rural classes, because of heavy soil pollution and unsatisfactory hygiene, are most afflicted. Infection is a household affair, the family being the unit of dissemination. Infected small children provide the chief source of soil contamination by their promiscuous defecation in dooryards and earthen-floored houses, where the resistant eggs remain viable for long periods.

The infective eggs are chiefly transmitted hand-to-mouth by children who have come in contact with contaminated soil directly, through playthings, or through dirt eating. In districts of Europe and in the Far East where night soil is extensively used for the fertilization of market gardens, human infection in all ages is also derived from vegetables (Fig. 49). Drinking water is rarely a source of infection.

Ascaris eggs are susceptible to desiccation, although they are more resistant than *Trichuris* eggs. A moist, loose soil with moderate shade provides a suitable environment; dryness is unfavorable for survival. Eggs may persist in garden soil up to 7 years, although only 10 percent survive. They are destroyed by direct sunlight within 15 hours and are killed at temperatures above 40° C, perishing within an hour at 50° C. Exposure to −8° to −12° C, although fatal to *Trichuris* eggs, has no effect on *Ascaris* eggs which, in the soil, can survive the ordinary freezing temperatures of winter. Eggs are resistant to chemical disinfectants and can withstand temporary immersion in strong chemicals. They survive for months in sewage or night soil.

Pathology and Symptomatology.   The usual infection, consisting of 10 to 20 worms, often goes unnoticed by the host, and is discovered only on a routine stool examination or by the discovery of an adult worm passed spontaneously in the stool. The most frequent complaint of patients infected with *Ascaris* is vague abdominal pain. An eosinophilia is present during the larval migration, but patients harboring the adult worms may exhibit little or no eosinophilia. During the lung migration, the larvae may produce host sensitization which results in allergic manifestations such as pulmonary infiltration, asthmatic attacks, and edema of the lips. Some instances of Loeffler's syndrome and tropical eosinophilia have been attributed to migrating *Ascaris* larvae. Instances of endophthalmitis have been observed for which the eye was removed, and the sections revealed nematode larvae which were probably *Ascaris*. Koino ingested 2,000 embryonated *Ascaris* eggs of human source at one time and thereby demonstrated that large numbers of larvae simultaneously migrating through the lungs may cause a serious hemorrhagic pneumonia (Fig. 48). In Nigeria, Fiske attributes the high bronchopneumonia rate in children of over 5 months of age to the migration of *Ascaris* larvae. Encephalitis and meningitis have been reported in *Ascaris*-infected patients, suggesting that the migrating larvae may reach the brain.

Serious and sometimes fatal effects of ascariasis are due to the migrations of the adult worms. They may be regurgitated and vomited, escape through the external nares, or, rarely, be inhaled into a bronchus. Many instances of invasion of the bile ducts, gallbladder, liver, and appendix have been reported. They may occlude the ampulla of Vater and cause acute hemorrhagic pancreatitis. The worms may carry intestinal bacteria to these sites and stimulate the production of abscesses. The worms may penetrate the intestinal wall, migrate into the peritoneal cavity, and produce peritonitis. Continuing their migration, they may come out through the body wall, usually at the umbilicus in children and the inguinal region in adults. Intestinal volvulus, intussusception, and obstruction may also result from *Ascaris* infection. Fever and certain drugs are two of the causative factors of *Ascaris* migration.

Even when the worms cause little or no traumatic damage, the by-products of living or dead worms may produce marked "toxic" manifestations in sensitized persons, such as edema of the face and giant urticaria, accompanied by insomnia and loss of appetite and weight.

Young pigs infected with *Ascaris* do not gain weight normally, and it is possible that the human *Ascaris* may affect undernourished children similarly. This action

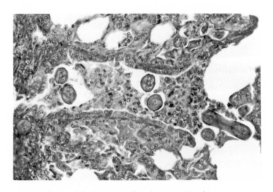

Fig. 48. *Ascaris* larvae in lung. Note extensive hemorrhagic verminous pneumonia. ($\times$ 200)

may be due to the food actually consumed by the worms or to the trypsin-inhibiting substance that they produce which interferes with the host's protein digestion. It has been shown that 20 adult worms consume 2.8 g of carbohydrate and 0.7 g of protein daily. Hence, heavy infections, running into the hundreds, would consume a significant proportion of their host's diet.

As a rule, prognosis is favorable, and the infection responds readily to treatment. It is serious in acute enteritis and intestinal obstruction in young children or when the adult parasite has invaded vital organs.

Diagnosis. The clinical symptoms of intestinal ascariasis are indistinguishable from those of other intestinal helminthic infections. *Ascaris* pneumonitis, although the symptoms are fairly characteristic, is usually mistaken for an atypical pneumonia. Diagnosis is made by finding the fertile or infertile eggs in the feces. The numerous fertile eggs are detected in the direct coverglass mount. If direct examination is negative, concentration technics (Page 324) may be employed. Infertile eggs are more easily missed by the examiner than any other nematode eggs, and virgin ascariasis is often overlooked. Egg production is fairly constant and egg-counting methods (Page 325) give a fairly reliable index of the number of worms. The adult worm may be detected radiologically (Fig. 47). This is obviously the only way an infection with only immature and male worms may be detected.

Treatment. Piperazine salts (see under *Treatment* for *Enterobius vermicularis*, above) are safe and very effective in ascariasis; a single dose will cure 75 to 85 percent of the infections. A dose on 2 consecutive days will eliminate approximately 95 percent of the infections. Piperazine can be given at any time of day, since the presence of food in the digestive tract has little, if any, effect on its activity against *Ascaris*. Purgation is not required. The dosage schedule for 1- and 2-day treatment of ascariasis with piperazine citrate is as follows:

Patient's weight (lb)	Daily dose of citrate syrup (ml)	Daily dose of hexahydrate (g)
30–50	20	2.0
51–100	30	3.0
101 +	35	3.5

Piperazine acts on the transmembrane potential of *Ascaris* muscle, temporarily relaxing it. The worm thereby loses its urge to move upstream and to press against the sides of its host's intestine in order to maintain its position. Peristalsis carries it out while it is relaxed.

Piperazine citrate syrup has been used successfully in partial intestinal obstruction due to ascariasis, combined with abdominal decompression with a Levin tube and supportive therapy. If, in addition to *Ascaris*, hookworms are also present, bephenium hydroxynaphthoate (Alcopara) (See Page 128) or thiabendazole (See Page 120) may be used as they are effective against both parasites. Hexylresorcinol (See Page 128) has long been the accepted chemotherapeutic agent from the standpoint of efficiency and safety. The parasites are eliminated in 70 to 80 percent of the patients after one treatment and in 93 to 98 percent after two treatments. It is less convenient to administer than piperazine citrate.

Stilbazium iodide is very effective against *Ascaris*, but awaits approval of the Food and Drug Administration.

Prevention. Since ascariasis is essentially a household and dooryard infection and is intimately associated with family hygiene, prophylaxis depends upon the sanitary disposal of feces and upon health education. Anthelmintic treatment is ineffective because of repeated reinfection in endemic areas. Control is difficult because of ignorance, poverty, and inertia among the people most afflicted. The installation of sanitary latrines is ineffective unless accompanied by an educational campaign designed to promote their use, especially by children. This educational program calls for the concerted efforts of schools, civic organizations, home economic educators, and public health workers. Night soil should not be used as fertilizer unless treated by compost manuring or chemicals. (Fig. 49).

FAMILY TRICHOSTRONGYLIDAE

The members of the family TRICHOSTRONGYLIDAE are thin worms in which the buccal capsule is absent or rudimentary. The male bursa has two large lateral lobes and a small dorsal lobe with well-developed rays. These worms are intestinal parasites of ruminants and, less frequently, of man and other mammals. The species parasitic in man belong to the genera *Trichostrongylus* and *Haemonchus*.

Several species of the genus *Trichostrongylus* are natural parasites of mammals. They are small nematodes, 4 to 7 mm, that inhabit the jejunum and upper ileum of man. At times the biliary passages may be invaded. The parasites have a more-or-less cosmopolitan distribution in man in Africa (Egypt), Asia Minor, Asia, Japan, Indonesia, Australia, and, rarely, the United States. Their prevalence is variable; high incidences have been reported in selected groups in Asia and the Far East. The several species include; *T. colubriformis* with a high incidence in Indonesia and Iraq; *T. orientalis,* with a high incidence in Japan and Korea. The rhabditiform larvae (Fig. 44); characterized by a minute knob at the tip of the tail, develop into pseudofilariform larvae in 3 to 4 days in the soil. A high humidity, warm temperature, abundant shade, and grass or carpet vegetation are necessary for their extracorporeal development. Ingested with contaminated green vegetation, the larvae burrow into the intestinal wall and then erupt as adolescent worms into the intestinal lumen to become adults in about 21 days. Infections are usually so light that no objectional symptoms are produced. Heavy infections may cause a secondary anemia and, sometimes, signs of cholecystitis. Eosinophilia is transient. Diagnosis is based upon finding in the feces or duodenal contents ellipsoidal greenish eggs (Fig. 141) that are larger and more pointed at one end than hookworm eggs. Bephenium

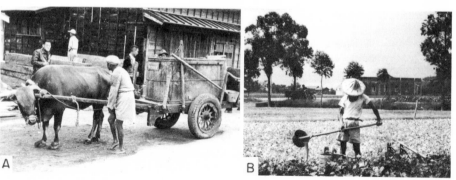

Fig. 49. Use of nightsoil as fertilizer. A, collection from homes. B, diluted nightsoil applied to vegetables with TLC.

(Alcopara) and thiabendazole (Mintezol) are effective against *Trichostrongylus*. The worms are resistant to tetrachlorethylene; some reported therapeutic failures in hookworm infection may be due to mistaking *Trichostrongylus* eggs for those of hookworm. Prevention depends upon avoiding the consumption of raw plants.

The sheep wireworm, *Haemonchus contortus*, a cosmopolitan parasite of economic importance in sheep, cattle, and other ruminants, has been reported as an incidental parasite of man in Brazil and Australia. It measures 10 to 30 mm in length and has an attenuated anterior end. The elongated eggs resemble those of *Trichostrongylus* and can only be differentiated by cultivation of the larvae. Development is direct, with a single host and a free-living larval stage. Infection takes place through the digestive tract. Heavy infections produce an anemia resembling that of hookworm infection.

FAMILY STRONGYLIDAE

The members of the family STRONGYLIDAE are parasites of the digestive tracts of mammals. The well-developed buccal capsule is without teeth or cutting plates, but bears a crown of chitinous leaf-like processes. The male has two prominent copulatory spicules; the vulva is located in the posterior half of the female. Man is an incidental host of three species.

Ternidens deminutus, which resembles the hookworm, is found in monkeys. It has been reported in natives of Africa and Asia. The worm, which may be found anywhere from the duodenum to the colon, at times produces cystic nodules or ulcers, but gives rise to no particular symptoms other than anemia during heavy infection. Therapy with piperazine is effective. *Oesophagostomum apiostomum,* a common parasite of monkeys and gorillas, has been reported from man in Africa. The encysted larvae produce exudative and proliferative nodular fibrous tumors in the cecum, from which the immature worms emerge to complete their growth. *Oesophagostomum stephanostomum* was found once in man in Brazil. The immature worms form fibrous nodules in the ileum, cecum, and colon.

FAMILY PHYSALOPTERIDAE

The members of the family PHYSALOPTERIDAE have a cuticular cephalic collar, two large triangular denticulated lips, and no buccal capsule. The caudal end of the male has pedunculated papillae and large asymmetrical alae that join ventrally. The female deposits smooth, transparent, thick-shelled embryonated eggs. The life cycle probably involves intermediate arthropod hosts. Various species are parasitic in the digestive tracts of birds, reptiles, and mammals.

Physaloptera caucasia, the only species parasitic in man, was discovered in the Caucasus. *P. mordens,* recorded from Africa, is believed to be the same species. It is a natural parasite of monkeys and sometimes of man. It is found attached to the walls of the esophagus, stomach, and small intestine. The maximum length of the male is 5 cm, and that of the female 10 cm.

ACANTHOCEPHALID WORMS

The ACANTHOCEPHALA, or thorny-headed roundworms, form a unique group by reason of their structure and extreme parasitic habits. These worms are common parasites of fish and birds and, less frequently, of other vertebrates. Although superficially resembling the roundworms, they differ in several fundamental characteristics from the NEMATODA, and perhaps more nearly resemble the CESTOIDEA. These distinctive features are absence of digestive tract, a more-or-less flattened body, a spinous retractile proboscis, a protonephridial excretory system, and embryonic hooklets. These parasites are included here with intestinal nematodes merely for convenience.

The worms are mostly small, but range from a few millimeters to over 60 cm in length. The elongate nonsegmented body is roughly cylindrical or spindle-shaped. The surface is irregularly roughened by transverse ridges. There is a sheathed retractile proboscis armed with rows of recurved hooks. The sexes are separate, the male being distinguished by its much smaller size and muscular copulatory bursa. The life cycle of the ACANTHOCEPHALA involves alternation of hosts. The parasites of aquatic animals probably have crustaceans or larval insects as intermediate hosts, and those of terrestrial animals have various insects. Two species have been found in man.

Macracanthorhynchus hirudinaceus has a cosmopolitan distribution. The worm has a rugose appearance with pseudosegmentation and a retractile proboscis with five to six rows of spines. The length of the female is 20 to 65 cm, and that of the male 5 to 10 cm. The eggs are fully embryonated at oviposition. The larva is enclosed in three embryonic envelopes and has hooklets on the anterior end. The natural definitive hosts are hogs, wild boars, peccaries, and, less frequently, dogs and cats. Man is an accidental host. The intermediate hosts are species of larval beetles. Human infections, possibly spurious, have been reported once in Bohemia and once in southern Russia, diagnosis being made from eggs in the feces.

Moniliformis moniliformis has a cosmopolitan distribution. The adult worm resembles a confluent beaded chain of pseudosegments. The length of the female is 10 to 27 cm, and that of the male 4 to 5 cm. The cylindrical proboscis has 12 to 15 rows of recurved hooks. The ellipsoidal eggs, 85 to 118 μ, have three envelopes and four hooklets. The definitive hosts are rats, mice, hamsters, dogs, and cats. Man is an incidental host. The intermediate hosts are beetles and cockroaches. Single cases of natural infection in man have been reported from Italy, the Sudan, and British Honduras. Experimental infection in man indicates that the parasite, when present in considerable numbers, may produce acute abdominal pain, diarrhea, and exhaustion. Prevention involves the protection of food from beetles and cockroaches.

NEMATODE PSEUDOPARASITES OF MAN

Other rhabditoid worms have been reported as pseudoparasites or accidental parasites of man. *Meloidogyne (Heterodera) radicicola,* a root parasite of vegetables, once attained considerable prominence as a human parasite under the name *Oxyuris incognita,* because its eggs were confused with those of *Enterobius,* hookworm, and *Trichostrongylus* (Fig. 141) and were found in human feces.

Three species of the genus *Rhabditis* and *Turbatrix aceti,* the vinegar eel, are probably accidental contaminants.

7

Blood and Tissue Nematodes of Man

The parasitic nematodes of the blood and tissues may be arranged in three groups: (1) the filarial worms and the guinea worm; (2) the larva migrans invasion of the skin, subcutaneous tissue, and viscera by larval nematodes; and (3) the rare parasites of the liver, kidneys, lungs, eyes, and subcutaneous tissues.

FILARIAL PARASITES OF MAN

Filariae

The slender filarial worms of the family FILARIIDAE are parasites of the circulatory and lymphatic systems, muscles, connective tissues, or serous cavities of vertebrates. The principal species parasitic in man are: *Wuchereria bancrofti, Brugia malayi, Onchocerca volvulus, Loa loa, Acanthocheilonema perstans,* and *Mansonella ozzardi*. Microfilariae identical with those of *Dipetalonema streptocerca,* a parasite of the chimpanzee, have also been found in man. A few infections with *Dirofilaria* of animals have been reported in man. The filarial parasites of man are highly host specific; only two have been reported in other primates: *A. perstans* in the gorilla and *Loa loa* in the baboon.

The filiform, creamy-white worms (Fig. 50) range from 2 to 70 cm in length, the female being not more than twice the size of the male. The simple mouth is usually without definite lips, and the buccal cavity is inconspicuous. The esophagus is cylindrical, has no cardiac bulbus, and is usually divided into an anterior muscular and a posterior glandular portion. In some species the males possess caudal alae; in others they are absent; there are two copulatory spicules.

A distinctive feature of filarial worms is that the viviparous female gives birth to prelarval microfilariae (Fig. 51). Their morphology, location in the host, and type of periodicity are of value in differentiating species. A sheath of unknown significance is present in *W. bancrofti, B. malayi,* and *Loa loa*. It is a delicate close-fitting membrane, which is derived from the original eggshell and is only detectable as it projects beyond the head or tail. The cuticle has transverse striations. A column of cells with deeply staining nuclei, which represents the rudiments of the intestine and perhaps other organs, extends nearly the whole length and occupies almost the entire width of the body. Its absence or presence at the tip of the tail varies in the different species. Size is so variable that it cannot be used alone for the differentiation of species. A fungus conidia of the genus *Helicosporium,* which when airborne may contaminate blood smears, resembles a microfilaria, al-

141

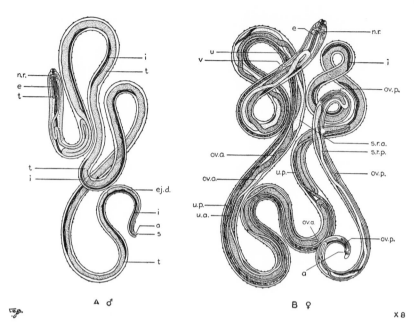

Fig. 50. Morphology of *Loa loa*, A, male; B, female.

a, anus; e, esophagus; ej.d., ejaculatory duct; i, intestine; ov.a., anterior ovary; ov. p., posterior ovary; n.r., nerve ring; s, spicules; s.r.a., anterior seminal receptacle; s.r.p., posterior seminal receptacle; t, testis; u, uterus; u.a., anterior uterus; u.p., posterior uterus; v. vulva. (Redrawn from Looss, 1904.)

though it is much smaller; this may confuse the unwary and untutored (Fig. 52).

The microfilariae do not appear in the host until some months after infection, the latent, or prepatent, period corresponding to the growth of the worms to maturity and to the birth and escape of the microfilariae into the blood and tissues. The average time after infection that the microfilariae of *W. bancrofti* are found in appreciable numbers in the blood is about 1 year. These microfilariae reach the blood by migration through the walls of the lymphatics to the neighboring small blood vessels, or by way of the thoracic duct. They remain for several months in the host after the destruction of the adult female worms by chemotherapeutic agents or surgical removal. When microfilariae are injected intravenously into an uninfected nonimmune host, their survival varies with the species—from weeks to years. Of course they develop no further unless ingested by the insect vector.

The periodicity of microfilariae in the peripheral blood varies with the species. Nocturnal periodicity is a prominent characteristic of the microfilariae of *W. bancrofti* in the Western Hemisphere. They are found in the blood chiefly at night, the number increasing to a maximum about midnight and then decreasing to a minimum about midday. Nocturnal periodicity is only relative, since a few microfilariae are present in the blood during the day. In the islands of the South Pacific east of longitude 170° E, they are nonperiodic, being present both day and night. In the Philippines there is a modified periodicity, the number during the day being about one-third that during the night.

The nocturnal periodicity of the microfilariae of *W. bancrofti* was first described by Manson. The experimental infection of monkeys and dogs with mammalian species of filariae that show nocturnal periodicity indicates that the microfilariae are concentrated in the small blood vessels of the lungs during the day and

MICROFILARIAE OF MAN

DIAGNOSTIC CHARACTERISTICS

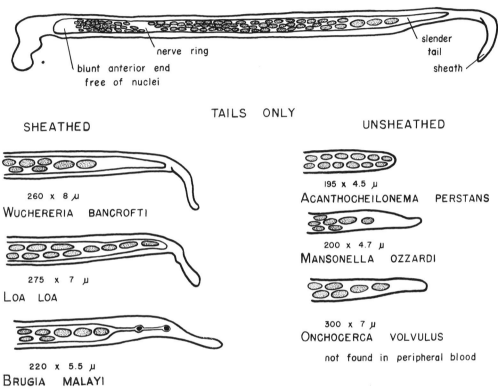

nerve ring

slender
tail

blunt anterior end
free of nuclei

sheath

TAILS ONLY

SHEATHED   UNSHEATHED

260 x 8 μ

WUCHERERIA   BANCROFTI

195 x 4.5 μ

ACANTHOCHEILONEMA   PERSTANS

275 x 7 μ

LOA LOA

200 x 4.7 μ

MANSONELLA   OZZARDI

220 x 5.5 μ

BRUGIA   MALAYI

300 x 7 μ

ONCHOCERCA   VOLVULUS

not found in peripheral blood

Fig. 51. Microfilariae of man.

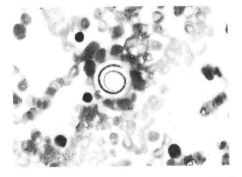

Fig. 52. *Helicosporium* sp., filiform-coiled conidia (helicospore) of air-borne fungus, occasionally found contaminating blood smears and confused with microfilariae. (× 500)

are liberated into the peripheral circulation at night. The stimulus that initiates this
migration has not yet been identified. Increased oxygen pressure by hyperventilation
or exercise may be a possible stimulus that causes the microfilariae of *W. bancrofti*
to leave the peripheral circulation for the lungs, but *Loa loa* with a diurnal

periodicity is not affected by changes in oxygen pressure. Periodicity in a patient with *W. bancrofti* has been reversed by altering the sleeping hours. Periodicity is a phenomenon associated with species; the microfilariae, when transfused into a new host, show the same periodicity as in the donor.

The life cycle of the filarial worm involves: (1) the ingestion of the microfilaria from the blood or tissues by a bloodsucking insect; (2) the metamorphosis of the microfilaria in the intermediate insect host first into a rhabditoid and then into an infectious filariform larva; and (3) the transference of the infective larva to the skin of a new host by the proboscis of the biting insect, and the development of the larva, after entry through the bite wound, into a mature worm at its selective site. Within a few hours after ingestion by a suitable insect, the microfilaria penetrates the wall of the midgut and makes its way to the thoracic muscles where it undergoes metamorphosis. In 1 to 3 weeks it reaches the infective stage. When the insect bites the definitive host, the larvae probably escape from the tip of the proboscis to the skin near the bite wound through which they enter the body.

There are little data concerning natural or acquired immunity of man to filarial infections, although the high percentage of asymptomatic cases of wuchereriasis suggests host resistance.

Filarial worms have species-specific and group-specific antigens, which give cross-reactions between the different species and also with other nematodes. Thus, satisfactory antigens for serologic and intracutaneous diagnostic tests in man may be prepared from the more accessible filarial parasites of dogs and cotton rats.

The detection of sensitizing antibodies by the intracutaneous injection of antigens has been extensively used as a diagnostic procedure in wuchereriasis, loasis, and onchocerciasis. The interpretation of a positive cutaneous reaction is based on the size of the erythema, the wheal, or the swelling. A delayed reaction is usually present in persons who show an immediate positive reaction, and occasionally occurs when there is no immediate reaction. The test is not species specific, does not detect all infections, and gives about 10 percent falsely positive reactions in noninfected persons; this reaction may be due to past infection, possible previous exposure to nonhuman species of filariae, or general sensitization to dog proteins or the diluting fluid of the antigen. This test is especially valuable in making the diagnosis in patients in whom microfilaria cannot be found in the peripheral blood.

Wuchereria bancrofti

Disease.   Bancroftian filariasis, wuchereriasis, elephantiasis.

Life Cycle.   Man is the only known definitive host. Transmission of infection requires a suitable species of mosquito (Fig. 53). The adult worms are located in the lymphatics, and the microfilariae are found in the blood and lymph. Adults of both sexes lie tightly coiled in the nodular dilatations of the lymphatic vessels and sinuses of the lymph nodes. The length of life of *W. bancrofti* in man is considered to be about 5 years as estimated from the duration of the microfilariae in the blood of persons after departure from endemic regions.

The microfilariae ingested by the mosquito with its blood meal migrate to its muscles. After 6 to 20 days of development, the larvae force their way out of the muscles, causing considerable damage, and migrate to the proboscis. Observers have found that three microfiariae per cubic millimeter of blood will produce

WUCHERERIA BANCROFTI

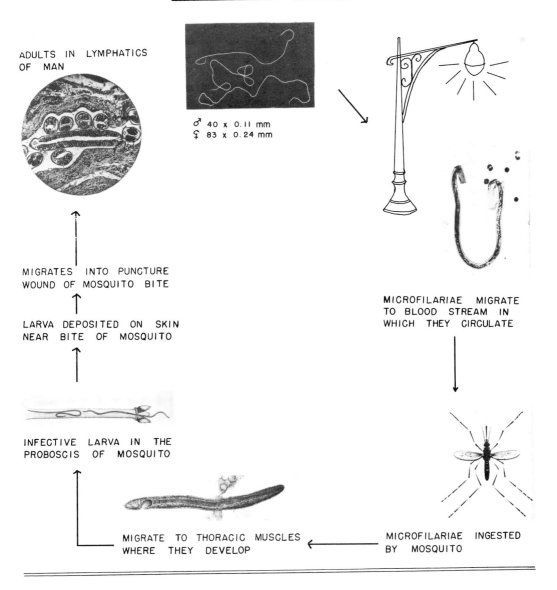

ADULTS IN LYMPHATICS
OF MAN

♂ 40 x 0.11 mm
♀ 83 x 0.24 mm

↑

MIGRATES INTO PUNCTURE
WOUND OF MOSQUITO BITE

↑

LARVA DEPOSITED ON SKIN
NEAR BITE OF MOSQUITO

↑

INFECTIVE LARVA IN THE
PROBOSCIS OF MOSQUITO

↑

MIGRATE TO THORACIC MUSCLES
WHERE THEY DEVELOP

MICROFILARIAE MIGRATE
TO BLOOD STREAM IN
WHICH THEY CIRCULATE

↓

MICROFILARIAE INGESTED
BY MOSQUITO

←

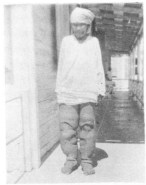

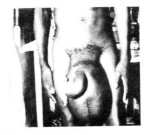

ELEPHANTIASIS

Fig. 53. Life cycle of *Wuchereria bancrofti*.

145

optimal infections in the mosquito, that 0.5 will fail to infect, and that 10 will kill the mosquito. Perhaps individuals with heavy microfilaremia should not be treated but should be allowed to serve as sources of lethal meals for mosquitoes! During the blood meal the developed larvae emerge from the proboscis onto the skin of the new host. On penetrating the skin through the bite wound, the larvae pass to the lymphatic vessels and nodes where they grow to maturity in about a year. The adult worms tend to frequent the varices of the lymphatic vessels of the lower extremities, the groin glands and epididymis in the male, and the labial glands in the female. The microfilariae migrate from the parent worm through the walls of the lymphatics to the neighboring small blood vessels or are carried in the lymphatic circulation to the blood stream.

Epidemiology. The parasite has a worldwide range in tropical and subtropical countries, extending as far north as Spain and as far south as Brisbane, Australia. In the Eastern Hemisphere it is present in Africa, Asia, Japan, Taiwan, the Philippines, Indonesia, and the islands of the South Pacific. In the Western Hemisphere it is found in the West Indies, Costa Rica, and northern South America. The infection in the United States, which was introduced by African slaves to Charleston, South Carolina, died out over 40 years ago. The incidence of periodic filariasis is correlated with density of population and poor sanitation, since *C. quinquefasciatus,* the principal vector, breeds mainly in water contaminated with sewage and decaying organic matter. In the South Pacific the incidence of nonperiodic filariasis is as high or higher in the rural districts as in the large villages, since its chief vector is *Aëdes polynesiensis,* a brush mosquito. Incidence varies with race, age, and sex, largely due to environmental factors. Europeans, who are better protected against mosquitoes, have a much lower incidence than natives.

The principal vector in the Western Hemisphere is *Culex quinquefasciatus* (= *fatigans*), and in the South Pacific *Aëdes polynesiensis.* The former is a night-biting domesticated and urban mosquito, and the latter is a day-biting sylvatic nondomesticated mosquito. At least 48 species of mosquitoes, including *Aëdes, Anopheles, Culex,* and *Mansonia,* are natural or experimental vectors.

The designation of the specific name *W. pacifica* for the nonperiodic filaria of the South Pacific by Manson-Bahr has led to an academic controversy as to whether this form should be considered a separate species or a variety of *W. bancrofti.* In the South Pacific nonperiodic filariasis differs from the periodic in its geographic distribution—e.g., Fiji and Samoa vs. Micronesia and Melanesia; in its sylvan instead of urban foci, in its vector *Aëdes polynesiensis* as opposed to *Culex quinquefasciatus,* and *Anopheles farauti* and *A. punctulatus;* and in somewhat questionable minor morphologic differences in the adult worms. Periodicity is reported to be retained even when infected populations are transferred to non-periodic regions. Also, a Fijian strain of *Culex quinquefasciatus,* susceptible to periodic microfilariae, has proved refractory to nonperiodic microfilariae.

Pathology and Symptomatology. Filarial symptoms are caused by the adult worms, living as well as dead and degenerating. Microfilariae, which appear about a year after the initial infection, apparently cause slight or no pathology, although they have been tentatively associated with tropical pulmonary eosinophilia, granulomas of the spleen, and allergic reactions following their destruction. The adult worms lie in the dilated lymphatics or in the sinuses of the lymph nodes. The pseudotubercular granulomatous reaction around the trapped worms becomes pronounced on their death. It occludes the small lymphatics, narrows the larger, and ultimately walls off the necrotic tissues surrounding the degenerating worms. The early cellular reactions and edema give way to vascular hyperplasia, fibroblastic proliferation, and caseation. Finally, there is absorption and replacement of the parasite by hyalinized, or even calcified, scar tissue. The lymphatics become varicose, collateral branches open up, and lakes of lymph develop in the sinuses of the lymph nodes. The living and dead worms and microfilariae early evoke an infiltration of eosinophilic leukocytes in the inflamed tissues.

Because bancroftian filariasis may run its course over many years, it varies greatly in its clinical manifestations. The human reaction to filarial infection is varied and manifold, and it is impossible to delimit specifically the disease stages. It is possible, however, to classify broadly the results of filarial infection into the asymptomatic, inflammatory, and obstructive types.

ASYMPTOMATIC FILARIASIS.   In endemic areas children are exposed to infection at an early age, and by the age of 6 years they exhibit microfilariae in their blood without experiencing symptoms referable to their infection. On physical examination the patient may exhibit a moderate generalized enlargement of lymph nodes, especially of the inguinal lymph region. Blood examination discloses numerous microfilariae and a low-grade eosinophilia. In time the adult worms die, and the microfilariae disappear without the patients being aware of the infection.

INFLAMMATORY FILARIASIS.   The inflammatory filarial infection is an allergic phenomenon due to sensitivity to the products of the living and dead adult worms. Superimposed streptococcal and fungal infections may be involved occasionally. Recurrent attacks are characterized by funiculitis, epididymitis, orchitis, retrograde lymphangitis of the extremities, and localized areas of swelling and redness of the arms and legs. Fever, chills, headache, vomiting, and malaise may accompany these attacks, which last from several days to several weeks. The lymphatics of the legs and genitalia are chiefly affected. In males acute lymphangitis of the spermatic cord (funiculitis) with tender, thickened cord, epididymitis, orchitis, and scrotal edema are common. The red blood cells, hemoglobin, and sedimentation rate are unchanged. There is a leukocytosis up to 10,000, and an eosinophilia of 6 to 26 percent. Somewhat similar acute attacks may occur at monthly or longer intervals in patients with or without elephantiasis. Usually the affected extremity becomes red, hot, and very painful. Therapy with antimicrobial drugs is usually unsuccessful, suggesting a verminous rather than bacterial etiology. Abscesses of the pelvis of the kidney, epididymis, retroperitoneal tissues, inguinal nodes, and iliopsoas muscles may result from the dead and degenerating worms. These abscesses may be sterile, but frequently pyogenic bacteria are present. The acute granulomatous reaction in the lymphatics to the worms and their toxic products, which is manifest by local inflammation and systemic allergic symptoms, gradually merges into a chronic proliferative overgrowth of fibrous tissue around the dead worms that produces lymphatic obstruction, recurrent attacks of lymphangitis, and, at times, elephantiasis.

OBSTRUCTIVE FILARIASIS.   Elephantiasis is the dramatic end result of filariasis (Fig. 53). Many mistakenly believe that it is the inevitable termination of every filarial infection, but, fortunately, the grossly enlarged scrotum or leg is the exception rather than the rule. Elephantiasis has been reported in 1 to 70 percent of infected natives in various parts of the world, many of whom are exposed to infective mosquitoes from birth. Obstructive filariasis develops slowly, usually follows years of continuous filarial infection, and is preceded by chronic edema and often by repeated acute inflammatory attacks. In the chronic stage the cellular reaction and edema are replaced by fibroblastic hyperplasia; there is absorption and replacement of the parasite by proliferative granulation tissue; and extensive lymph varices are produced. The high protein content of the lymph stimulates the growth of dermal and collagenous connective tissue, and, gradually over a period of years, the enlarged affected parts harden, producing chronic elephantiasis. The site of the obstructive inflammation determines the parts of the body affected. Obstruction of the thoracic duct or the median abdominal lymph vessels may affect the scrotum and penis of the male and the external genitalia of the female, while infection of the inguinal glands may involve the extremities and external genitalia. Elephantiasis commonly affects the legs and genitalia and may result in excessive deformity. It is uncommon in persons under 30 years of age. There is little correlation between the presence of microfilariae in the blood and elephantiasis, since microfilariae disappear after the death of the worms. Rupture of the lymphatics of the urinary bladder or kidney may produce chyluria; those of the tunica vaginalis, hydrocele or chylocele; and those of the peritoneum, chylous ascites. The most common features are hydrocele and lymphangitis of the genitalia and recurrent attacks of lymphangitis with fever and pain. Thus, recurrent lymphangitis, and even elephantiasis, may be accentuated or in some cases even produced by superimposed streptococcal infections.

Prognosis is good in light infections. The prognosis once elephantiasis has developed is poor unless surgery is successful.

Diagnosis. The diagnosis of filariasis will depend upon a history of exposure to mosquitoes in an endemic area, in conjunction with the clinical findings discussed above. The blood should be examined for microfilariae by placing a drop, obtained at night, on a slide and examining it under the low power of the microscope for actively moving microfilariae. To determine the species of microfilariae, thin or thick blood smears stained with Wright or Giemsa stain will bring out the diagnostic characteristics. To detect light infections, 1 ml of night blood is laked in 10 ml of a 2 percent formalin solution. The sediment is examined directly or may be allowed to dry on a slide and then stained (Page 326). The blood of patients with clinical filariasis does not always contain microfilariae. Approximately a year elapses from the time of infection until the worm matures and produces microfilariae; hence, during the early months of clinical inflammatory filariasis, microfilariae will not be found in the blood. Likewise, late in the disease, by the time elephantiasis has developed, the adult worms and microfilariae may both have died. The intradermal test using *Dirofilaria* antigen, and the complement-fixation, hemagglutination, and flocculation tests are of diagnostic value when microfilariae cannot be found in the blood. The microfilariae of *Wuchereria bancrofti,* which may occur in the urine when chyluria is present, are easily separated by centrifuging.

Treatment. It is common knowledge in endemic filarial areas that rest and moving to a cool climate reduce the number and severity of the acute inflammatory attacks. Diethylcarbamazine (Hetrazan), which is given orally, is quickly lethal to microfilariae and either kills the adult females or permanently sterilizes them. The dosage is 2 mg per kilogram of body weight three times daily, for 7 to 14 days. Headache, dizziness, nausea, and fever may be encountered during therapy. Antimicrobial drugs are useful in recurrent lymphangitis caused by secondary streptococcal infection.

The massive edema that precedes and accompanies elephantiasis of the legs may be alleviated by pressure bandaging. Administration of steroids to patients with elephantiasis may be followed by diuresis and an increased number of microfilariae in the blood stream. Both effects are ascribed to a lessening of the inflammatory reaction around the adult worms which allows freer lymphatic drainage from the smaller limb. Various operative measures have been tried in elephantiasis. The removal of the enlarged scrotum is usually successful and results in permanent cure. The repair of enlarged legs, attempting to provide anastomosis between the deep and superficial lymphatics, is not entirely satisfactory.

Prevention. The prevention of wuchereriasis in endemic areas includes the control of mosquitoes and human sources of infection. The residual spraying of houses and the use of larvicides, successful against *Culex quinquefasciatus* and other domesticated mosquitoes (Page 275), are not effective against sylvan mosquitoes such as *Aëdes polynesiensis*. The mass administration of Hetrazan to destroy the microfilariae in the blood of carriers and the use of insecticides to control the mosquitoes has proven successful on St. Croix, Virgin Islands, and Tahiti. The protection of the individual by screened quarters, bed nets, mosquito repellents, and protective clothing is an educational and economic problem.

Brugia (Wuchereria) malayi

Disease. Malayan filariasis.

Life Cycle. Man is the only definitive host. The fine, white, thread-like adult worm closely resembles *W. bancrofti,* the female being 55 by 0.16 mm, and the male 23 by 0.09 mm. The nocturnal periodicity of the morphologically distinct, sheathed microfilariae (Fig. 51) is less absolute than that of *W. bancrofti*. The intermediate hosts are *Mansonia, Anopheles,* and *Armigeres*. The microfilaria in the mosquito develops into an infective larva in 6 to 12 days.

Epidemiology. The extensive geographic distribution of this parasite includes Ceylon, Indonesia, the Philippines, Southern India, Asia, China, Korea, and a small focus in Japan. It is the predominant filarial infection in Southern India and Ceylon. Its distribution in the flat alluvial areas along the coast corresponds to that of its principal insect hosts, *Mansonia* mosquitoes. It is most prevalent in low regions with numerous ponds infested with water plants of the genus *Pistia,* which are essential for the breeding of these mosquitoes. When *Mansonia* mosquitoes are the vectors, the disease is essentially rural in distribution, but when *Anopheles* mosquitoes are the vectors it tends to be urban or suburban.

Pathogenicity. The parasite, like *W. bancrofti,* produces lymphangitis and elephantiasis. It differs from *W. bancrofti* in that persons with clinical filariasis show a much higher microfilarial rate than those without symptoms. In Malaya there are about five times as many symptomless carriers as those suffering from elephantiasis. Malayan filariasis is characterized by superficial lymphadenopathy and a high eosinophilia (7 to 70 percent).

Diagnosis. Identification of microfilariae in blood (Fig. 51). The "knotting" of the microfilaria, an agonal phenomenon during drying of the film, may be prevented by adding chloroform or menthol to the blood.

Treatment. Similar to *W. bancrofti* (see above).

Prevention. The principal means of prevention is the control of *Mansonia* mosquitoes by destruction or removal of the water plant *Pistia stratiotes*. Phenoxylene 30 (sodium and ammonium salts of methyl chlorphenoxyacetic acid) is a cheap satisfactory herbicide.

Onchocerca volvulus

Disease.   Onchocerciasis, onchocercosis.

Life Cycle.   Man is the only definitive host, although closely allied species occur in other mammals. The adult worms are found in the subcutaneous tissues, usually encapsulated in fibrous tumors, within which the worms are intricately coiled. The tumors contain a variable number of worms and microfilariae. Occasionally, the unencapsulated worms migrate in the tissues. The liberated microfilariae (Fig. 51) are present in the nodules, subcutaneous tissues, lymphatics, and skin, rarely in the blood or internal organs.

The principal intermediate hosts are the black flies of the genus *Simulium*. The metamorphosis to an infective larva in *S. damnosum* requires 6 to 10 or more days in the thoracic muscles, from which the mature larvae migrate to the proboscis of the fly. When the infected black fly bites, larvae escape to the skin of the new host and penetrate the bite wound. The worm becomes an adult in less than a year and lives for at least 5 years.

Epidemiology.   In Africa onchocerciasis occurs on the West Coast from Sierra Leone to the Congo Basin, extending eastward through the Congo, Angola, and the Republic of the Sudan to East Africa. In the Americas it is found in the highlands of Guatemala, in the states of Oaxaca and Chiapas in Mexico, and in northeastern Venezuela. Endemic areas in Central America are confined to the highlands, usually at 1,000 to 4,000 feet above sea level, along streams and river courses where black flies are abundant. In Africa the infection is common below 1,000-foot elevation. The disease is confined to the neighborhood of rapidly flowing streams, the incidence falling markedly after a distance of 5 miles owing to the distribution of the insect vectors, which breed in clear swift streams and rarely travel over 2 to 3 miles from the water courses. Man is the only source of infection. On clear days the female bites most frequently in the early morning and evening, but at all hours in the shade or when the sky is overcast.

In Africa the disease is uncommon in children under 10 years of age, but in America it is more frequent—about one-sixth of all cases. The incidence is highest in young and middle-aged adults. The disease is more prevalent in men than in women because of greater occupational exposure. It is less prevalent in Europeans in Africa than in the natives because of better protection against black flies.

Pathology and Symptomatology.   Onchocerciasis is a chronic infection of the subcutaneous tissues, skin, and eyes. Its lesions are produced by the adult worms and microfilariae, augmented by the allergic response of the host. The nodules, 5 to 25 mm in size, may appear in any part of the body, but in Africa they are seen most commonly on the trunk, thighs, and arms (Fig. 54), and in the Americas on the head and shoulders. The cause of this distribution is exposure of the whole unclothed body in tropical Africa, and only the head, feet, and hands in the cool upland endemic areas in the Americas. The number of nodules per patient is usually three to six, although as many as 150 have been reported.

The histologic appearance of the tumor varies according to age and size. The early nodules show an initial inflammatory reaction with vascular dilatation and later a foreign-body granulomatous reaction around the worms, with granulocytes, endothelial cells, small round cells, and, occasionally, plasma cells and lymphocytes.

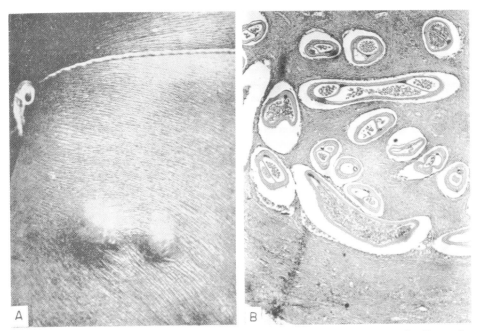

Fig. 54. *Onchocerca volvulus.* A, nodules on hip. (After Blacklock, 1926.) B, section through nodule showing adults containing microfilariae. ($\times$ 30)

Microfilariae are present in the nodule and neighboring tissues. The late nodules contain fibroblasts, endothelial cells, and often giant cells. There is a fibrous capsule with a grayish-white, collagenous periphery and a soft, yellowish, grumous, inner portion. The nodules gradually undergo caseation, fibrosis, and calcification.

In Africa the first manifestation of the disease, especially in children, is often a skin infection, which may disappear or persist throughout life. The earliest change is a diminution of the subepidermal elastic fibers, which is followed by a progressive reduction in the subepidermal and dermal elastic fibers. The final "burned out" stage is characterized by absence of elastic fibers, depigmentation, thickening of epidermis, and proliferation of connective tissue in the subepidermal layers. The chronic cutaneous manifestations take the form of xeroderma, lichenification, achromia, atrophy, and a pseudoichthyosis with thick wrinkled skin, leading in some instances to "hanging groin" (genital elephantiasis). Superimposed on this condition may be a pruriginous dermoepidermitis, the so-called filarial itch (Fig. 55). It may start as an acute febrile erysipelas or as a slowly progressive myxedematous thickening of the skin, at times accompanied by keratitis and iritis. The second type chiefly affects the face but may also involve the arms and, less often, the legs. The skin is thickened and hyperpigmented, and there is intense itching. In the third type there are papulovesicular excoriated lesions sometimes impetiginous or there may be papillomatous, verrucose, and hyperkeratotic patches on the arms, hand, and neck. Microfilaria may be found in scrapings from these lesions.

During the incubation period of several months to a year, there is an eosinophilia and transient urticaria. The tumors are well tolerated although at times painful. A slight fever and insomnia may be present. The eosinophilia varies from 15 to 50 percent.

Ocular involvement represents the most serious clinical manifestations of the

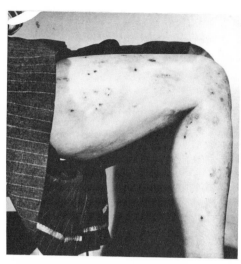

Fig. 55. Onchocercal skin lesions. Microfilariae were found in scrapings from the lesions. (Patient is a missionary from Portuguese Angola.)

disease; is responsible for much blindness; and is related to the site, intensity, and duration of the infection. The eye acts as a trap for the penetrating microfilariae, which may be found in all the ocular tissues, but seems to have a predilection for the cornea, choroid, iris, and anterior chambers. Numerous living and dead microfilariae may be observed in the vitreous humor. They can always be found in any ocular lesion and not infrequently are observed in eyes without lesions. The production of ocular pathology has been variously attributed to: (1) the mechanical action or secretory products of the living microfilariae, (2) toxins from dead microfilariae, (3) toxins from the adult worm, and (4) supersensitivity of the patient. The first ocular symptoms are photophobia, lacrimation, blepharospasm, and sensation of a foreign body.

The conjunctiva contains many microfilariae, especially at the limbus. Some persons show no reaction and others a chronic conjunctivitis with small nodules, dilated blood vessels, and brown spots on the limbus. The ocular changes are due to a slow and insidious sclerotic process that first manifests itself clinically 7 to 9 years after the initial infection. The earliest and most typical corneal lesion is a superficial punctate keratitis that is visible by the corneal microscope. Later refractile, "snowflake" opacities, 1 to 2 mm in diameter and composed of corneal infiltrations of leukocytes or dead microfilariae, may be observed, and still later superficial and deep vascularization. The lesions become serious when a diffuse plastic iritis that affects vision develops. The iris becomes thickened, and adhesive synechiae give the pupil an irregular pear shape. Finally the iris becomes adherent to the anterior surface of the lens capsule and undergoes atrophy with depigmentation and "pumice stone" appearance. Except in patients with serious ocular involvement, prognosis is favorable. Chemotherapy and early removal of nodules may check the progress of ocular lesions. There is no evidence of the existence of natural or acquired immunity.

Diagnosis. The presence of subcutaneous nodules, eosinophilia, cutaneous manifestations, and ocular lesions in persons in endemic regions is suggestive of onchocerciasis. The development of allergic symptoms, especially pruritus, following the administration of diethylcarbamazine is often of diagnostic value. The microfilariae may be obtained by teasing slices of skin on a slide in a drop of physiologic sodium chloride solution, or in the dermal lymph collected by pressing a fold of skin between the blades of a forceps until pitted, and puncturing the middle of the fold to a depth of 1 mm with a fine needle. Microfilariae may be found when no nodules are detectable and may be present in clinically healthy skin. Repeated examination may be necessary. The scapular region is the area of choice for obtaining specimens.

Treatment. Surgical removal of the encysted adult parasites is an established procedure, but it is difficult to locate all the parasitic nodules. It is not an effective method of treatment for ocular onchocercosis, since the microfilariae may survive for 4 to 8 months after the destruction of the adult worms. Diethylcarbamazine (see *Treatment* for *Wuchereria bancrofti,* above) destroys the microfilariae; however, it has little effect on the adult worm, since the microfilariae and the skin lesions reappear in 2 to 4 months. The destruction of the microfilariae produces pronounced allergic reactions which take the form of intense pruritus, dermatitis, edema, conjunctivitis, adenopathy, fever, and intestinal colic. The allergic symptoms are so pronounced that the use of diethylcarbamazine as a diagnostic agent has been advocated, and careful administration of the drug is required in ocular onchocerciasis. An initial dose of 25 mg, which can be increased gradually, and at the same time steroids should be administered to reduce inflamation. Suramin (Page 52, *Treatment* for *Trypanosoma gambiense*) acts upon the adult worm, and the microfilariae begin to disappear in about 4 months, while in 2 months the nodules show degenerated worms. The initial dose is 0.5 g and then 1.0 g is given at weekly intervals for 5 weeks. Suramin is contraindicated in patients with severe ocular involvement. The logical approach is to treat first with Suramin or surgery to eliminate the adult worms and then with diethylcarbamazine to destroy the microfilariae.

Prevention. Prevention of onchocerciasis includes the removal of nodules, the source of infection, control of the vector, and the protection of susceptible persons. Treatment of the infected persons is important. A combination of surgical removal of the adult worms and the destruction of the microfilariae by diethylcarbamazine reduces the infectivity of carriers, but this method of control alone is not completely effective. Control of the vectors depends upon the destruction of the aquatic larvae by larvicides especially during the dry seasons, and the spraying of riparian vegetation with insecticides, since residual spraying of houses is ineffective as *Simulium* does not invade them. The individual may be protected by fly-proof clothing, headnets, and especially by repellents.

Loa loa

Disease. Loasis, eye worm, fugitive swellings, Calabar swellings.

Life Cycle. Man and, possibly, monkeys are the only definitive hosts. The adult, thread-like, cylindrical worms (Fig. 50) inhabit the subcutaneous tissues. The sheathed microfilariae (Fig. 51) usually have a diurnal periodicity in the blood. The length of life of the worm in man has been variously reported as 4 to 17 years. The principal intermediate insect hosts are *Chrysops silacea* and *C. dimidiata.* The ingested microfilaria passes through a cyclic development in these flies in 10 to 12 days. Man, when bitten by the fly, is infected by the escape of the infective larvae from the membranous labium to the skin near the bite wound. Within an hour the larvae penetrate to the subcutaneous and muscular tissues, where they become adult worms in about 12 months.

Epidemiology.   Loasis is limited to the African equatorial rain forest and its fringe. Incidence in endemic areas varies greatly (8 to 75 percent), depending on the prevalence of and exposure to *Chrysops* flies, which breed in muddy streams and swamps. It is found in tropical West Africa from Sierra Leone to Angola, the watershed of the Congo River, the Congo Republic, Cameroon, and Southern Nigeria. Occasionally Europeans are infected, but usually they are well protected from the flies. The incidence of natural infection in flies is 1 to 35 percent in the various localities. Man is usually bitten during the daytime by the flies (Page 280) that shun bright sunlight and that frequent woodland, particularly forest swamp land; they seem to bite Negroes more readily than whites. In the tropical rain forests a complex host-parasite-vector relationship may exist between man, monkeys, and several species of *Chrysops*.

Pathology and Symptomatology.   The parasite usually causes no serious damage to the host. The adult worms migrate through the subcutaneous tissues, the maximal recorded rate being an inch in 2 minutes. They have been removed from all parts of the body, but they are particularly troublesome when passing in the orbital conjunctiva or across the bridge of the nose. Involvement of the eye (Fig. 56) causes irritation, congestion, pain, tumefaction of the eyelids, and impaired vision. Temporary inflammatory reactions, known as fugitive or Calabar swellings, are characteristic of the infection. These painless, nonpitting, subcutaneous swellings, which may reach the size of a hen's egg, are most frequently observed on the hands, forearms, and in the vicinity of the orbit. They appear spontaneously at irregular intervals, disappear in about a week, and are probably manifestations of supersensitiveness to the parasite or its products.

The experimental injection of a minute amount of *Dirofilaria* antigen into the skin of a patient with *Loa loa* results in the production of a large Calabar swelling. At times the skin shows papules, becomes infiltrated, and later is lichenified. Aggregations of microfilariae may produce an eosinophilic inflammation and fibrosis in the spleen. During the incubation period of 1 or more years, there may be vague symptoms of slight fever, pain in limbs, paresthesia, pruritus, and sometimes urticaria. Infected persons comprise symptomless carriers and patients with allergic manifestations including edema, pruritus, and eosinophilia, with or without demon-

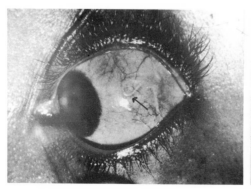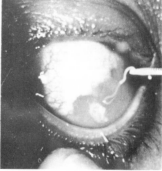

Fig. 56. *Loa loa* in the eye. (*Arch. Ophthal.,* 76:877, 1966. Courtesy of P. Fenton and R. J. H. Smith.)

strable adult worms or microfilariae. The first signs of the disease may be the development of Calabar swellings or the appearance of the worm under the conjunctiva. Infected persons have a wide variety of clinical symptoms attributable to the wandering worm. There may be an urticarial dermatitis, soreness from indurated tendon sheaths, and abscesses from secondary pyogenic infection. There is an eosinophilia of 12 to 70 percent.

Diagnosis. Diagnosis is based on observing the worm under the conjunctiva, Calabar swellings, eosinophilia, and finding the characteristic microfilariae in the blood during the day (Fig. 57). Microfilariae are detectable only in 20 to 30 percent of patients. Intracutaneous and complement-fixation tests with *D. immitis* antigen are helpful when other diagnostic methods fail.

Treatment. Surgical removal of the adult filarial worms, when accessible, is an accepted method of treatment. A favorable time is during their migration across the nose or conjunctiva. Chemotherapy with diethylcarbamazine (See Page 148, *Treatment* for *Wucheria bancrofti*) is effective.

Prevention. Protective measures include the control of *Chrysops* with larvicides as far as practicable, the elimination of carriers by treatment with diethylcarbamazine, and the protection of persons from the flies by nets, screens, and repellents.

Acanthocheilonema perstans

Disease. Acanthocheilonemiasis, dipetalonemiasis.

Life Cycle. The adult female worm is 80 mm in length, the male 45 mm. The adult is found in the mesentery, the retroperitoneal tissues, the pleural cavity, and the pericardium. The microfilariae (Fig. 51) are found in the peripheral blood

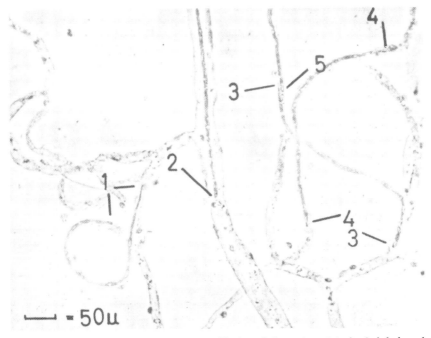

Fig. 57. Five microfilariae of *Loa loa* in capillaries of the retina. (*Arch. Ophthal.,* vol. 74, 1965. Courtesy of Drs. D. Toussaint and P. Danis.)

and capillaries of the lungs. In different localities they exhibit either a diurnal or, more commonly, a nocturnal periodicity, but they are essentially nonperiodic.

Man is the chief definitive host. The same species, or closely related ones, have been found in the chimpanzee and the gorilla. The intermediate hosts are the blood-sucking midges of the genus *Culicoides*. After a 7- to 10-day metamorphosis in the midge, the infective larva is transferred to the skin of a new host by the biting insect.

Epidemiology.   This parasite is found mainly in tropical Africa, although reported in North Africa and also in South America. Human infection is very common in endemic areas where intermediate hosts are abundant. The incidence is much less in Europeans, who are better protected than the natives against the night-biting *Culicoides*.

Pathogenicity.   The encysted worms usually occur singly and cause little tissue reaction. The incubation period is unknown. Usually there are no symptoms other than minor allergic phenomena, although edema, Calabar swellings, and lymphatic varices have been attributed to its presence. Microfilariae have been found in enlarged painful livers; treatment with a trivalent antimony compound reduced the number of microfilariae and the symptoms abated. Diethylcarbamazine does not appear to be effective against this worm.

Diagnosis.   Diagnosis is made by finding the characteristic microfilariae in the blood.

Prevention.   Preventive measures include the control of the vector, protection of the individual, and residual spraying of houses.

Mansonella ozzardi

Disease.   Mansonelliasis ozzardi, Ozzard's filariasis.

Life Cycle.   The adult worm inhabits body cavities, mesentery, and visceral fat. The sharp-tailed microfilaria is unsheathed and nonperiodic (Fig. 51). Man is the only known definitive host. *Culicoides furens* is a definite vector in which the larvae become infective by the sixth day, and by the eighth day migrate to the proboscis.

Epidemiology.   This parasite is found in parts of Central and South America and some of the islands of the West Indies.

Pathogenicity.   The adult worms cause little damage to the connective tissue of the peritoneum. Occasionally a hydrocele or enlarged lymph node is noted. No particular symptoms are attributed to this worm.

Prevention.   Prophylaxis depends on the control of the vectors and protection of persons from their bites.

Dipetalonema streptocerca

Found in Ghana and the Republic of the Congo in Africa.

The adult worm is unknown in man, but has been found in the connective tissues of chimpanzees. The unsheathed microfilariae, which are found in the skin of man and chimpanzees, have the appearance of a walking stick with a crooked handle. Man and chimpanzees are definitive hosts. Its intermediate insect host is *Culicoides grahami,* in which infective forms are produced by the eighth day. This worm is probably nonpathogenic, but it may cause cutaneous edema and elephantiasis. Most infected persons are symptomless. Diethylcarbamazine causes the disappearance of the microfilariae.

Dirofilaria Infections of Man

Human infections with various animal *Dirofilaria* were reviewed by Beaver and Orihel in 1965. Although these infections are cosmopolitan, the majority have been reported from southern United States, many apparently originating in Florida. These wandering worms have been found primarily in adults and, for some unknown reason, much more frequently in females than in males. A single worm is common, and microfilariae are not present in the blood.

Dirofilaria immitis lives in the right ventricle and pulmonary artery of the dog. The adult female worm is approximately 25 cm in length, and the male 15 cm. Several genera of mosquitoes serve as vectors of this parasite. Thirty-seven human infections with worms morphologically indistinguishable from *D. immitis* have been found in the heart (2 cases) or in infarct lesions in the lungs. The majority of the worms were dead, and identification was made from microscopic cross sections of them. The most common symptoms experienced by those infected were cough and chest pains. The two cardiac infections were incidental findings at autopsy.

Dirofilaria conjunctivae is the name given to a filarid worm of uncertain origin first reported from a conjunctival tumor. Nodules containing this type of worm have been found on the eyelid, neck, hand, arm, chest, and leg. A total of 50 infections have been reported from the United States. The nematode-containing nodules, 1 to 2 cm in diameter may be painless or painful, and of weeks' or months' duration. It appears that the *D. conjunctivae* infections reported from southeastern United States are caused probably by *D. tenuis* of raccoons, *Procyon lotor*.

Treatment of these infections consists of careful surgical removal.

Dracunculus medinensis

Disease. Dracontiasis, dracunculosis, dracunculiasis, fiery serpent of the Israelites.

Life Cycle. The female is 500 to 1,200 by 0.9 to 1.7 mm, and the male 12 to 29 by 0.4 mm. The adult worm inhabits the cutaneous and subcutaneous tissues and attains sexual maturity as early as 10 weeks. The life span of the female is 12 to 18 months. The fate of the male is unknown. In about a year the gravid female migrates to the subcutaneous tissues of the leg, arm, shoulders, and trunk, parts most likely to come in contact with water. When ready to discharge the larvae, the cephalic end of the worm produces an indurated cutaneous papule, which soon vesiculates and eventually forms an ulcer. When the surface of the ulcer comes in contact with water, a loop of the uterus, which has prolapsed through a rupture in the anterior end of the worm, discharges the motile larvae into the water. Repeated contacts with water evoke successive discharges of larvae (Fig. 58).

The slender rhabditiform larvae with long filiform tails move about in water and are ingested by species of *Cyclops,* in which they metamorphose in the body cavity into infective forms within 3 weeks. Numerous species of *Cyclops* are suitable hosts. The infective larva is actively motile in the body cavity of *Cyclops* during the first month and then becomes inactive and tightly coiled. Ordinarily only one to three larvae are present, and more than five cause the death of the crustacean. The cycle is completed when the infected copepods are ingested in drinking water by susceptible definitive hosts, such as man or domesticated and wild furbearing animals. The larvae penetrate the wall of man's digestive tract and migrate to the loose connective tissues. Multiple infections occur.

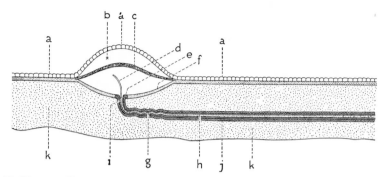

Fig. 58. Diagram illustrating relationship of *Dracunculus medinensis* to blister and sheath. a, skin; b, blister fluid; c, fibrogelatinous layer; d, filamentous coil of uterus; e, central eschar; f, granulomatous base; g, convoluted portion of worm; h, straight portion of worm; i, anterior end of worm; j, connective tissue sheath; k, subcutaneous tissues. (Adapted from Fairley and Liston, 1924.)

Epidemiology.   Stoll estimates that 48 million persons are infected. In man the parasite is found in North, West, and Central Africa; southwestern Asia; northeastern South America; and the West Indies. *D. insignis* is present in fur-bearing animals in North America and China.

In western India a high percentage of the inhabitants, mostly under the age of 20 years, have been infected by drinking water from step-wells. These wells are not provided with a bucket and rope, but people stand ankle or knee deep while filling containers. During this time the parent worm ejects her larvae and at the same time previously infected *Cyclops* are withdrawn with water.

Pathology and Symptomatology.   If the worm fails to reach the skin, it dies and either disintegrates, is absorbed, or becomes calcified (Fig. 59). Their presence in the mesenteric tissues may explain certain pseudoperitoneal syndromes and allergic manifestations.

When the worm reaches the surface of the body, it liberates a toxic substance that produces a local inflammatory reaction in the form of a sterile blister with serous exudation. The worm lies in a subcutaneous tunnel with its anterior end beneath the blister, which contains a clear yellow fluid (Fig. 58). Its course may be marked by induration and edema. The blisters may appear at any location that favors the escape of the larvae to the water, the usual distribution being legs,

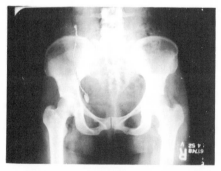

Fig. 59. X-ray showing calcified *Dracunculus medinensis* in abdominal wall of African studying in New York City. There were numerous scars on her feet from removal of worms.

ankles, and feet especially between the toes, and less frequently the arms and trunk. The contamination of the ruptured blister may produce abscesses, cellulitis, extensive ulceration, and necrosis.

The onset of symptoms occurs just previous to the local eruption of the worm. The early manifestations of urticaria, erythema, dyspnea, vomiting, pruritus, and giddiness are of an allergic nature. Symptoms usually subside with the rupture of the worm, but sometimes they recur during the operative removal of the worm, probably from the escape of the secretions into the tissues. There is a slight-to-moderate increase in eosinophils. If the worm is broken during extraction and the larvae escape into the subcutaneous tissues, a severe inflammatory reaction ensues, and secondary bacterial infection may result in abscess formation and sloughing of the tissues. The prognosis is usually good, unless extensive secondary infection follows.

Diagnosis.   Diagnosis is made from the local lesion, worm, or larvae. The outline of the worm under the skin may be revealed by reflected light. Calcified worms may be located by roentgenologic examination. The discharge of larvae may be stimulated by cooling the ulcerated area. Positive reactions may be obtained in a high percentage of patients using intracutaneous tests with antigenic extracts of the worm.

Treatment.   Treament comprises the removal or the destruction of the Guinea worm. The ancient method of rolling up the worm on a stick so as to remove a few centimeters per day is still employed in Asia and Africa. Severe inflammation and sloughing results if the worm is ruptured during this procedure. Surgical removal under procaine anesthesia by multiple incisions after localization of the worm by roentgen rays and collargol injections is preferable.

Thiabendazole, 50 to 100 mg/kg daily for 1 to 3 days is reported to be effective against *Dracunculus*. Niridazole (Ambilhar), 30 mg/kg, orally, daily for 10 days caused a high percentage of the worms to be eliminated spontaneously, or it eased their manual removal. Side effects of therapy were not common or severe. Trimelarsan is reported to be effective.

Prevention.   Lack of education makes it difficult to institute prophylactic measures in many localities. The native religious practice of ablution favors contamination of the waters with resulting infection of *Cyclops*. In order to protect the sources of drinking water, wells and springs should be surrounded by cement curbings, and bathing and washing in these waters should be prohibited. Suspected water should be boiled and, whenever possible, supplies should be taken from running water, a source relatively free from *Cyclops*. The destruction of *Cyclops* may be achieved by treating water supplies with chlorine or copper sulfate, or by planting fish that are destructive to these crustaceans. Immature worms are destroyed by Diethylcarbamazine when this drug is used prophylactically.

LARVA MIGRANS

Larva migrans is the term applied to the migration of larval nematodes in unsuitable hosts. The larvae, unable to complete their normal development, are distributed in the tissues and eventually die and are destroyed by the cells of the host. Larva migrans in man may be separated into three groups: (1) cutaneous, largely due to the filariform larvae of the dog and cat hookworms; (2) visceral, chiefly from *Toxocara* larvae that enter through the intestinal tract; and (3) subcutaneous and visceral, by the invasion of advanced stages of spiruroid larvae. Similar conditions are encountered in the cutaneous lesions of nonhuman schistosome cercariae, the sparganosis of the diphyllobothriid tapeworms, and the myiasis of larval flies.

Visceral Larva Migrans

Disease. Visceral larva migrans is a clinical syndrome resulting from the invasion of human viscera by nematode larvae, usually the adults of which are parasitic in lower animals. Dog and cat ascarids of the genus *Toxocara* are apparently the most common cause of the disease. Aberrant human *Ascaris, Strongyloides,* and hookworm larvae may occasionally produce the syndrome.

Life Cycle. The dog and cat *Toxocara canis* and *T. cati* are widely distributed throughout the world, and undetected human infections with their larvae are probably more widespread than the reports from the United States, England, Europe, Philippines, Hawaii, Australia, Mexico and Puerto Rico would indicate. The adult female worms are 10 to 12 cm in length and pass numerous eggs into their host's feces. In moist soil the eggs become embryonated in several weeks. When ingested by dogs or cats, the larvae hatch in the small intestine, migrate through the intestinal mucosa, and by way of the bloodstream reach the liver, lungs, bronchial tree, and trachea. They are swallowed again and mature in the small intestine of these animals. In man, an aberrant host, the larvae hatching from ingested embryonated *Toxocara* eggs penetrate the intestinal mucosa and are carried by the bloodstream to the liver, lungs, and other organs; here they wander for weeks and months causing inflammation and stimulating the production of eosinophilic granulomata.

Pathology and Symptomatology. The characteristic lesion has most frequently been encountered in the liver and consists of a gray, elevated, circumscribed area approximately 4 mm in diameter. Microscopically, these granulomatous lesions consist of eosinophils, lymphocytes, epithelioid cells, and giant cells of foreign-body type surrounding the larva. Extensive hepatic parenchymal necrosis may be present, and Charcot-Leyden crystals may be seen. Eosinophilic granulomatous lesions without larvae are numerous and are encountered in practically every organ of the body. They may be due to larval migration through the area or represent the site of the death and distintegration of the larva. Lesions containing *Toxocara* larvae have been found in the liver, brain, eye, spinal cord, lungs, cardiac muscle, kidney, and lymph nodes (Fig. 60).

To date the disease has been recognized largely in children from 1 to 4 years of age. A history may be elicited of close contact with the soil, dogs, or cats and dirt eating. The disease frequently follows a benign, asymptomatic course characterized by a marked persistent eosinophilia of 20 to 80 percent and hepatomegaly. Intermittent pain, dermatitis, and neurologic disturbances may be present in more severe infections. Pneumonitis is occasionally present, and pulmonary infiltration may be seen in roentgenograms of the chest. The liver and spleen may be enlarged. Skin rashes on the lower extremities have been reported.

A number of the children have exhibited marked anemia accompanied by a high white blood cell count. There is usually a marked increase in blood globulins, largely gamma globulin. The liver function tests are often normal, although the cephalin flocculation test may be positive. The erythrocyte sedimentation rate may be elevated. Albumin may be present in the urine. The larvae of several nematodes including *Toxocara* may cause choroiditis, iritis, hemorrhage. Studies of the eyes of

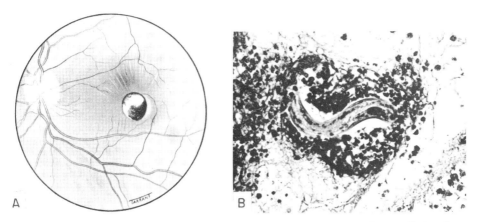

Fig. 60. Visceral larva migrans (*Toxocara canis*) in eye. A, tension lines radiating from granuloma. (*Brit. J. Ophthal.,* 45:793, 1961. Courtesy of I. M. Duguid.) B, larva surrounded by eosinophiles in vitreous chamber. (*Trans Amer. Acad. Ophthal. Otolaryng.,* 55:99, 1950. Courtesy of H. C. Wilder.)

children (aged 3 to 13 years) removed because of a clinical diagnosis of retinoblastoma, a malignant tumor with definite hereditary characteristics, revealed nematode larvae in a number of them.

The varied clinical manifestations are due to the number of larvae, their location, and the individual patient's allergic response to their presence. One patient with a severe infection was found to harbor 60 larvae per gram of liver, 5 per gram of muscle, and 3 to 5 per gram of brain tissue. Repeated infections with larval nematodes in abnormal hosts frequently result in the development of allergic reactions. Hence, the infection may become especially clinically significant in hypersensitive individuals.

Diagnosis. The diagnosis of larval *Toxocara* infections is usually established on clinical grounds with the triad of marked eosinophilia, hepatomegaly, and hyperglobulinemia. In severe infections, liver biopsy and the demonstration of typical eosinophilic granulomatous lesions and larvae confirm the diagnosis. Skin tests and serologic reactions employing antigens prepared from various nematodes have given promising, although equivocal, results. High anti-A and anti-B titers have been reported.

The differential diagnosis may include trichinosis, hepatitis, eosinophilic leukemia, Loeffler's syndrome, familial eosinophilia, miliary tuberculosis, asthma, whooping cough, retinoblastoma, endophthalmitis, and liver invasion by adult *Capillaria hepatica,* a nematode.

Treatment. As only a few infections with visceral larva migrans have been recognized, therapy is still in the experimental stage. Steroids may be of value in ameliorating hypersensitivity reactions. Broad-spectrum antibiotics are suggested for pulmonary involvement. Treatment at present is largely supportive and symptomatic including anti-anemic measures.

Prevention. Small children should be protected against contact with infected dogs and cats, especially kittens and puppies, which are more commonly and heavily infected and may carry *Toxocara* eggs on their fur. Animals under 6 months should be dewormed with piperazine every month and older ones every 2 months. Worms passed as a result of treatment should be destroyed. Dog and cat stools passed in children's play areas should be buried, and sand boxes, which offer an attractive defecating area to cats, should be covered when not in use. There is no satisfactory chemical for killing the eggs in soil.

Cutaneous Larva Migrans, Creeping Eruption

Disease.   Creeping eruption is a dermatitis characterized by serpiginous intracutaneous lesions. Among the nematode larvae, the hookworm *Ancylostoma braziliense* is most commonly incriminated, although other species of hookworms—*A. caninum, Uncinaria stenocephala,* and *Necator americanus*—occasionally are the etiologic agents. *Strongyloides stercoralis* may also cause similar lesions. Another nematode with larvae that causes creeping eruption is *Gnathostoma spinigerum,* found in the Orient. Creeping eruption due to fly larvae (maggots) is a dermal myiasis, due primarily to the larvae of the horse bot *Gasterophilus.*

Epidemiology.   Creeping eruption, which is prevalent in many tropical and subtropical countries of the world and in the United States especially along the Gulf and southern Atlantic states, is caused by the filariform larvae of *A. braziliense,* which lives as an adult in the intestine of man's two close animal friends, dog and cat; hence, their feces are ever available to pollute the human environment. Sea bathers who bask in the sun on the beach, plumbers who work in close contact with larva-infested soil, and children whose castles are made in sand boxes that are open to cat and dog pollution are most commonly infected. All of these environments supply the moist, sandy soil required for the development of hookworm larvae.

Pathology and Symptomatology.   At the points of larval invasion, indurated, reddish, itchy papules develop and in 2 to 3 days narrow, linear, slightly elevated, erythematous, serpiginous, intracutaneous tunnels, 1 to 2 mm in diameter, are produced by the migratory larvae (Fig. 61). They move from a fraction of an inch to over an inch per day, but rarely pass beyond a few inches from the original site of entry. Vesicles form along the course of the tunnels, and the surface becomes dry and crusty. Local eosinophilia and round-cell infiltration may be present. The itching is intense especially at night, and the resultant scratching may lead to secondary infection. The feet, legs, and hands are most commonly involved, but infection of any portion of the body exposed to infested soil may occur. Plumbers are most commonly infected on their knees, elbows, buttocks, and shoulders; secondary infection in them may be extensive. The larval infection may persist for weeks or even as long as a year. The author, who as a student was given an experimental infection of five larvae by Drs. White and Dove (who unraveled the mysteries of this disease in 1926), noted the decease of the first larva in 2 weeks and the last in 8 weeks. At the site of their demise a red papule was formed. A few patients with cutaneous infections develop a transitory infiltration of the lungs with a high eosinophilia of the blood and sputum, which is either the result of pulmonary migration of the larvae or an allergic reaction of the host.

Treatment.   Light infections with only several larvae can be cured by freezing an area in the active portion of the lesion with ethyl chloride or carbon dioxide snow. Numerous chemotherapeutic agents have been tried, but there is little evidence that they provide any less favorable environment for the larvae than does the normal human skin. Thiabendazol (See Page 120), 25 mg twice daily for 2

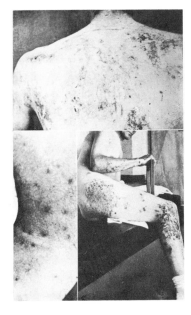
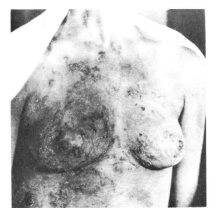
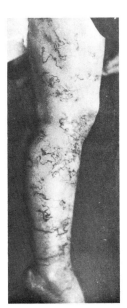

LESIONS SECONDARILY INFECTED AND   UNINFECTED

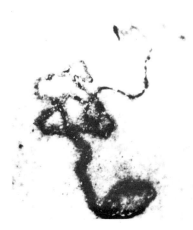
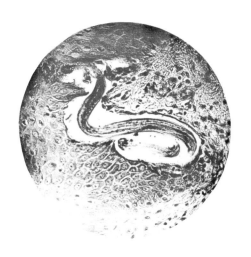

TYPICAL SERPIGINOUS LESION   SECTION OF LARVA IN SKIN

Fig. 61. "Creeping eruption"–cutaneous larva migrans caused by the larva of *Ancylostoma braziliensis*. (After Kirby-Smith, Dove and White, 1926.)

to 4 days, has proven successful in a small number of cases. Application of a 10 percent aqueous suspension of thiabendazole to the lesions of 15 patients gave relief from pruritis in 3 days, and 160 of 164 lesions cleared in 1 week. The secondary bacterial infection should be treated with suitable antibiotics.

Prevention. Control of creeping eruption of hookworm origin consists of avoiding skin contact with soil which has been contaminated with dog or cat feces. Keeping dogs and cats off beaches and from beneath houses, where plumbers may work, and anthelmintic treatment of dogs and cats will prevent contamination of the soil. Children's sand boxes should be covered when not in use. Skin infection with *Necator* and *Strongyloides* can be prevented by proper disposal of human excreta.

Larva Migrans of *Gnathostoma spinigerum*

Disease.   Gnathostomiasis.

Life Cycle.   The adult worm, which lives in tumors of the intestinal wall in fish-eating mammals, is a large reddish nematode, the male being 11 to 25 mm and the female 25 to 54 mm. The egg, 69 by 37 μ, has a sculptured shell with a transparent knob at one end.

Man is an unnatural host in whom the worms do not reach maturity. The life cycle involves two intermediate hosts, *Cyclops* and a fish, reptile, or amphibian. The eggs, which erupt into the intestinal tract and are passed in the feces, in water produce motile, ensheathed rhabditiform larvae, which are ingested by species of *Cyclops*. In order to become infective to the definitive hosts the larvae require further development in a second intermediate host.

Epidemiology.   This parasite is found in Southeast Asia, Thailand, China, Japan, the Philippines, and Indonesia. Man probably acquires the infection, like the natural mammalian hosts, by ingestion of fish, although, since the worms are immature, the possibility of infection from *Cyclops* in drinking water cannot be ruled out.

Pathology and Symptomatology.   In natural hosts one or more adult worms are enclosed in indurated nodules in the wall of the stomach and at times in the wall of the intestine. In man the immature worms may locate in the internal organs or near the skin, where they produce local, transitory or persistent, inflammatory swellings and abscesses. They are able to migrate through the tissues of the host and tunnel horizontally through the dermal tissues, producing a type of creeping eruption. Invasion of the eye, with iritis, uveitis, hemorrhage, and orbital cellulitis, has been reported. Extensive hemorrhagic necrotic tracts are produced by the wormy migration through the spinal cord and brain. Among the signs and symptoms arising from the local inflammation are eosinophilia, hematuria, hemoptysis, edema of the pharynx with dyspnea, angioneurotic edema, and abscesses.

Diagnosis.   The subcutaneous swellings, marked eosinophilia, and residence in an endemic area suggest the possibility of infection, but final diagnosis depends upon the identification of the worm. Intracutaneous tests have been used.

Treatment.   Surgical removal of worm.

Prevention.   In endemic areas, thorough cooking of fish is desirable.

MINOR NEMATODES OF MAN

Capillaria hepatica

C. hepatica is a cosmopolitan parasite, primarily of the rat, and of other rodents, dogs, cats, peccaries, monkeys, and rarely, of man. The adult worm, which is named for the organ in which it lives, the hepar, resembles *Trichuris trichiura,* but has a shorter anterior portion. The lemon-shaped eggs, 51 to 68 by 30 to 35 μ have outer shells that are pitted, like a golf ball. The adult female worm deposits eggs in the liver where they remain undeveloped. When the infected liver of a rat is eaten through cannibalism by another rat, the eggs escape in the feces to become embryonated in the soil from which infective eggs are ingested. In rodents and man the accumulations of eggs cause an inflammatory reaction in the liver with the production of fibrous connective tissue and, in heavy infections, extensive tissue destruction and hepatic cirrhosis. A fatal infection in a child was characterized by enlarged liver, ascites, anemia, and eosinophilia.

Diagnosis is possible only by microscopic examination of the liver. Numerous observers have reported eggs in human feces, but these are spurious cases from eating infected animal livers.

Capillaria philippinensis

C. philippinensis was first described in 1964 from a male patient from Ilocos Norte who, after a year of recurrent ascites, emaciation, and cachexia, died after months of intractable diarrhea. The worms, embedded in both the small and large intestine, measured 2.5 to 4.3 mm for the female and 2.3 to 3.17 mm for the male. As of 1969, over 1,200 cases and 100 deaths have been reported. Apparently all of the victims have unusual food habits, eating dishes containing organs of various small mammals. The female worm is unusual in that it contains normal Trichuris-like eggs, some with thin-shelled eggs and embryos and some with developing larvae which suggests that autoinfection is possible. Thiabendazole appears to be effective against this parasite. Fluid and electrolyte replacement is important.

Dioctophyme renale

D. renale, the kidney worm, is found in Europe, North and South America, and China. The female 200 to 1,000 by 5 to 12 mm, is a large reddish nematode; the male measures 140 to 400 by 4 to 6 mm. The brownish-yellow barrel-shaped eggs, 66 by 42 μ, have thick, pitted shells.

The parasite is most frequently found in the dog and mink, but it has been observed in other wild and domesticated fish-eating animals. The eggs, passed in the urine, are ingested by annelids parasitic on fresh water crayfishes. When the annelids, with their encapsulated embryos, are eaten by fish, the larvae pass through a third and fourth stage in their mesentery. Mammals acquire the adult worms by consuming infected fish.

The parasite is usually found in the right kidney, less frequently in the abdominal cavity of mammals. It destroys the kidney substance leaving an enlarged cystic shell containing the coiled worm and purulent material. If both kidneys were invaded, the host would die, and the worm would become extinct. All 11 cases of human infection have been of the renal type, and the symptoms have been those of renal dysfunction or ureteral obstruction. Prognosis is grave, since the only treatment is removal of the infected kidney. Diagnosis is made by finding the eggs in the urine.

Gongylonema pulchrum

This is a cosmopolitan parasite of the upper digestive tract of ruminants, equines, hogs, and other mammals, and, accidentally, of man's buccal cavity. The variously named species reported in man have been grouped under *G. pulchrum.* Some 20 human infections have been recorded, 9 in the United States. The long, slender, yellowish-white female nematode is 14.5 cm long. The males attain a maximal length of 6.2 cm. The eggs, 60 by 30 μ, have thick transparent shells. The embryonated eggs, passed in the feces, are ingested by species of dung beetles or by the cockroach, *Blattella germanica.* The liberated larvae develop within 4 weeks in the body cavity of the insect into infective forms about 2 mm in length. Upon ingestion by the definitive mammalian host, they probably burrow into the wall of the stomach or duodenum and then migrate to the esophagus and oral cavity, where they become adult worms in the mucosa or submucosa.

In man the thread-like worm has been found only in the mucosa and sub-dermal connective tissues in the vicinity of the mouth, where its migrations produce local irritation, inflammation, and reflex nervous symptoms. Surgical removal is the only therapy available.

As man is infected through the accidental ingestion of the insect host or through contaminated food or water, prophylaxis depends largely upon personal and house-hold hygiene, especially roach control.

Thelazia callipaeda

The members of the family THELAZIIDAE are parasites of the orbital, nasal, and oral cavities of mammals and birds, the air sacs of birds, and the air bladders and intestines of fish. The life cycles are incompletely known but probably involve an arthropod intermediate host. The species that have been reported from man, *Thelazia callipaeda* and *T. californiensis,* are parasites of the eyes of dogs and other mammals, the former in the Orient and the latter in California. The slender creamy-white adult worms are 5 to 17 mm in length, and the embryonate eggs are 57 by 35 μ. The adult worms inhabit the conjunctival sac and frequently crawl across the corneal conjunctiva, giving rise to lacrimation and severe pain, and at times to nervous manifestations and paralysis of the ocular muscles. Diagnosis depends upon the identification of the worm after removal from the anesthetized eye. No method of prevention, other than the avoidance of ingesting arthropods (e.g., flies) and raw water, is known.

Syngamus laryngeus

The members of the family SYNGAMIDAE are parasites of the respiratory tract of birds and mammals.

Man is an accidental host of *S. laryngeus,* a parasite of the upper respiratory passages of ruminants. Some 22 cases of human infection have been reported from Brazil, the West Indies, and the Philippines. The adult worms, attached to the laryn-geal mucosa, produce coughing and sometimes hemoptysis. Its life cycle is un-known. Diagnosis is established by finding the adult worm in the sputum, or eggs in the sputum or feces.

Metastrongylus elongatus

Species of the family METASTRONGYLIDAE are parasites of the respiratory and circulatory tracts of mammals.

M. elongatus, the porcine lungworm, is a filariform flesh-colored nematode, 12 to 50 mm in length. It is a common parasite of hogs and, at times, of deer, sheep, and cattle; it has been reported three times in man. The eggs are evacuated in the sputum or swallowed and passed in the feces. The larvae are ingested by earthworms, in which they develop to the infective stage. The definitive host is infected by the ingestion of infected earthworms or, less frequently, contaminated soil. Diagnosis is made from the eggs in the sputum or feces.

Angiostrongylus cantonensis

A. cantonensis, a nematode which lives in the pulmonary arterioles of the rat, produces an eosinophilic meningoencephalitis in man. The young adult worms removed at autopsy measured: male 7.7 mm, female 12.8 mm.

Life Cycle. The adult female worms pass unsegmented eggs which are discharged into the bloodstream and lodge as emboli in the smaller vessels. These eggs develop and their larvae break into the respiratory tract, migrate up the trachea, and pass out of the rat in the feces.

Various snails of the genera *Achatina, Pila,* as well as slugs, a planarian and fresh-water shrimp, either eat the larvae or are penetrated by them. The larvae then undergo two molts and reach the third or infective stage. The third-stage larvae remain viable for long periods of time within the molluscan host, probably as long as the latter lives. When rats or man eat these infected hosts, the larvae migrate to the brain. In man they remain in the brain, but in rats they migrate by the venous system to the lungs. Fresh water prawns, land crabs, and planarians may serve as paratenic intermediate hosts.

Epidemiology. Although the life cycle of *Angiostrongylus* in the rat and its intermediate hosts has been demonstrated, the modes of human infection need further study. Human infection probably results from ingestion of infected intermediate hosts or larvae deposited by them in contaminated water and on vegetables.

Although *Angiostrongylus* in rats has a wide geographic distribution, in man it has been found in Taiwan, Thailand, Cambodia, Vietnam, Indonesia, Tahiti, Hawaii, and a number of other Pacific islands.

Pathology and Symptomatology. The clinical picture in man varies with the portion of the brain involved, but so few well-documented cases have been reported that a general description is impossible. A 15-year-old boy who presumably died as a result of a central nervous system infection with *Angiostrongylus* complained of continuous, severe headache. There was nuchal rigidity, positive Kernig's sign, and generalized hyperesthesia. Spinal fluid pressure was 280/180 mm of water with 528 cells per cu mm, 50 percent of which were eosinophils. Male and female worms were recovered from the spinal fluid.

A 50-year-old male spent several years in a mental hospital with increasing confusion, incoherence, and disorientation; he died in coma. Immature *Angiostrongylus cantonensis* male and female worms were found in the cerebrum, cerebellum, and vessels of the meninges. The infiltration around the living worms consisted of eosinophils, monocytes, and foreign-body giant cells, while areas of tissue necrosis surrounded the dead worms (Fig. 62).

This aberrant, incidental parasite of man has also been found in the eyes, and no doubt will be found elsewhere in the body.

Diagnosis. In the widely dispersed areas from the Pacific Ocean, Africa, and India to Ceylon, where *Angiostrongylus* is present in rats, patients with symptoms of central nervous system lesions may have this parasite. The white blood cell count is 10,000 to 15,000 per cu mm, eosinophils 25 to 50 percent with a relative

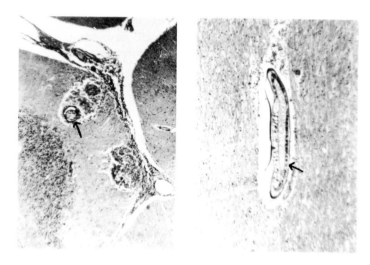

SECTION OF <u>ANGIOSTRONGYLUS</u> IN THE BRAIN

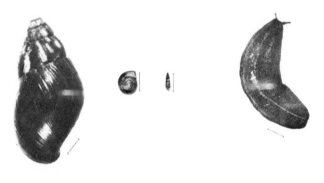

SNAIL   AND   SLUG HOSTS

Fig. 62. *Angiostrongylus cantonensis* and molluscan hosts. Scale = 1 cm. (Courtesy of Dr. J. E. Alicata.)

lymphocytosis. Cerebral cysticercosis, hydatid disease, trichinosis, and visceral larva migrans (*Toxocara*) should also be considered. The eosinophilia of the peripheral blood and spinal fluid would help rule out a virus infection. A skin test, using *Angiostrongylus* antigen, apparently is useful in diagnosis.

Treatment.   No specific treatment is available at present.

Prognosis.   Although *Angiostrongylus* infections may cause death, clinically it appears that there are many infections that cause only a temporary disability.

Prevention.   Boiling infected snails or prawns for 2 minutes kills the larvae, as does refrigeration at −15° C for 24 hours.

8

Cestoda

The tapeworms are parasitic worms of the class CESTODA of the phylum PLATYHELMINTHES. The adults inhabit the intestinal tract of vertebrates, and the larvae inhabit the tissues of vertebrates and invertebrates. These elongated, ribbon-like worms, generally flattened dorsoventrally, have no alimentary or vascular tracts and are usually divided into segments or proglottides which, when mature, contain both male and female sets of reproductive organs. The anterior end is modified into an organ of attachment, the scolex, armed with suckers and often with hooks. The important pathogenic species are: *Diphyllobothrium latum, Hymenolepis nana, Taenia saginata, T. solium, Echinococcus granulosus,* and *E. multilocularis.*

Morphology. The adult tapeworm consists of: (1) a *scolex* equipped for attachment; (2) a *neck,* the posterior portion of which is the region of growth; and (3) the *strobila,* a chain of progressively developing segments or *proglottides.* The length of the different species varies from 3 mm to 10 meters, and the number of proglottides from 3 to 4,000.

The globular or pyriform scolex has one of three types of organs for attaching the worm to the intestinal wall of the host: (1) elongated suctorial grooves or bothria (*Diphyllobothrium latum*), (2) cup-like sucking discs (*Taenia saginata*), and (3) in addition to suckers a rostellum armed with chitinous hooks (*Taenia solium*).

The proglottides vary in number, size, and shape according to the species and stage of development. Each proglottid is essentially a functioning individual, a member of a colonial chain or strobila. They originate in the posterior part of the neck and become progressively more mature. Thus, the anterior undifferentiated segments gradually merge into large mature proglottides with completely formed sexual organs (Fig. 73), and these in turn into gravid proglottides, which consist essentially of a uterus distended with eggs (Fig. 73). The gravid proglottides either break off from the strobila or disintegrate while still attached. The shape and internal structure of the mature and gravid proglottid are useful for the differentiation of order, family, or even species.

The white body is covered with a homogenous, elastic, resistant cuticle, or tegument, which is continuous from one segment to another. Electron microscopic studies have shown that the tegument contains mitochondria, membranes, vacuoles, inclusion bodies, and hydrolytic and oxidative enzymes, and is connected by protoplasmic tubes to cells lying deep in the parenchyma. Pore canals extend from the surface to the base of the tegument. The surface is covered with microtriches, microvillus-like structures. In some species the proximal portions of the micro-triches are hollow, and the distal portions solid (Fig. 63). Beneath the tegument is a single layer of circular muscles and a thin layer of longitudinal muscles. Two layers of transverse fibers extend from side to side, enclosing a medullary portion that contains most of the organs. Dorsoventral fibers also pass from one surface to the other. The parenchyma fills the spaces between the organs and the muscular layers.

Usually dorsal and ventral longitudinal excretory canals extend along the lateral margins of the segments, from their anastomoses in the scolex to their open-ings at the posterior border of the terminal proglottid. A transverse canal connects the ventral longitudinal trunks in the posterior part of each proglottid. The main canals receive branches formed by the collecting tubules from the terminal flame cells distributed throughout the parenchyma.

In the scolex there are cephalic ganglia with commissures and several anterior ganglia that are connected by commissures to form a rostellar ring. The sensory and motor peripheral nerves of the anterior end of the worm arise from these ganglia. A main lateral, and two accessory longitudinal, nerve trunks extend on each side from the cephalic ganglia through the entire series of proglottides. In each proglottid these lateral trunks are connected by transverse commissures.

Most cestodes are hermaphroditic. Each mature proglottid contains at least one set of male and female reproductive organs. The vas deferens of the male and the vagina of the female have a common genital pore that opens on the ventral surface or on the lateral margin of the proglottid. The genital opening may be on the same side of each proglottid (*Hymenolepis*), irregularly alternate (*Taenia*), or bilateral when two sets of reproductive organs are present (*Dipylidium*).

The male reproductive organs (Fig. 73) are situated in the dorsal part of the

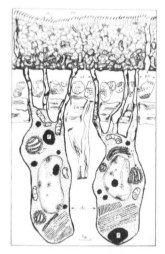

Fig. 63. Diagrammatic representation of a section through the tegument and neighboring structures of *Dipylidium*.
mi, microtrices; m, mitochondria; v, vacuoles; pc, pore-canal; bm, basement membrane; ct, connecting tube between dark cell (dc) and tegument; cm, circular muscle; lm, longitudinal muscle; n, nucleus; er, endoplasmic reticulum; pr, protein crystalloid; f, inclusions of fat or glycogen; op, opposed membranes; ipc, incomplete pore-canal. (*Quart. J. Micr. Sci.,* 103:139, 1962. Courtesy of L. T. Threadgold.)

proglottid. The minute ducts, *vasa efferentia,* which lead from the 3 (*Hymenolepis*) to 500 or more (*Taenia, Diphyllobothrium*) testes, join to form the *vas deferens,* which follows a convoluted course to the *cirrus,* a protrusile muscular organ enclosed in a thick-walled cirral pouch. The lower part of the vas deferens is often dilated to form the seminal vesicle. The cirrus opens anterior to the vagina into a common cup-shaped genital atrium.

The female reproductive organs (Fig. 73) lie toward the ventral surface of the proglottid. The *vagina,* a thin straight tube, extends inward and downward from its opening into the genital atrium, often expanding to form the *seminal receptacle.* The *ovary,* usually bilobed, is situated in the posterior part of the proglottid. The ova are discharged into the oviduct, which joins the *spermatic duct* from the *seminal receptacle* to form a common passage leading to the *ootype,* where the egg is formed. The *vitellaria* are concentrated in a single or bilobed mass or are diffusely distributed as discrete follicles throughout the proglottid. Their contents enter the ootype through the vitelline duct. Surrounding and opening into the ootype is a cluster of unicellular "shell" glands, *Mehlis' gland,* which is absent in some species. The *uterus* extends from the anterior surface of the ootype as a central tube of variable form.

Physiology.   Tapeworms lie in the intestinal lumen of the host with the scolex attached to the mucosa. The usual site is the ileum, but the worms may be present in the jejunum and, occasionally, in the colon. They have been reported from extraneous sites such as the gallbladder.

Evidently, cestodes must possess some form of anaerobic metabolism that enables them to live in a relatively oxygen-free intestinal tract. Under aerobic conditions oxygen is consumed, but the quantitative formation of acids is the same in both aerobic and anaerobic environments. Glycogen, which apparently plays the major role in metabolism, is evidently synthesized from dextrose.

Adult tapeworms obtain a good share of their nourishment by absorbing easily diffusible substances from the semidigested food of the host, but apparently part of their nourishment is derived directly from the host. The tegument is thought to be the main absorptive structure of cestodes, with the microtriches greatly increasing the surface area for absorption. Various enzymes are present in the tegument which participate in food absorption. The proximal portions of the microtriches probably serve for absorpton of food materials, some by simple diffusion, others by active transport. The distal portions of the microtriches may serve for attachment by interdigitating with the microvilli of the intestinal mucosa or may possibly be abrasive, thus freeing tissue fluids for absorption. Evidently, proteins are obtained largely from the intestinal mucosa of the host, whereas the greater part of the carbohydrates are absorbed from the intestinal contents. Thus, tapeworms are sensitive even to partial reduction of carbohydrates in the diet of the host. Starvation of the host and lack of vitamin B complex in the diet reduces the number of tapeworms, retards their growth, and curtails the production of ova. Larval cestodes absorb nourishment from the surrounding host's tissues.

The reproductive organs have attained an excessive development in order to overcome the hazards of completing the life cycle. Hermaphroditism and self-fertilization ensure fertility, although cross-fertilization between segments of the same or of other worms may take place. The spermatozoa are transferred to the vagina by the protrusile cirrus. Ova are fertilized in the ootype, then receive the yolk cells of the vitelline glands and acquire shells before they are finally stored in the uterus. Asexual reproduction in the intermediate host (*Echinococcus*) further increases the progeny.

Adult tapeworms such as *Taenia solium, T. saginata,* and *Diphyllobothrium latum* have a life span of 20 to 25 years, while some species are short-lived.

Life Cycle. With the exception of *Hymenolepis nana,* for which a single host suffices for both larva and adult, the common tapeworms of man require one or more intermediate hosts in which the larval worm develops after the ingestion of the egg. The definitive host acquires the adult worm by ingesting flesh containing the encysted larva. In most cestodes there is a high degree of species selectivity in both intermediate and definitive hosts—e.g., the definitive host of *Taenia solium* is man, and the intermediate host the hog. The egg of *T. solium,* however, when accidentally ingested by man, may develop into the larval *Cysticercus cellulosae.* Man is an intermediate host of *Echinococcus granulosus,* dogs and other canines being the definitive hosts.

When a uterine pore is present, the egg (Fig. 67) has an operculum, yolk material is abundant, development of the embryo takes place after leaving the host, and the fully developed embryo is ciliated. When no uterine pore is present, the thin-shelled egg (Fig. 73) has no operculum, yolk material is scanty, and embryonal development takes place in utero. This type of egg, on leaving the proglottid contains an *oncosphere,* or hexacanth embryo, with six hooklets enclosed in an inner covering, or *embryophore,* and a delicate outer shell that is often lost. The intervening space between these membranes is filled with fluid or semifluid material, at times containing yolk granules. In the TAENIIDAE the brownish embryophore is thick and radially striated.

The thick-walled eggs are quite resistant to heat and desiccation, and can survive for long periods on soil or vegetation contaminated with feces. Upon ingestion by a suitable intermediate host, the oncosphere, under stimulation of the digestive juices, escapes from the ruptured embryophore through its own exertions. Aided by its hooklets, it penetrates the intestinal wall, enters the lymphatic and vascular systems, and by active or passive migration gains access to selective tissues for its larval development. The life cycle is completed when the encysted larva is ingested by the definitive host. The larva, liberated by the digestive juices, attaches itself to the intestinal wall by the scolex and grows to an adult by the proliferation of proglottides.

There are two main classes of larvae: (1) solid, and (2) vesicular or bladder. The characteristic solid form is seen in *D. latum.* The ciliated larva, the *coracidium,* hatched out in water, is ingested by a freshwater crustacean, the first intermediate host, in the body cavity of which it becomes a small, spindle-like, solid *procercoid* larva with a cephalic invagination and a posterior spherical appendage containing the embryonal hooklets (Fig. 64A). When the infected crustacean is ingested by a second intermediate host such as a fish, the procercoid larva develops into a *plerocercoid,* a solid wormlike body without hooklets (Fig. 64B).

Characteristic vesicular larvae are seen in the other tapeworms of man. After the oncosphere migrates to the tissues of the intermediate host, its central cells liquefy, producing a spherical body with a peripheral lining of proliferating cells surrounding a collection of fluid. There are two types: the *cysticercoid* and the *cysticercus* or true bladder larva. The cysticercoid (Fig. 64C) has a slightly developed bladder that is usually reabsorbed or cast off and a solid posterior portion (*Dipylidium caninum*). The simple cysticercus (Fig. 64D) is formed by the enlargement

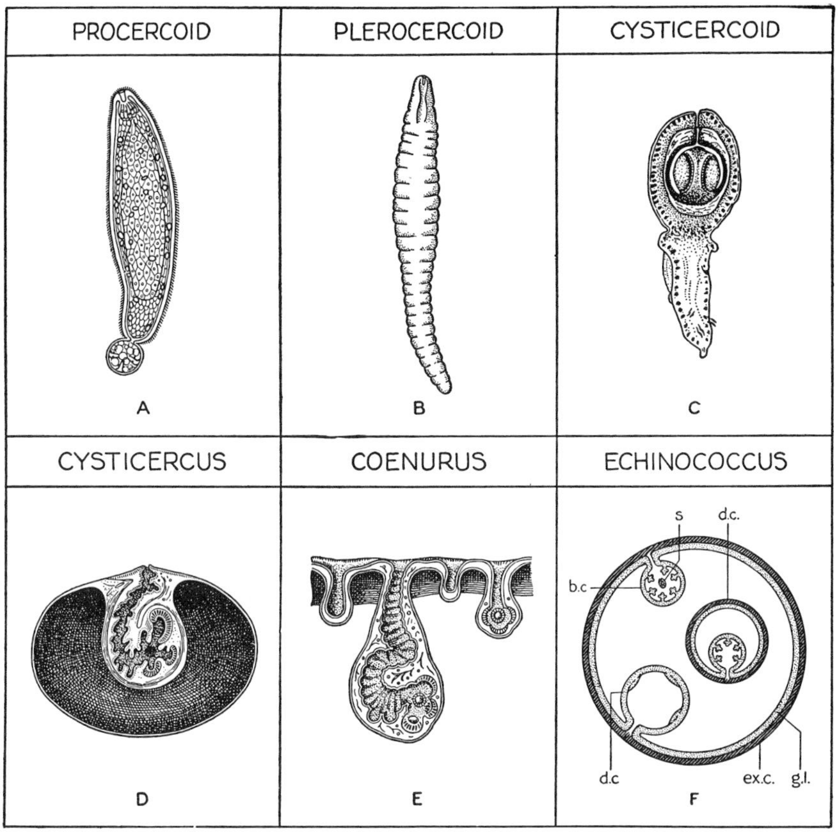

PROCERCOID	PLEROCERCOID	CYSTICERCOID
A	B	C
CYSTICERCUS	COENURUS	ECHINOCOCCUS
D	E	F

Fig. 64. Larval forms of tapeworms. b.c., brood capsule; d.c., daughter cyst; ex.c., external laminated cuticula; g.l., germinal or inner nucleated layer; s, scolex.

of the central cavity, the invagination of the proliferating wall, and the production of a scolex at the apex of the invaginated portion (*Taenia solium*). When a number of scolices develop from the germinal layer of the cyst wall, the cyst is known as a *coenurus* (Fig. 64E). When the germinal layer produces daughter cysts, or brood capsules which give rise to numerous scolices, the larval form is termed *echinococcus* or hydatid cyst (Fig. 64F). In the coenural and echinococcal forms, a single cyst, through asexual development, may give rise to numerous progeny, each capable of producing an adult worm.

Pathogenicity. The injury produced by the adult worm varies with the species. The size and number of the worms determine the systemic effects and the extent of intestinal irritation. The attachment of the scolices provides an avenue for bacterial invasion, and the presence of the strobila may induce temporary intestinal obstruction. All manner of vague gastrointestinal and nervous symptoms have been elicited. Lowered vitality and anemia have been associated with tapeworm infection, but usually no definite symptoms are manifest. Symptoms have been ascribed to the toxic products of the worm, to mechanical irritation, to depriving the host of food, and to the absorption of proteins, vitamins, and, possibly, hormones from the intestinal mucosa. The larval stages, however, may produce serious conditions. Cysticerci of *Taenia solium* in the brain and other organs where removal is difficult may cause marked symptoms. Echinococcal cysts produce symptoms of tumors and, because of the difficulty of removal in toto, may prove fatal.

Immunity.   Our knowledge of the immunity of cestode infections has been chiefly obtained from studies on the cestodes of lower animals. The adult tapeworms, which are not tissue invaders and as a rule do not cause appreciable intestinal damage, seldom evoke demonstrable immune reactions. On the other hand, intermediate hosts evidence definite immunity against the tissue-invading larval cestodes. In experimental animals the degree of immunity may be determined by the number and rate of growth of the surviving larval or adult worms.

Natural resistance is concerned chiefly with the obstacles confronting the invasion of the host by the cestode. It may be due to the habits of the host or to the protection obtained through evolution. Natural resistance varies in species, strains, and individuals. The insusceptibility of certain hosts to infection with the adult parasite may be due to the destructive action of digestive juices on the ingested eggs or larvae, and the failure of the scolex to evaginate from the cyst.

The production of immunity to adult cestodes by previous infection is debatable. Evidence of acquired immunity to larval cestodes is fairly conclusive. The mechanism of active resistance is not known, but it is probably dependent upon antibodies and cellular activity. Antibodies can be produced by active infection and, to a lesser degree, by the injection of worm antigens. Immunity against the larval tapeworm manifests itself by the early destruction of the unencysted larvae or the impentrability of the intestinal wall and the later destruction of the encysted larvae.

Antigens for immunization or for detecting antibodies may be prepared from chemical fractions of the whole adult or larval worms. Several types of larval antigens have been devised for serologic and intracutaneous diagnostic tests for *E. granulosus* infection. The chief antigenic constituents of larval antigens apparently reside in the polysaccharide and protein fractions. Group reactions permit the use of antigens from various species of cestodes for the serologic and intracutaneous diagnosis of specific larval tapeworm infections.

Diagnosis.   The diagnosis of intestinal taeniasis depends upon identifying the parasite by the characteristics of the proglottides, eggs, and, occasionally, the scolex.

9

Intestinal Tapeworms of Man

Diphyllobothrium latum

Disease. Diphyllobothriasis, bothriocephaliasis, dibothriocephalus anemia, fish tapeworm infection, broad tapeworm infection.

Life Cycle. The definitive hosts are man, dog, cat, and, less frequently, at least 22 other mammals including mongoose, walrus, seal, bear, fox, and hog.

The ivory or grayish yellow adult tapeworm (Fig. 65), the longest tapeworm of man, ranges from 3 to 10 meters in length and may have over 3,000 proglottides. The usual habitat of the worm is the ileum and sometimes the jejunum. It is attached to the mucosa by the suctorial grooves and has a sluggish movement. Its life span covers up to 20 years. Self-fertilization is the rule, but cross-fertilization between segments may occur.

The small, almond-shaped scolex (Fig. 67), 2 to 3 by 1 mm, has two deep dorsoventral suctorial grooves. The mature segments are broader than long—hence the name *latum*—and contain both male and female reproductive organs (Fig. 66). The male organs terminate in a muscular cirrus at the common genital pore. The female organs are characterized by a symmetrically bilobed ovary, a vagina that extends from the common genital pore, and a uterus that opens through the uterine pore in the midventral line a short distance behind the common genital pore. The dark, rosette-like, coiled uterus in the middle of the mature proglottid is a diagnostic characteristic. Daily, 1 million yellowish-brown eggs are discharged into the intestine from the distended uteri of the gravid proglottides, which, when egg laying is completed, disintegrate. The egg, 55 to 76 by 41 to 56 μ, has a single shell with an inconspicuous operculum at one end and often a small knob-like thickening at the other. The life cycle (Fig. 67) involves two intermediate hosts. The first inter-

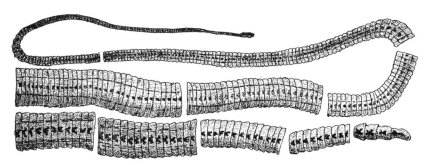

Fig. 65. Adult *Diphyllobothrium latum*. (Redrawn from Leuckart, 1863.)

175

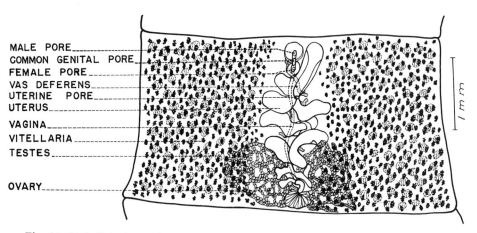

MALE PORE
COMMON GENITAL PORE
FEMALE PORE
VAS DEFERENS
UTERINE PORE
UTERUS

VAGINA
VITELLARIA
TESTES

OVARY

1 mm

Fig. 66. *Diphyllobothrium latum* proglottid.

mediate hosts are fresh-water copepods of the genera *Cyclops* and *Diaptomus;* the second are some of our finest fresh-water fishes: pike, salmon, trout, whitefish, and burbot.

At a favorable temperature the eggs hatch in 9 to 12 days after reaching water, the embryo in its ciliated embryophore escaping through the opercular opening. The free-swimming ciliated coracidium is ingested within 1 to 2 days by a suitable species of fresh-water crustacean, *Diaptomus* or *Cyclops,* in which it loses its cilia, penetrates the intestinal wall aided by its hooklets, and gains access to the body cavity. Here it increases in size from 55 to 550 μ to form an elongated procercoid larva.

When the infected copepod is ingested by suitable species of fresh-water fishes, it is digested and the procercoid larva penetrates the fishes' intestinal wall and enters the body cavity, viscera, fatty and connective tissues, and muscles. In 7 to 30 days it is transformed into a plerocercoid larva, an elongate, chalky, spindle-shaped, pseudosegmented organism, 10 to 20 by 2 to 3 mm. Carnivorous fishes may also obtain the plerocercoid larvae by ingesting small infected fishes, but in such transport hosts the plerocercoid larva undergoes no further development. A fish may contain numerous plerocercoids. When raw or insufficiently cooked fish is eaten by a susceptible mammalian host, the larva attaches to the intestinal wall and grows at an estimated rate of about 30 proglottides per day to reach maturity in 3 to 5 weeks.

Epidemiology.   The parasite is prevalent in regions of the temperate zones where fresh-water fish form an integral part of the diet. It is present in Europe in the Baltic countries, the lake region of Switzerland and adjoining countries, and Roumania and the Danube Basin; in Asia it is found in Russian Turkestan, Israel, northern Manchuria, and Japan; in South America, in Chile and Argentina; and in North America, in Michigan, Minnesota, California, Florida, and Alaska, (United States), and in central and western Canada. A few infections have been reported in Australia (mostly in immigrants), in East Africa and Malagasy, and in Ireland. The development of endemic foci in North America through infected immigrants, first recognized in 1906, illustrates the transplantation of an Old World parasite to a new environment.

Man is chiefly responsible for establishing and maintaining endemic foci. In endemic areas, dogs, cats, and, at times, wild fish-eating mammals are heavily in-

DIPHYLLOBOTHRIUM LATUM

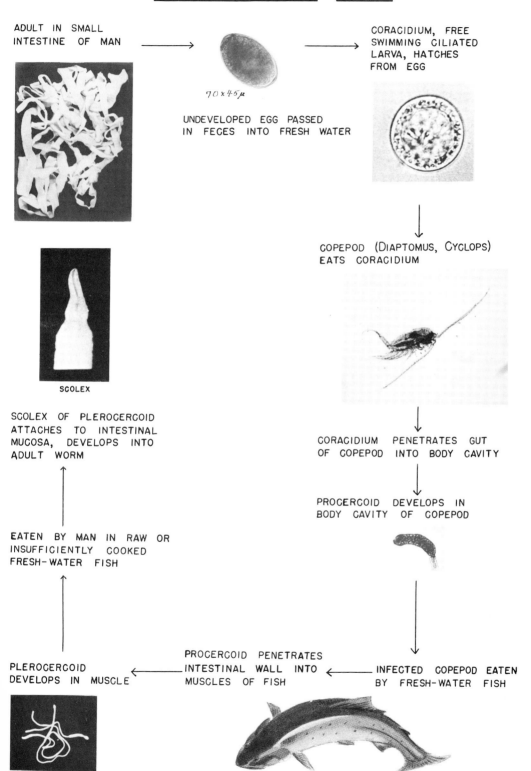

ADULT IN SMALL
INTESTINE OF MAN

$70 \times 45 \mu$

UNDEVELOPED EGG PASSED
IN FECES INTO FRESH WATER

CORACIDIUM, FREE
SWIMMING CILIATED
LARVA, HATCHES
FROM EGG

COPEPOD (DIAPTOMUS, CYCLOPS)
EATS CORACIDIUM

SCOLEX

SCOLEX OF PLEROCERCOID
ATTACHES TO INTESTINAL
MUCOSA, DEVELOPS INTO
ADULT WORM

CORACIDIUM PENETRATES GUT
OF COPEPOD INTO BODY CAVITY

PROCERCOID DEVELOPS IN
BODY CAVITY OF COPEPOD

EATEN BY MAN IN RAW OR
INSUFFICIENTLY COOKED
FRESH-WATER FISH

PLEROCERCOID
DEVELOPS IN MUSCLE

PROCERCOID PENETRATES
INTESTINAL WALL INTO
MUSCLES OF FISH

INFECTED COPEPOD EATEN
BY FRESH-WATER FISH

Fig. 67. Life cycle of *Diphyllobothrium latum.*

fected, but are relatively unimportant except in the spread of the infection in un-inhabited regions. Inadequate sewage disposal, the presence of suitable fresh-water intermediate hosts, and the custom of eating raw or semiraw fish are responsible for the establishment and maintenance of endemic areas. Epidemiologic studies indicate that the North American areas are becoming increasingly infected. The practice of allowing untreated sewage to enter fresh-water lakes is the most impor-tant contributing factor. The fishes of the lakes, other than the Great Lakes in north central United States and Canada, are frequently highly infected. The infection is most prevalent in Russians, Finns, and Scandinavians, who are accustomed to eating raw or insufficiently cooked fish. The Jewish housewife, in preparing Gefüllte fish, samples it as she adds condiments, thereby becoming infected. Her family who later eat the cooked dish do not become infected.

Pathology and Symptomatology.   Infection is usually limited to a single worm, although instances of intestinal obstruction by a large number of worms have been reported. The blood often shows a moderate eosinophilia. Many persons suffer no ill effects from the fish tapeworm, some, however, present a variety of clinical manifestations such as nervous disturbances, digestive disorders, abdominal discomfort and pain, loss of weight, weakness, malnutrition, and anemia. The indefinite digestive symptoms include hunger pains, epigastric fullness, loss of appetite, anorexia, nausea, and vomiting. The vague and varied symptoms are usually attributed to the absorption of the toxic secretions or byproducts of de-generating proglottides, or to the mucosal irritation caused by the worm.

The anemias associated with *D. latum,* particularly the pernicious hyperchromic type, have received considerable attention. It was first noted that anemia is more frequent in patients with a history of vomiting proglottides, and this in turn was shown to be due to the attachment of the worm high in the small intestine. It has now been demonstrated that *Diphyllobothrium* attached in the jejunum within 145 cm of the mouth competes very successfully with the host for the vitamin B_{12} that is ingested, and anemia results. If the worm is forced to retreat further down the intestine by chemotherapy, the anemia is relieved. The vitamin B_{12} content of *D. latum* is reported to be over 50 times that of *Taenia saginata. D. latum* has been shown to absorb as much as 80 to 100 percent of a single oral dose of radioactive vitamin B_{12} given the host. There is no evidence for a hemotoxin.

In North America there have been no reports of severe anemia in autochthonous cases, but the total number of infections is so small that the absence of anemia is not unexpected.

Diagnosis.   Diagnosis usually cannot be made from clinical symptoms, al-though residence in an endemic locality, a raw fish diet, and a pernicious type of anemia are suggestive. Laboratory diagnosis is based on finding the numerous operculated eggs or the evacuated proglottides in the feces or, at times, in the vomitus.

Treatment.   Treatment is essentially the same for all the tapeworms of man, but more persistent treatment is necessary for the numerous small tapeworms, *H. nana* and *H. diminuta,* than for the large tapeworms. In order to effect a cure, it is necessary that the scolex be expelled. Therefore, to check the results of treatment, careful search for the scolex in the feces should be made. If the scolex is not re-covered, it is necessary to wait for 3 months to ascertain that the patient is no longer passing proglottides or eggs.

Quinacrine hydrochloride (Atabrine) (See Page 93, *Treatment* for malaria) is the drug of choice against tapeworms. Oleoresin of aspidium is equally effective, but is potentially more toxic. Both of these drugs lose some of their effectiveness in children because of the frequent occurrence of vomiting following their administration. Either adults or children who vomit these drugs may be successfully treated by using a duodenal tube. Preparation of the patient is necessary before an anthelmintic is administered. On the day preceding treatment the patient should be placed on a liquid diet, and supper should be omitted except for black coffee, tea, or water. A soapsuds enema should be given in the evening to reduce the amount of fecal material that will be examined following treatment. A saline purgative should be given to patients under treatment for *Hymenolepis nana* the evening preceding treatment. The patient should remain in bed, and the following morning breakfast is omitted and the anthelmintic administered. Two hours after the administration of the last dose of anthelmintic, a saline purge is given to flush out the injured or dead worm. If the worm is not brought out by purgation or if the head is not recovered, a soapsuds enema should be given, since the worm or scolex may be lodged in the large intestine. Toilet paper used by the patient should not be placed in the bedpan as it makes the search for the tapeworm head very difficult. The large tapeworms are frequently removed (stained yellow) by a single course of therapy. *H. nana* infections are much more difficult to cure because of the large number of worms usually present.

The adult dose of *quinacrine hydrochloride* is 0.8 g. To prevent vomiting, the total dose may be divided into two portions and given at a half-hour interval. Children are given the following total dose: those weighing 40 to 75 pounds, 0.4 g; 76 to 100 pounds. 0.6 g; 100 pounds and over, 0.8 g.

If oral treatment is unsuccessful, a suspension of 0.8 g Quinacrine in 40 ml of distilled water is introduced through a duodenal tube, divided into two doses.

An emulsion consisting of 5.0 g or ml of *oleoresin of aspidium*, 8.0 g of acacia, and water made up to 60 ml is very effective. Half of the dose is given early in the morning, followed by the second portion 1 hour later. The total dose for children is 4.0 ml of the emulsion per 10 pounds of body weight.

Recent studies with the 4-aminoquinoline (Camoquin), dichlorophen, and niclosamide (Yomesan) indicate that they are of considerable value in cestode therapy.

Prevention. The prevention of fish tapeworm infection in an endemic region depends upon controlling the source of infection, the disposal of sewage, and the marketing of fish. Animal reservoir hosts may complicate the problem of controlling the sources of infection. The disposal of untreated sewage into bodies of fresh water should be prohibited. In spite of administrative difficulties, the sale of fish from heavily infested lakes should be prohibited. Freezing at $-10°$ C for 24 hours, thorough cooking for at least 10 minutes at $50°$ C, and proper drying and pickling of the fish will kill the larvae. The public should be educated as to the danger of eating raw or imperfectly cooked fish.

Hymenolepis nana

Disease. Dwarf tapeworm infection.

Morphology. The short worm (Fig. 68), averaging 20 by 0.7 mm, may have as many as 200 proglottides. The small globular scolex bears a short retractile rostellum with a single ring of small hooks and four cup-shaped suckers. The mature trapezoidal proglottid, about four times as broad as long, has a single genital pore on its left side, three round testes, and a bilobed ovary. In the gravid proglot-

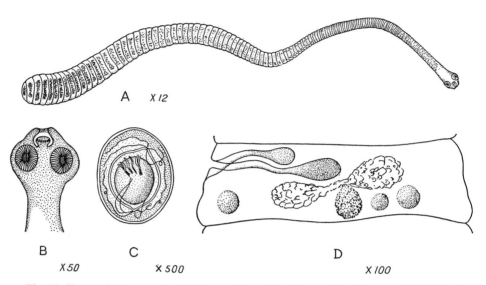

Fig. 68. *Hymenolepis nana.* A, adult worm; B, scolex; C, egg; D, mature proglottid showing reproductive organs. (A redrawn from Leuckart, 1863; B redrawn from Blanchard, 1886; C redrawn from Stiles, 1903; D redrawn from Leuckart, 1886.)

tid, the sacculate uterus contains 80 to 180 eggs. The oval or globular egg, 47 by 37 μ, has two membranes enclosing a hexacanth embryo with six hooklets. The inner membrane has two polar thickenings from each of which arise 4 to 8 slender polar filaments.

The habitat of the worm is in the upper two-thirds of the ileum. Its life span is several weeks. The morphologically indistinguishable murine species, *H. nana* var. *fraterna,* is found in rats and mice.

Life Cycle.   The natural definitive hosts are man, mice, and rats. No intermediate host is required for its life cycle (Fig. 69). The murine *H. nana* var. *fraterna* uses fleas and beetles as intermediate hosts, and infection of the definitive host results from their ingestion. The gravid proglottides of *H. nana* rupture in the intestine setting free the eggs, which are immediately infective when passed in the feces. When ingested by a new host, the oncosphere is liberated in the small intestine and penetrates a villus where it loses its hooklets and, in 4 days, becomes a cercocystis. Then it breaks out of the villus into the intestinal lumen, where it attaches itself to the mucosa and becomes a strobilate worm in 10 to 12 days. In about 30 days after infection, eggs appear in the feces. Internal autoinfection may occur at times and results in heavy infections; the egg, instead of passing from the host in the feces, may hatch in the intestinal tract, the freed oncosphere penetrates a villus and repeats its cyclic development.

Epidemiology.   It is estimated that over 20 million persons throughout the world are infected. Surveys reveal an incidence by countries of 0.2 to 3.7 percent, although in certain areas 10 percent of the children are infected. In the southern United States the incidence is 0.3 to 2.9 percent. The infection is largely confined to children under 15 years of age. The incidence is slightly higher in boys than in girls, and the infection rate in Negroes is about half that in the white race.

Transmission is dependent upon immediate contact, since the feebly resistant eggs, which are susceptible to heat and desiccation, cannot long survive outside

HYMENOLEPIS NANA

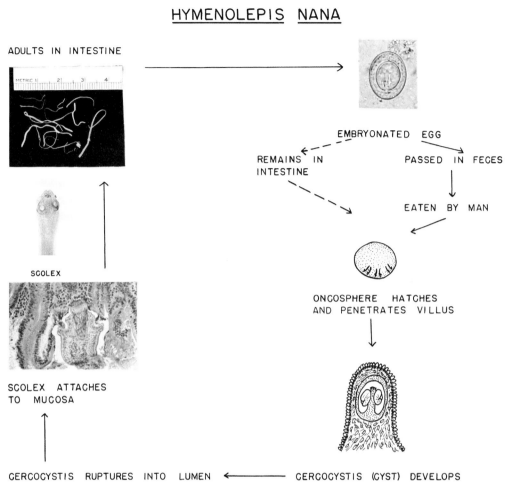

Fig. 69. Life cycle of *Hymenolepis nana.*

the host. Infection is transmitted directly from hand to mouth and, less frequently, by contaminated food or water. The unhygienic habits of children favor the prevalence of the parasites in the younger age groups. Man is the chief source of infection, although occasional infections may arise from rodent sources. Mice and rats have been infected with *H. nana,* and children have been infected with the murine strain *H. nana* var. *fraterna,* although certain differences in the facility of development in the reciprocal hosts have been noted.

Pathogenicity.   Ordinarily there is no material damage to the intestinal mucosa, but a catarrhal enteritis may be produced by heavy infections, as many as 2,000 worms having been reported. Light infections produce either no symptoms or vague abdominal disturbances. In fairly heavy infections, children may show asthenia, loss of weight, lack of appetite, insomnia, abdominal pain with or without diarrhea, anorexia, vomiting, dizziness, headache, nervous disturbances, and, if supersensitive, allergic manifestations. There may be a secondary anemia and an eosinophilia of 4 to 16 percent. Since children can readily reinfect themselves, infections occasionally may assume serious proportions, with bloody diarrheic stools, abdominal pain, and severe systemic symptoms.

Diagnosis.   By finding eggs in the feces.

Treatment.   Quinacrine (Atabrine) is the drug of choice (See Page 178). Antitaenial drugs are less successful than with the large tapeworms.

Prevention.   Prevention is difficult, since transmission is direct and only a single host is involved. Control is chiefly dependent upon improving the hygienic habits of children. Treatment of infected persons, environmental sanitation, safeguarding of food, and rodent control also may be undertaken.

Hymenolepis diminuta

This cosmopolitan cestode of the small intestine of rats and mice has been reported in man over 200 times, usually in children under 3 years of age. The adult worm, 10 to 60 cm by 3 to 5 mm, is larger than *H. nana* and has 800 to 1,000 proglottides. The club-shaped scolex has a rudimentary apical unarmed rostellum and four small suckers. The mature proglottides, 0.8 by 2.5 mm, resemble those of *H. nana*. The gravid proglottid contains a saccular uterus filled with egg masses. The egg, 58 by 86 μ, differs from the egg of *H. nana* in the absence of polar filaments on the inner membrane (Fig. 141).

The principal intermediate hosts are the larval rat and mouse fleas and the adult mealworm beetle, although other species of fleas, myriapods, cockroaches, beetles, and lepidopterans may also serve as hosts. In these insects the hatched embryo develops into a cercocystis which, when ingested by a natural definitive host, becomes a mature adult in about 18 to 20 days. Man is infected accidentally by food or hands contaminated with infected insects. Infections in man are light, and the cestode's life span in him is short, experimental infections in an adult man lasting only 5 to 7 weeks. Diagnosis is made by finding the eggs in the stool. Treatment is with Quinacrine, as in other tapeworm infections (See Page 178).

Dipylidium caninum

Disease.   Dipylidiasis, dog tapeworm infection.

Life Cycle.   The definitive hosts are dogs, cats, and wild carnivora. Man is an occasional host. The adult worm, which inhabits the small intestine, ranges from 15 to 70 cm in length and has 60 to 175 proglottides. The rhomboidal scolex has four prominent oval suckers and a retractile conical rostellum armed with 30 to 150 rose-thorn-shaped hooks arranged in transverse rows. The vase-shaped mature proglottid has a double set of reproductive organs and a genital pore midway on each lateral margin. The gravid proglottid, 12 by 2.7 mm, is packed with membranous egg capsules, containing 15 to 25 eggs. The globular egg, 35 to 60 μ in diameter, contains an oncosphere with six hooklets (Fig. 70).

The gravid proglottides separate from the strobila singly or in groups of two or three, and are capable of moving several inches per hour. They either creep out of the anus or are passed in the feces. The eggs are expelled by the contractions of the proglottid or by its disintegration outside (rarely inside) the intestine, some becoming imbedded in the host's fur, especially in the perianal region.

The intermediate hosts are larval fleas of the dog, cat, and human, and the dog louse *Trichodectes canis*. When ingested by the larval flea, the oncosphere escapes

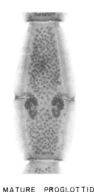

MATURE PROGLOTTID

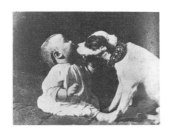

CLUSTER OF EGGS
IN UTERINE CAPSULE

GRAVID PROGLOTTID

CHILD RECEIVES INFECTED FLEA
FROM MAN'S BEST FRIEND, THE DOG

Fig. 70. *Dipylidium caninum.* (Dog kissing child from Riley, W. A., and Johannsen, O. A. *Medical Entomology,* 2nd ed., New York, 1938. Courtesy of McGraw-Hill Book Company.)

from its covering, penetrates the wall of the gut, and develops into a pear-shaped infective cysticercoid larva in the adult flea. When the infected flea is ingested by a definitive host, the cysticercoid larva is liberated in the small intestine and in about 20 days becomes an adult worm.

Epidemiology. Several hundred human infections have been reported. Most infections occur in children under 8 years and about one-third are in infants under 6 months of age. Transmission results from the accidental swallowing of infected fleas or lice from dogs or cats, either through the contamination of food or by hand-to-mouth. A high percentage of dogs are infected.

Pathogenicity. Dogs and cats experience no ill effects except in heavy infections, when they may become weak, emaciated, and subject to nervous and digestive disorders. Man, who rarely harbors more than one parasite, seldom shows symptoms. Children may manifest slight intestinal discomfort, epigastric pain, diarrhea, and pruritus, reflex symptoms, and, occasionally, allergic reactions. Rarely, a patient may show pronounced epigastric pain, emaciation, and loss of weight. The drug of choice for therapy is Quinacrine (See Page 93).

Diagnosis. By finding the characteristic proglottides or, infrequently, clusters of eggs in the perianal region or feces.

Prevention. Small children should not be allowed to fondle dogs and cats infected with fleas and lice. The picturesque and touching habit of kissing a canine by adults and children should not be encouraged. (Fig. 70). These household pets should be given anthelmintic and insecticidal treatments.

Taenia saginata

Disease.   Taeniasis, beef tapeworm infection.

Life Cycle.   The life cycle (Fig. 72) involves an intermediate host. Man is the only definitive host. The adult worm (Fig. 71), is 4 to 10 meters in length and is sometimes longer. It has 1,000 to 2,000 proglottides. Abnormalities of proglottid morphology are frequently encountered. The pyriform scolex, 1 to 2 mm in diameter, has four prominent hemispherical suckers, but no well-developed rostellum or hooks. The mature proglottides, about 12 mm broad and somewhat shorter, have irregularly alternate lateral genital pores and differ from those of *T. solium* in having twice as many testes and a bilobed ovary. The gravid proglottides, 16 to 20 by 5 to 7 mm, are differentiated from those of *T. solium* by the more numerous lateral branches (15 to 30 on each side) of the uterus (Fig. 73). The gravid uterus, which has no uterine pore, contains about 100,000 eggs. The yellow-brown eggs (Fig. 73) cannot be distinguished from those of *T. solium*. The radially striated embryophore, 30 to 40 by 20 to 30 μ surrounds a hexacanth embryo. In the uterus the egg is covered by an outer membrane with two delicate polar filaments, which is lost soon after it leaves the proglottid.

The habitat of the adult worm is the upper jejunum. Roentgenograms reveal that the location of the worm is usually in the upper jejunum below a level of 40 to 50 cm from the duodenojejunal juncture, and that only about 6 percent of the worms are in the lower jejunum. Its life span covers up to 25 years. The proglottides, usually detached singly, may force their way through the anus by their movements or may be carried out in the stool, and when first passed, are quite active and assume various shapes. Almost immediately after passage the proglottides expel a milky fluid full of eggs from their anterior border, where the forward branches of the uterus have ruptured with the separation of the proglottid from the strobila. Thus, the liberation of the 100,000 eggs from the proglottid is not wholly dependent upon its disintegration.

Cattle are the most important intermediate hosts, but other herbivora such as camels are often infected. The eggs, infective when evacuated, are ingested from

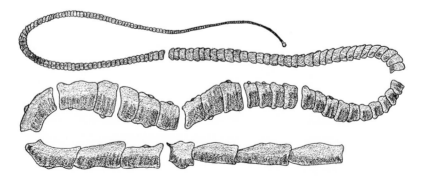

Fig. 71. Adult *Taenia saginata*. (Redrawn from Leuckart, 1863.)

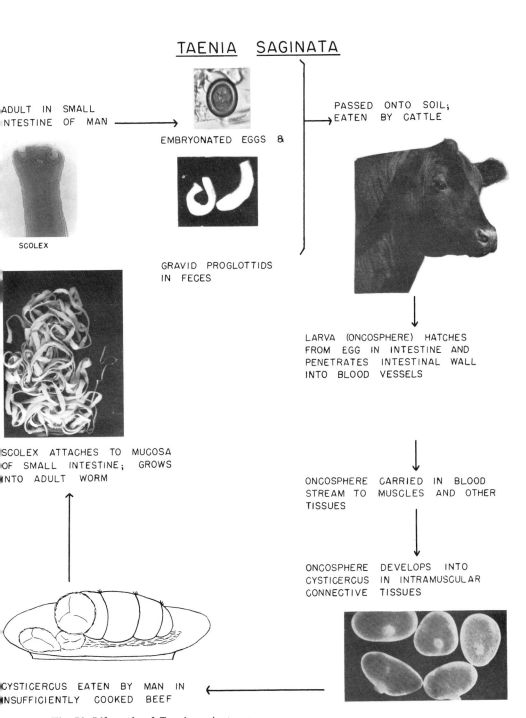

Fig. 72. Life cycle of *Taenia saginata*.

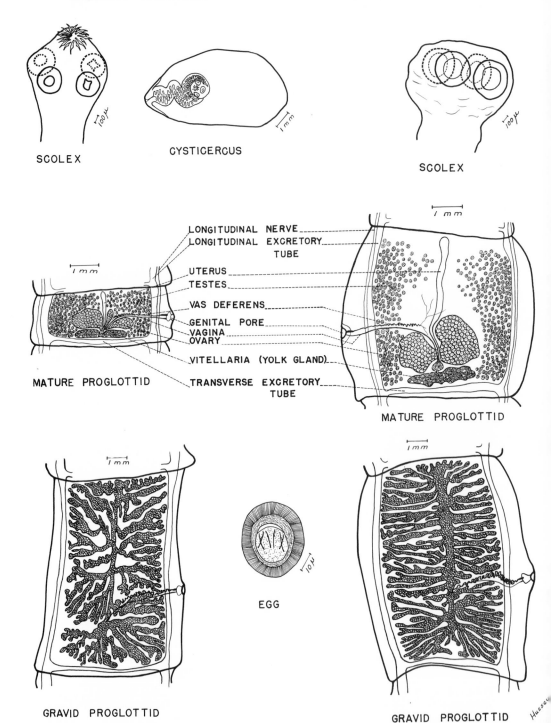

TAENIA SOLIUM   TAENIA SAGINATA

SCOLEX   CYSTICERCUS   SCOLEX

LONGITUDINAL NERVE
LONGITUDINAL EXCRETORY
          TUBE
UTERUS
TESTES
VAS DEFERENS
GENITAL PORE
VAGINA
OVARY
VITELLARIA (YOLK GLAND)
TRANSVERSE EXCRETORY
          TUBE

MATURE PROGLOTTID   MATURE PROGLOTTID

GRAVID PROGLOTTID   EGG   GRAVID PROGLOTTID

Fig. 73. *Taenia solium, T. saginata,* diagrammatic.

the ground or vegetation by these hosts. Hatching requires pretreatment with the gastric juices before the intestinal juices can effect the disintegration of the embryophore and the activation of the embryo. The hexacanth embryo escapes from its shell, penetrates through the intestinal wall in 10 to 40 minutes into the lymphatics or blood vessels, and is carried to the intramuscular connective tissues, where it develops into a mature bladder worm, *Cysticercus bovis* (Fig. 64D), in 12 to 15 weeks. The masseters, hind limbs, and humps of cattle are the selective sites, but the cysticerci may be found in other muscles and viscera. The mature pinkish cyst, about 5 by 9 mm, has an opaque invaginated neck and a scolex with four suckers. It undergoes degeneration and calcification in about a year, although living cysticerci have been found 150 weeks after experimental infections of cattle. When the living cysticercus is ingested by man, the scolex evaginates and attaches itself to the mucosa of the jejunum, and a mature worm develops in 8 to 10 weeks. Usually only a single adult worm is present, but as many as 28 have been reported.

Epidemiology. This parasite is cosmopolitan in beef-eating countries. Man acquires the infection from eating raw or imperfectly cooked beef containing the cysticerci. Cattle are infected from grazing land contaminated by human pollution, through fertilization with night soil or through sewage-laden water. Flooded pastures along the rivers are important sources of bovine cysticercosis. In these pastures the eggs may remain viable 8 or more weeks.

Symptomatology. The adult worm rarely causes symptoms of significance. Infected persons, especially those who know they harbor this large tapeworm, may complain of epigastric pain, vague abdominal discomfort, nervousness, vertigo, nausea, vomiting, diarrhea, or increased or loss of appetite. There usually is no appreciable loss of weight. There may be a moderate eosinophilia.

Gravid proglottides that lodge in the appendiceal lumen may cause slight mucosal lesions and initiate a secondary appendicitis. Very rarely a mass of tangled strobila may cause acute intestinal obstruction, or the penetration of the worm into the duct of Wirsung may lead to pancreatic necrosis.

The migration out of the anus of the muscular, active, gravid proglottides give the patient the feeling that he is having an unsolicited stool, causing considerable consternation. The finding of actively moving proglottides in the underclothing, in bed, or on a freshly passed stool is also disturbing.

Prognosis is good, although it is sometimes difficult to eradicate the scolex. There is slight if any risk of cysticercosis, since only three instances have been reported: two in the skeletal muscles and one in the mesenteric lymph nodes.

Diagnosis. Diagnosis is based on the recovery of the gravid proglottides or the eggs from the feces or perianal regions. Specific diagnosis is made from the 15 to 30 lateral uterine branches on each side of the main uterine stem in the gravid proglottid or from the hookless scolex recovered after therapy. Perianal swabbing with cellophane tape swabs, gives a much higher recovery of eggs than examining the feces by direct smears and concentration methods, as eggs may not be present in the stool.

Treatment. See Page 178. Drug of choice, quinacrine hydrochloride (Atabrine).

Prevention. Prophylactic measures comprise: (1) removal of sources of infection by treating infected individuals, and prevention of contamination of soil with human feces; (2) inspection of beef for cysticerci; (3) refrigeration of beef;

and (4) thorough cooking of beef. Cysticerci may be destroyed by freezing at −10° C for 5 days, heating above their thermal death point of 57° C, and pickling in 25 percent salt solution for 5 days. The most practical safeguard is to cook beef thoroughly until it has lost its reddish tinge.

Taenia solium

Disease.   Taeniasis; pork tapeworm infection.

Life Cycle.   Man is the only definitive host, and, unfortunately, he is also a host of the cyst. The adult worm is 2 to 4 meters (occasionally 8) in length, and when fully developed contains 800 to 1,000 segments. The globular scolex (Fig. 74), about 1 mm in diameter, is equipped with four cup-shaped suckers and a low cushioned rostellum with a double crown of 25 to 30 hooks. The mature proglottid (Fig. 73) is roughly square with unilateral or irregularly alternate genital pores on consecutive segments. The trilobed ovary consists of two lateral lobes and one small lobe. *T. solium* may be distinguished from *T. saginata* by its gravid uterus with 7 to 12 thick lateral branches on each side of the main uterine stem. The mature egg, indistinguishable from that of *T. saginata,* contains a hexacanth embryo with six hooklets surrounded by a light brown, thick, striated spherical or subspherical shell, 30 to 40 μ in diameter.

The habitat of the worm is the upper part of the jejunum. Its life span is long, up to 25 years. Nourishment is obtained from the intestinal contents. The terminal, gravid, motile proglottides separate, from time to time, from the strobila in groups of five or six. The gravid proglottid liberates about 30,000 to 50,000 eggs by its rupture before or after leaving the host.

The usual intermediate hosts which harbor the cyst are hogs and wild boars; sheep, deer, dogs, and cats are less frequently infected, and man and other primates only occasionally. The eggs, extruded by the definitive host, are ingested in food or water by a susceptible intermediate host. The hexacanth embryo escapes from its shell, penetrates the intestinal wall into lymphatics or blood vessels, and is carried to various organs of the body. The mature cysticercus, known as *Cysticercus cellulosae,* is an ellipsoidal translucent cyst, 10 by 5 mm, with an opaque invaginated scolex equipped with suckers and hooks. The lingual, masseteric, mucosal, diaphragmatic, and cardiac muscles are chiefly affected, but the liver, kidneys, lungs, brain, and eye may also be involved. When infected "measly" pork is eaten by man, the cyst is dissolved by action of the digestive juices and its evaginated scolex attaches to the jejunal mucosa and develops into an adult worm in several months.

Epidemiology.   The incidence of *T. solium* infection in man varies throughout the world. The adult parasite is extremely rare in man in the United States largely because hogs do not have access to human feces. Food preparation habits and religious customs concerning meat affect the incidence of this parasite. The incidence in hogs, in some countries 25 percent, is highest where insanitation and faulty methods of fecal disposal are prevalent.

Symptomatology.   The adult parasite, usually a single specimen, causes only slight local inflammation of the intestinal mucosa from the mechanical irritation of the strobila and the attachment of the scolex. Rare instances of intestinal perforation with secondary peritonitis and gallbladder infection have been reported. Serious lesions, however, result from infection with the larval cysticercus (Fig. 80).

TAENIA SOLIUM

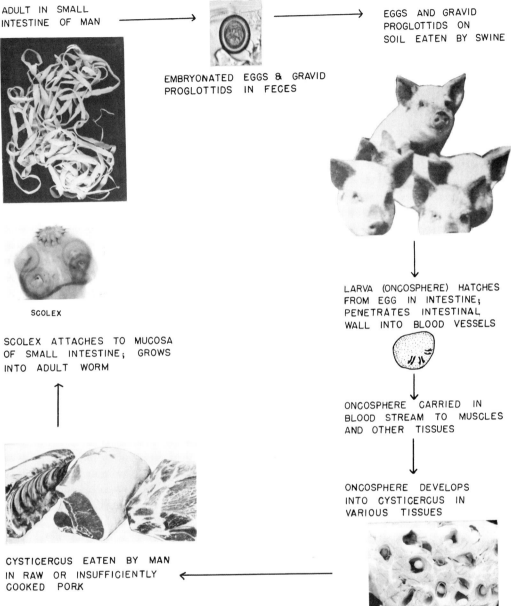

ADULT IN SMALL
INTESTINE OF MAN

EMBRYONATED EGGS & GRAVID
PROGLOTTIDS IN FECES

EGGS AND GRAVID
PROGLOTTIDS ON
SOIL EATEN BY SWINE

SCOLEX

SCOLEX ATTACHES TO MUCOSA
OF SMALL INTESTINE; GROWS
INTO ADULT WORM

LARVA (ONCOSPHERE) HATCHES
FROM EGG IN INTESTINE;
PENETRATES INTESTINAL
WALL INTO BLOOD VESSELS

ONCOSPHERE CARRIED IN
BLOOD STREAM TO MUSCLES
AND OTHER TISSUES

ONCOSPHERE DEVELOPS
INTO CYSTICERCUS IN
VARIOUS TISSUES

CYSTICERCUS EATEN BY MAN
IN RAW OR INSUFFICIENTLY
COOKED PORK

Fig. 74. Life cycle of *Taenia solium*.

Most infected persons show no appreciable symptoms. There may be mild chronic digestive disorders such as irregularities of the appetite, headache, vague abdominal pains, alternate constipation and diarrhea, and faulty nutrition. In children and debilitated persons these symptoms may be more pronounced and may be accompanied by languor, weakness, anemia, and nervous manifestations. There may be a variable eosinophilia as high as 28 percent and a leukopenia.

The prognosis for intestinal taeniasis is good, but the infection should be terminated to reduce the risk of cysticercosis.

Diagnosis. Proglottides or eggs are often observed in the feces or perianal region. Specific diagnosis is made by the identification of the proglottides, since the eggs cannot be differentiated from those of *T. saginata*. The gravid proglottid is distinguished from that of *T. saginata* by the smaller number, 7 to 12, pairs of the lateral branches of the uterus (Fig. 73).

Treatment. See Page 178. Drug of choice, quinacrine hydrochloride, (Atabrine). CAUTION! To prevent vomiting by the patient and possible regurgitation of eggs or proglottides into the stomach leading to cysticercosis, prochlorperazine (Compazine) should be given as an antiemetic before the quinacrine.

Prevention. The control of *T. solium infection* comprises: (1) treatment of infected persons, (2) sanitation, (3) inspection of pork, and (4) thorough cooking and processing of pork. The prompt treatment of infected persons not only reduces the sources of infection, but also eliminates the danger of autoinfection with cysticerci. In endemic areas human feces should not be deposited in areas accessible to hogs. Governmental meat inspection has lowered the incidence of human infection in countries where raw or insufficiently cooked pork is consumed, but it is impossible to guarantee freedom from infection by any system of inspection. Thorough cooking is the most effective means of prophylaxis. Cysticerci are killed by heating at 45 to 50° C, but pork should be cooked for at least one-half hour for every pound or until grey. Cysticerci are killed below −2° C; but at 0 to −2° C, they survive for nearly 2 months; and at room temperature for 26 days. Freezing at −10° C for 4 days or more is an effective but expensive procedure. Pickling in brine is not always successful.

MINOR TAPEWORMS OF MAN

Genus Bertiella. Species of the genus *Bertiella* have a large globular scolex without a definite rostellum or hooks and a relatively large strobila. The embryophore has a bicornuate process. The life cycle is not completely known, but certain species of mites are proved experimental hosts. The species that have been reported as incidental parasites of man are natural parasites of primates. *B. studeri* has been found in man several times in Asia and neighboring islands and in the West Indies, and *B. mucronata* twice in the West Indies and Brazil.

Genus Inermicapsifer. There are two species of the genus *Inermicapsifer* that have been found in man. *I. cubensis* is a fairly common parasite of very young children in Cuba, 70 cases having been reported. It is about 30 cm in length and has about 350 proglottides. Its eggs, 49 to 55 μ, are encased in groups of 6 to 11 in capsules in the gravid proglottid. *I. arvicanthides,* a parasite of African rodents, has been found three times in children.

Genus Mesocestoides. *M. variabilis,* a parasite of carnivorous animals, has been reported twice in children, in Texas and in Denmark, and another species of *Mesocestoides* once in the Republic of the Congo.

Genus Raillietina. Species of the genus *Raillietina* have a cushion-shaped rostellum armed with a double row of small hammer-shaped hooks and four suckers usually equipped with minute hooklets. Their natural definitive hosts are probably rodents. *R. madagascariensis* has been reported 13 times in man and *R.*

celebensis twice, chiefly in the Eastern Hemisphere, while *R. demerariensis* of South America has been found several times.

Several species of adult taenial worms, other than the beef and pork tapeworms, have been occasionally reported in man. These species are often variations or aberrant forms of *T. saginata,* characterized by the absence of external segmentation, or perforated or fenestrated proglottides. *T. confusa* has been identified seven times in man in the United States and has also been reported in Africa and Japan. It is probably identical with *T. bremneri* described by Stephens in northern Nigeria. *T. africana* from an East African native, is distinguished by an unarmed scolex with a small extra apical sucker and a gravid uterus with radiating unbranched arms.

In veterinary practice three common taenial worms may be mentioned: (1) *T. pisiformis* of dogs with the rabbit as an intermediate host; (2) *T. ovis* of dogs with sheep as intermediate host; and (3) *T. taeniaeformis,* often known as *T. crassicollis,* of cats, with mice and rats as intermediate hosts in which the cysticercus is often associated with sarcomatous growths in the liver. *T. taeniaeformis* has been reported from a child in Argentina.

10

Extraintestinal Larval Tapeworms of Man

The tapeworms capable of producing human infection in their larval stages include: (1) the hydatid cysts of *Echinococcus,* (2) the cysticercus of *Taenia solium,* (3) the spargana or plerocercoid larvae of several species of diphyllobothriids, (4) the coenuri of species of *Multiceps,* and (5) *Hymenolepis nana* cysts. These larval infections, except those of *H. nana,* produce serious symptoms, and, with the exception of *Multiceps,* are not uncommon in certain areas of the world.

Hydatid Cyst of *Echinococcus granulosus*

Disease. Echinococcosis, hydatid disease, hydatid cyst.

Life Cycle. The adult worm (Fig. 75) lives in the small intestine of dogs, wolves, jackals, coyotes, foxes, rarely in cats, and in other carnivora. These hosts acquire the adult tapeworm by devouring various organs of herbivores which contain the cyst stage with its numerous protoscolices (Fig. 76). It is the smallest tapeworm (2.5 to 9.0 mm) of medical importance. The globular scolex bears a

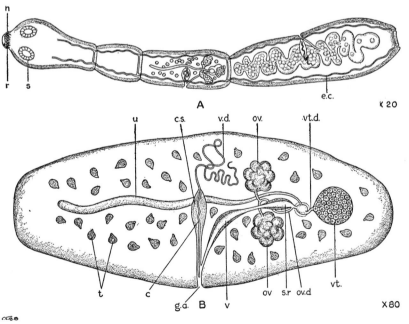

Fig. 75. *Echinococcus granulosus.* Adult worm. e.c., excretory canal; h, hooklets; r, rostellum; s, sucker. (Composite drawing.)

prominent rostellum with a double crown of 30 to 36 hooks and four prominent suckers. The first of the three proglottides contains immature sexual organs, the more elongated middle proglottid has fully developed reproductive organs, and the last or gravid proglottid has a median uterus with 12 to 15 branches distended with some 500 eggs. The egg, 30 to 38 μ, resembles those of the other taenia. Its life span is about 5 months, although it may live over a year. Except for a catarrhal inflammation of the intestine during heavy infections, it does not harm the canine host.

Hydatid Cyst. When the egg, from the feces of an infected dog or various carnivores, is ingested by an intermediate host, including man, the liberated embryo penetrates the intestinal wall, passes into the lymphatics or mesenteric venules, and is carried by blood stream to various parts of the body (Fig. 78). If not destroyed by phagocytic cells, it loses its hooklets, undergoes central vesiculation, and becomes a cyst of about 10 mm in diameter in 5 months. The common intermediate host is the sheep, but cattle, horses, other herbivora, and hogs may be infected. Man also may harbor the cyst stage, much to his detriment, but he does not participate in the complete cycle, as his infected organs are not eaten by dogs.

In man hydatid cysts are of three types: (1) unilocular, (2) osseous, and (3) alveolar of *E. multilocularis.* The unilocular cyst is the most common form in man and lower animals. The unilocular cyst grows slowly and requires several years for development. In man the completely developed cysts, if uninfluenced by pressure, are more or less spherical, and are usually 1 to 7 cm in diameter, but may reach 20 cm. The cyst has: (1) an external, laminated, nonnucleated, hyaline, supporting cuticula, 1 mm thick; (2) an inner, nucleated, germinal layer, 22 to 25 μ thick; (3) colorless or light-yellow sterile fluid that causes distention of the limiting membranes; (4) brood capsules, which have only the germinal layer,

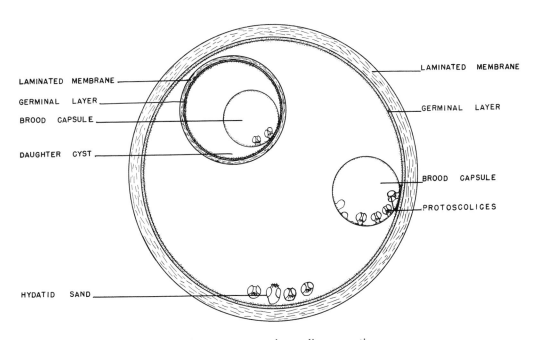

Fig. 76. Hydatid cyst of *Echinococcus granulosus;* diagrammatic.

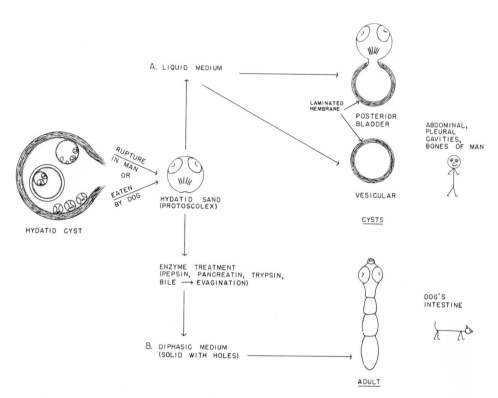

Fig. 77. Differentiation of protoscolices of *Echinococcus granulosus*. A, unevaginated protoscolices form hydatid cysts; B, strobilization occurs in diphasic medium (canine intestine). (After Smyth, Howkins and Barton, 1966.)

containing protoscolices; and (5) daughter cysts, which are replicas of the mother cysts. The external elastic cuticula, which is secreted by the germinal layer, permits the entry of nutritive substances, but excludes substances inimical to the parasite. When ruptured it contracts, thus facilitating the dissemination of the contents of the cyst. The inner surface of the internal germinal layer is studded with small papillary brood capsules in various stages of development (Fig. 76). As these vesicles enlarge, small oval buds that become protoscolices develop on the inner surface. When the brood capsule ruptures, the protoscolices escape into the hydatid fluid, where they are known as "hydatid sand" (Fig. 76). It is estimated that an average fertile cyst contains 2 million protoscolices, which when eaten by a dog would produce innumerable mature adult tapeworms in about 7 weeks. Hydatids without brood capsules and protoscolices are known as sterile or acephalocysts. The protoscolices are most remarkable for when (1) they are ingested by carnivores they evaginate in the intestine and develop into adult tapeworms; and (2) if the cyst ruptures within the host, the protoscolices develop into daughter cysts (Fig. 77).

The endogenous daughter cyst with a thin transparent wall develops in the cystic fluid and at times may produce granddaughter cysts. Opinions differ as to its chief derivation from protoscolices, brood capsules, or broken bits of germinative tissue. In the bones, growth of the hydatid cysts follows the line of least resistance along the bony canals, with erosion of the osseous tissues and invasion of the

ECHINOCOCCUS GRANULOSUS

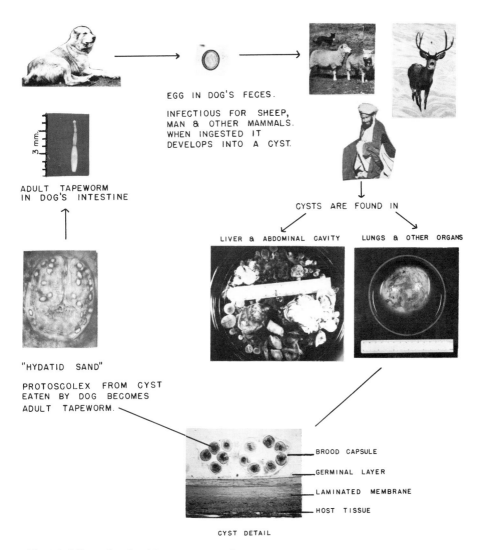

EGG IN DOG'S FECES.

INFECTIOUS FOR SHEEP, MAN & OTHER MAMMALS. WHEN INGESTED IT DEVELOPS INTO A CYST.

ADULT TAPEWORM IN DOG'S INTESTINE

CYSTS ARE FOUND IN

LIVER & ABDOMINAL CAVITY   LUNGS & OTHER ORGANS

"HYDATID SAND"

PROTOSCOLEX FROM CYST EATEN BY DOG BECOMES ADULT TAPEWORM.

BROOD CAPSULE

GERMINAL LAYER

LAMINATED MEMBRANE

HOST TISSUE

CYST DETAIL

Fig. 78. Life cycle of *Echinococcus granulosus*.

medullary cavity. The bony structure is slowly permeated with a gelatinous infiltration and is replaced with small semisolid cysts with little or no fluid and no scolices. Osseous cysts occur most frequently in the upper ends of the long bones, ilium, vertebrae, and ribs.

Epidemiology. The prevalence of human echinococcosis depends upon the intimate association of man with infected dogs. Lebanese Christians are infected with hydatid disease at about twice the rate of Lebanese Moslems, suggesting that the Moslems' belief in the uncleanliness of dogs may be responsible for their lower infection rate. The risk of infection of dog owners was 21 times that of non-dog owners; 10 percent of the infected Armenians had allowed their dog to share their bed. The percentage of infected dogs in grazing countries throughout the world is 20 to 50 percent and depends upon the canine consumption of infected offal and carcasses. The incidence of hydatid cysts in such countries is variable but runs 30 percent or more in sheep and cattle, and 10 percent in hogs. In certain countries goats, camels, and water buffaloes are infected. Cattle are not a potent reservoir hazard, since their cysts are mostly sterile. The incidence of infection is high in man in grazing countries where association with dogs is intimate. In North America there have been relatively few autochthonous cases reported, but in recent years echinococcosis has been found among the Indians of Canada and Alaska. In Canada the moose and caribou are the intermediate hosts, and the wolf the most important definitive host. Indians infect their dogs by feeding them the lungs of moose and caribou, and the dogs in turn infect man.

Infection often takes place in childhood, the period of unhygienic habits. There is little difference in the infection rate between the sexes. Transmission is by ingestion of the eggs, chiefly a hand-to-mouth affair. Man obtains eggs on his hands from the soil or the fur of infected dogs or from uninfected dogs that have contaminated their fur by rolling on ground soiled by dog feces. Eggs are killed rapidly by direct sunlight, but they may remain alive for months in moist shady places. Thus, infection may be acquired from water and vegetables. Canine digestive juices are inimical to the oncosphere; hence, the dog is seldom infected with the cyst. If the dog harbored both the adult worm and the cyst Echinococcus would probably be an extinct species.

Pathology and Symptomatology.   The pathology in man depends upon the location of the cyst. The distribution of cysts in man is approximately: liver including secondary peritoneal invasion 66 percent, lungs 22 percent, kidneys 3 percent, bones 2 percent, brain 1 percent, and other tissues 6 percent (muscles, spleen, eye, heart, thyroid).

The unilocular cyst evokes an inflammatory reaction of the surrounding tissues that produces an encapsulating fibrous adventitia. The impairment of the organs by the common unilocular cyst is chiefly due to pressure. Erosion of blood vessels leads to hemorrhage, and torsion of the omentum to vascular constriction. The neighboring tissue cells, depending upon the density of the tissues, undergo atrophy and pressure necrosis as the cyst increases in size.

The symptoms, comparable to those of a slowly growing tumor, depend upon the location of the hydatid cyst. In the abdomen the cysts give rise to increasing discomfort, but symptoms do not appear until the cysts have obtained a considerable size. A remarkable feature is the extent of the involvement of the organs and the long existence of the cyst before symptoms may be detected.

Hepatic cysts are essentially primary. Over three-fourths of them are found in the right lobe, mostly toward the inferior surface, so that they extend downward into the abdominal cavity. Cysts of the dome of the liver grow slowly, persisting even as long as 30 years before producing marked symptoms. Pressure on bile ducts may cause obstructive jaundice.

Rupture of a cyst sets free protoscolices, bits of germinal membrane, brood capsules, and daughter cysts, which may reach other tissues through the blood or by direct extension and development into secondary cysts. In this respect, this infection with its metastases is like cancer. Rupture may occur from coughing, muscle strain, blows, aspiration, and operative procedures. After rupture of a cyst, signs of secondary echinococcosis may not appear for 2 to 5 years. Hepatic cysts usually rupture into the abdominal cavity, but they may also discharge into the gall-bladder, biliary ducts, or pleural cavity. The rupture of a primary cyst of the right heart may produce metastases in the lung, and of the left heart metastases in the brain, spleen, kidney, liver, and other organs. The peribronchial cysts that discharge into a bronchus occasionally may undergo spontaneous cure, but in the majority of cases rupture is incomplete, and a chronic pulmonary abscess results. The patient has a sudden attack of coughing usually accompanied by allergic symptoms, and the sputum contains frothy blood, mucus, hydatid fluid, and bits of membrane. Secondary infection with *Salmonella* or pyogenic bacteria may occur. The first evidence of the presence of pulmonary cysts, often symptomless until complications develop, may be of an allergic character. Among the more common early symptoms are slight hemoptysis, coughing, dyspnea, transient thoracic pain, palpitation, tachy-cardia, and pruritus. In the brain, the tumors produce symptoms of intracranial pressure and Jacksonian epilepsy. A renal cyst may cause intermittent pain, hema-turia, and kidney dysfunction; and in case of rupture, hydatid material may be present in the urine. A splenic cyst may cause a dull pain and bulging of the ribs, while spotty areas of dullness and resonance on percussion may be demonstrated with pelvic cysts. Spinal involvement may result from vertebral cysts.

The mortality rate is higher in secondary and infected cysts than in primary, uncomplicated cysts. When a cyst ruptures, the escape of fluid may give rise to allergic manifestations, usually in the form of an urticarial rash and pruritus. Rup-ture may be accompanied by an irregular fever, gastrointestinal disturbances, ab-dominal pain, dyspnea, cyanosis, syncope, delirium, and mania. If considerable hydatid material suddenly enters the blood stream, serious anaphylactic symptoms or even sudden death may result.

The osseous cyst produces a pseudotuberculous reaction with foreign-body giant cells. In the diaphysis it causes destruction of the trabeculae, necrosis, and spon-taneous fracture with thickening of cortex and distortion of the cancellous tissues. The slow insidious growth of osseous cysts renders diagnosis difficult, and they are often in locations where surgical removal is impossible.

Prognosis. Many patients live for years—the cyst dies and calcifies and remains silent. Prognosis is good when the primary cyst is accessible to surgical treat-ment; is less favorable when secondary infection is present; and is grave in in-operable cases, secondary echinococcosis, and osseous lesions.

Diagnosis. Clinical diagnosis is based upon the presence of a slowly growing cystic (especially hepatic) tumor, history of residence in an endemic area, and close association with dogs. Hydatid cysts require differentiation from malignancies, ab-scesses, hepatic cirrhosis, tuberculosis, and syphillis. Roentgenologic examinations are useful especially for pulmonary cysts and calcified cysts in any location (Fig. 79). A scintiscan of the liver may detect an uncalcified cyst.

Laboratory diagnosis is made by finding the protoscolices, brood capsules, or daughter cysts in the cyst after surgical removal, or hydatid fragments from a rup-tured cyst in the sputum or urine. An eosinophilia is suggestive, but many infected persons have a normal number of these cells. The indirect hemagglutination (IHA) and bentonite flocculation test (BFT) are the serologic tests of choice be-cause of the ease of performance, as well as the accuracy. Titers of over 1:400 in the IHA, and 1:5 or higher in the BFT, are considered to be positive tests. Approximately 82 percent of the liver infections give positive serology while only

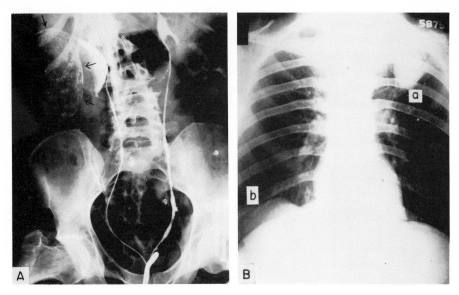

Fig. 79. A, *Echinococcus* cyst of the kidney, undergoing calcification. B, *Echinococcus* cysts of the lungs; a, spontaneously ruptured cyst; b, intact cyst (shown also in figure 78).

33 to 50 percent of the lung infections are positive. Hepatic cirrhosis, lupus, nephrosis, and multiple myeloma all may result in falsely positive tests. Complement fixation is positive in 80 to 90 percent of cases of human echinococcosis. It is of value in detecting residual cysts in patients after operation, since the titer falls after their removal. The intracutaneous test, first used by Casoni, yields about 86 percent of positive reactions in human echinococcosis, but it may show as high as 18 percent falsely positive results in uninfected persons. An immediate negative reaction is good evidence of freedom from the disease, but a positive reaction may persist for years after the removal, or death and calcification, of the cysts.

Treatment.   The treatment of the accessible unilocular hydatid cyst is surgical, the location of the cyst determining the exact surgical procedure. Chemotherapy and roentgen rays are ineffective. Whenever possible the cyst should be enucleated, but its intimate fusion with the surrounding tissues often makes enucleation difficult. Removal of cyst fluid and its replacement by 10 percent formalin to give a final concentration of 2 percent will kill the protoscolices and germinal membrane. When the cyst is large or infected, or closure is impossible, marsupialization is the operation of choice. Primary cerebral cysts require operative interference, but secondary cysts are inoperable. Pulmonary cysts should be removed whenever possible. Extreme caution should be used to prevent the rupture and discharge of the cyst into the tissues. Allergic symptoms should be treated wih epinephrine or antihistaminic drugs. For inoperable or multiple secondary cysts, the so-called biologic therapy, based on the injection of hydatid fluid antigens, has been used in South America. Improvement in subjective symptoms and the gradual atrophy of the cysts have been reported.

Prevention.   Preventive measures should be directed toward reducing infection with the adult parasite in dogs and with the larval worm in sheep and hogs. In endemic areas dogs should be barred from slaughterhouses and should not be fed uncooked offal; the refuse from slaughtered animals should be sterilized; stray dogs should be destroyed. All dogs should be given taeniafuges once or twice a year. In Iceland this proved most effective in eliminating the infection from the country. Food should be prepared under hygienic conditions, and in certain localities vegetables should be cooked and drinking water boiled. The public should be informed regarding the method of transmission, warned concerning the danger of intimate contact with dogs, and instructed in personal cleanliness.

Alveolar Hydatid Cyst of *Echinococcus multilocularis*

The alveolar cyst is the larval stage of *E. multilocularis.* The adult tapeworm is found in foxes and cats, and the cysts in their prey—mice and voles. Dogs represent a potential source of infection for man if they feed on rodents. Both adult and larval stages differ from those of *E. granulosus.*

This cyst is found in man, and occasionally in cattle, in the Bavarian-Tyrolean region, Jura, Russia, Siberia, and Alaska. The adult worm has recently been reported from foxes in North Dakota. The cyst, due to the very thin laminated membrane, is not sharply defined from the surrounding tissues. It is a porous spongy mass of small irregular cavities filled with a jelly-like matrix; the cavities are separated from each other by connective tissue. In man the cyst is usually sterile, and may undergo central necrosis and even calcification while continuing growth at the periphery. Its growth is neoplastic and metastases occur by direct extension or through the blood or lymph. It is found most frequently in the liver. Man may be infected by eating raw plants contaminated with feces of infected foxes, cats, or dogs, thus ingesting eggs which develop into cysts. In Alaska, the infection is acquired from the feces of sled dogs. Man is apparently not a favorable host, for the cysts usually do not complete normal development and lack protoscolices.

Operation offers the only hope for treatment, but complete extirpation of the cyst tissue is difficult.

Cysticercus cellulosae

Man may be both the definitive and the intermediate host of *T. solium* and thus harbor either the adult worm or the cyst. The larval stage of *T. solium* is called *Cysticercus cellulosae,* and the infection in man is known as cysticercosis cellulosae.

Morphology. The mature cysticercus (Fig. 64D) is an oval, translucent cyst with an opaque invaginated scolex bearing four suckers and a circlet of hooks. It is usually enclosed in a tough host-tissue adventitious capsule, but in the vitreous humor of the eye and in the pia mater or ventricles of the brain it may be unencapsulated. It attains its full size in about 10 weeks. The cysts are oval and about 5 mm in diameter, but in the brain they may grow to a large size, several centimeters in diameter.

Life Cycle. See Figure 80.

Epidemiology. Man may acquire the cyst from the eggs in three ways: (1) the ingestion of food or water contaminated by infected human feces, (2) oral transmission by the unclean hands of carriers of the adult worm, and (3) internal autoinfection by the regurgitation of eggs into the stomach by reverse peristalsis. About 25 percent of patients harboring cysts give a history of having harbored the adult worm at some time. Human cysticercosis is probably more common than indicated by its low reported incidence, since many infections escape detection. It is a disease of adult life and is more prevalent in males than in females. It is associated with insanitary surroundings and poor personal hygiene.

Pathology and Symptomatology. The cysticerci, often multiple and even numbering into the thousands, may develop in any tissue or organ of the human body. The most common sites are striated muscles and the brain, but they also occur in the subcutaneous tissues, eye, heart, lung, and peritoneum. The growing cyst produces a foreign-body inflammatory reaction that results in the production of a fibrous capsule. On the death of the larva, which may survive up to 5 years, there is an increase of the cystic fluid and a pronounced tissue response to the toxic proteins. The degenerating parasite usually undergoes calcification. The pathology depends upon the tissue invaded and the number of cysticerci. Invasion of the brain and eye causes serious damage, while that of the subcutaneous tissues and striated muscles is of little consequence.

During the stage of invasion there may be no prodromal symptoms or only slight muscular pain and a mild fever. The cysticerci are well tolerated in the muscles and subcutaneous tissues, and even in heavy infections there may be no symptoms. Muscular pains particularly in the back of the neck, weakness, fatigue, cramps, loss of weight, and nervousness may be present. In the muscles there is degeneration and atrophy in the immediate vicinity of the parasite. Eosinophilia of varying degrees is usually present.

The serious manifestations of the disease occur in cerebral cysticercosis, usually associated with an unrecognized general cysticercosis. Cysticerci may be present in the cerebral cortex, meninges, ventricles, and, less often, in the cerebral substance. They are usually found near the surface of the brain over the frontal and parietal lobes and along the middle cerebral arteries; they are found occasionally in the occipital region and the cerebellum. Cerebral edema and pressure are produced, but there is a relative tolerance while the parasite is alive. Encapsulation results from the proliferation of neuroglia and cellular granulation tissue with inflammatory vascular changes. The neuroglia and nerve cells show pressure or toxic changes. Eventually the parasite may be absorbed and replaced by fibrous tissue that may lead to the late manifestations of epilepsy. At times calcification and incomplete absorption of the parasite occur.

Definite symptoms usually do not occur for 5 to 8 years or even 20 years, until the death of the parasite evokes toxic inflammatory reactions. Symptoms may be caused earlier by pressure of the cysts and obstruction of cerebrospinal fluid. The patient, however, may show symptoms within a year if the cysticerci are located in the areas governing motor function. The most prominent late manifestations are irregularly recurrent epileptic attacks of the Jacksonian type, associated with fibrotic dead or calcified larvae. These attacks range from petit mal, with or without loss of consciousness, to various stages of major epilepsy with aura. Periods of unconsciousness without convulsions may be the only manifestations. Cysticerci in various parts of the brain produce a variety of focal motor, sensory, and mental symptoms. There may be symptoms of brain tumor, meningitis, encephalitis, hydrocephalus, and disseminated sclerosis. Transitory paresis, failing vision, sudden headaches, vomiting, and disordered mentality may be leading symptoms. The most obvious symptoms are psychic—e.g., confusion, irritability, insomnia, anxiety, changed personality, lack of concentration, hallucinations, and, occasionally, mental deterioration. Involvement of the spinal cord may produce hyperesthesia and altered reflexes. Increased intracranial pressure may cause papilledema and optic atrophy. A branching, unencapsulated, racemose type of larva in the subarachnoid spaces and choroid plexus may give rise to symptoms of generalized cerebral disease.

CYSTICERCOSIS
TAENIA SOLIUM

ADULT WORM ATTACHED
TO MUCOSA OF SMALL
INTESTINE OF MAN →

EGGS IN STOOL OR FROM
SOIL EATEN BY MAN
OR

EGGS OR PROGLOTTIDS IN
INTESTINAL TRACT ARE
CARRIED TO STOMACH BY
REVERSE PERISTALSIS

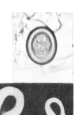

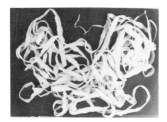

SCOLEX

LARVA (ONCOSPHERE) HATCHES
FROM EGG IN INTESTINE;
PENETRATES INTESTINAL
WALL INTO BLOOD VESSELS

ONCOSPHERE CARRIED IN
BLOOD STREAM TO MUSCLES
AND OTHER TISSUES

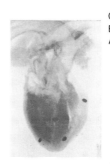

ONCOSPHERE DEVELOPS
INTO CYSTICERCUS

HEART
CALCIFIED CYSTS

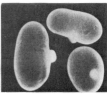

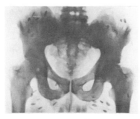

MUSCLES
CALCIFIED CYSTS

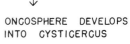

CYSTS IN BRAIN

Fig. 80. Cysticercosis; *Taenia solium.*

201

The spinal fluid presents no consistent characteristic changes. There may be increased pressure, increased cells—mostly lymphocytes and large mononuclears, a variable percentage of eosinophils, and a decrease in glucose. About 10 percent of the patients with cerebral cysticercosis show an eosinophilia of the blood.

In the eye (Fig. 81) the cysticercus, usually single, is subretinal or in the vitreous humor. The grayish unencapsulated cysticercus in the vitreous is continually changing shape. Often damage other than discomfort is minimal, but sometimes the retina may be detached, the vitreous fluid clouded, the parasite surrounded by an inflammatory exudate, and the iris inflamed. The patient may experience intraorbital pain, flashes of light, grotesque shapes in the visual field, and blurring and loss of vision. Death of the parasite may lead to iridocyclitis.

Involvement of the cardiac muscle may cause tachycardia, dyspnea, syncope, and abnormal heart sounds.

Diagnosis. Clinical diagnosis of cerebral cysticercosis is made from epileptiform convulsions or other nervous manifestations in a person who has resided in an endemic area, especially if there has been a history of subcutaneous nodules. Idiopathic epilepsy usually begins in childhood; verminous epilepsy begins later in life. Differential diagnosis from other neurologic diseases is necessary. Biopsy of palpable subcutaneous cysts gives a definite diagnosis. Roentgen ray examination of the infected muscles or brain may be diagnostic if the cysts have calcified. Ventriculograms at times are helpful. The location of the tentative cysticercus for ex-

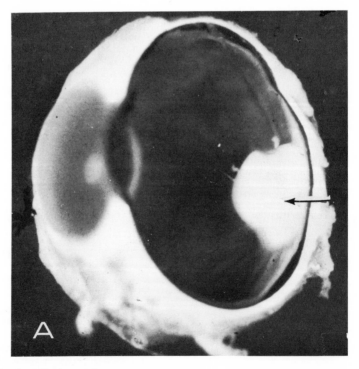

Fig. 81 Taenia solium cyst in eye.
A, gross. (Courtesy of Dr. J. A. C. Wadsworth, Institute of Ophthalmology, N.Y.)

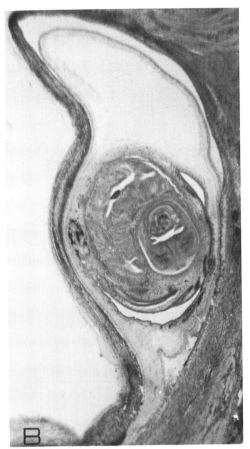
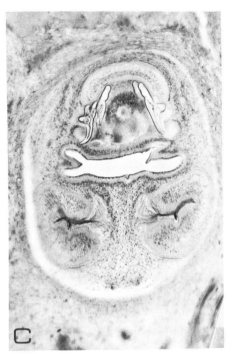

Fig. 81 (cont.). *Taenia solium* cyst in eye. B, cyst embedded in retina; C, section of scolex showing suckers and hooks. (Courtesy of Dr. J. A. C. Wadsworth, Institute of Ophthalmology, N.Y.)

ploratory incision may be made by encephalography and study of the visual fields. In the eyes the larva may be detected with the ophthalmoscope. Complement-fixation, hemagglutination, and intracutaneous tests are of value.

Treatment. Treatment is surgical. The parasite in the eye should be removed as soon as possible. Removal of a solitary cysticercus from the brain gives complete or partial recovery, but surgery is impossible when numerous cysts are present.

Prognosis. Favorable if the infection is limited to the subcutaneous tissues and muscles. Unfavorable if the cysticerci are present in the brain, heart, or important viscera.

Prevention. Prevention requires prompt treatment for the removal of the adult worms from patients. Personal hygiene and environmental sanitation are important.

SPARGANOSIS

The plerocercoid larvae of several species of diphyllobothriid tapeworms have been found in man. They are known as spargana, and the disease as sparganosis. The adult worms are either found in the lower mammals or are unknown.

Nonbranching Spargana

The spargana of several species of *Spirometra* (*Diphyllobothrium*) have been described in man.

Life Cycle. The adult worm *Spirometra mansonoides* resembles *D. latum,* but is smaller. The definitive hosts are dogs, cats, and wild carnivora. The primary intermediate hosts are species of *Cyclops,* and the secondary intermediate hosts include various small animals, snakes, and frogs. The life cycle follows the same pattern as that of *D. latum.*

Epidemiology. This parasite is found in east and southeast Asia, Japan, Indochina, and to a lesser extent in Africa, Europe, Australia, and North and South America.

Man may acquire sparganosis by: (1) the ingestion of infected *Cyclops,* containing the procercoid, in drinking water, (2) by consuming frogs, snakes, or rodents harboring the plerocercoid, or (3) by the penetration of cutaneous lesions by pleroceroids from poultices made of the infected flesh of frogs, snakes, or possibly, warm-blooded animals. The spargana are white, up to several centimeters in length, a few millimeters wide, and exhibit considerable muscular activity.

Pathogenicity. In man the larvae may be found in any part of the body, especially in and about the eyes; in the subcutaneous and muscular tissues of the thorax, abdomen, and thighs; in the inguinal region; and in the thoracic viscera. The spargana may migrate through the tissues. The elongating and contracting larvae within a slimy matrix cause an inflammatory and painful edema of the surrounding tissues. Degenerated larvae cause intense local inflammation and necrosis, but no fibrous tissue formation. Infected persons may show local indurations, periodic giant urticaria, edema, and erythema accompanied by chills, fever, and high eosinophilia. Ocular infection, of relatively frequent occurrence in southeastern Asia, produces a painful edematous conjunctivitis with lacrimation and ptosis.

Prognosis depends upon the location of the parasite and its successful removal. Miliary sparganosis has a grave prognosis.

Diagnosis. The diagnosis of sparganosis is made by finding the larvae in the lesions, but the identification of species requires lengthy feeding experiments to experimental animals.

Treatment. Surgical removal of the larva.

Prevention. In endemic areas drinking water should be boiled or filtered and the flesh of possible intermediate hosts thoroughly cooked. The native practice of applying the flesh of frogs and other vertebrates to inflamed mucocutaneous areas should be discouraged.

Branching Spargana

A budding larval tapeworm, designated as *Sparganum proliferum,* has been reported several times in Japan and once in the United States. The adult worm and its life cycle are unknown. The larva is characterized by irregular, lateral, supernumerary processes, which may bud off as new spargana in the tissues. Diagnosis is made by finding the larvae in the chylous nodular lesions.

GENUS *MULTICEPS*

The adult tapeworms of the genus *Multiceps* are found in the intestines of dogs and wild canines. The larval worm, which is known as a coenurus (Fig. 64 E), develops in the tissues of herbivorous or omnivorous animals. The infection is known as coenurosis, and the condition is usually serious. The identification of the particular species of *Multiceps* is extremely difficult.

Multiceps multiceps. *M. multiceps,* a common adult parasite of dogs has a cosmopolitan distribution in sheep-raising countries. It is 40 to 60 cm in length and has a pyriform scolex with a double crown of 22 to 32 large and small hooks. The intermediate hosts are sheep and goats and, less frequently, other herbivora. The coenuri develop chiefly in the central nervous system, causing fatal "blind staggers" in sheep, although other tissues may be invaded. At least 24 cerebral infections have been reported in man, who becomes infected by ingesting the tapeworm egg from the dog's stool. The larval worm is usually single, although as many as 20 have been obtained from an infant. The globular-to-sausage-shaped cysts, which range in size up to 20 mm or more, contain multiple small invaginated scolices that arise from the germinal wall. The symptoms, requiring several years to develop, depend upon the exact location of the coenurus. Usually there are symptoms of increased intracranial pressure including loss of consciousness, convulsions, temporary anesthesia, paresis, occasional diplopia, staggering gait, and a positive Romberg. The cellular content and protein of the spinal fluid are increased. Diagnosis can only be made by the surgical recovery of the larva. Prognosis is grave. In endemic areas prevention requires the protection of food and hands from the feces of dogs.

Multiceps serialis. *M. serialis* as an adult inhabits the intestine of dogs and wild CANIDÆ. The coenuri develop in the intermuscular connective tissue of rodents. Human infections have been reported three times.

Multiceps glomeratus. Only the larval form of *M. glomeratus* in African rodents is known. It has been reported three times in African natives.

TREMATODA OR FLUKES

11

Trematoda

The flukes are parasitic worms of the class TREMATODA of the phylum PLATY-HELMINTHES. Their parasitic existence has brought about a specialized development of the organs of reproduction and attachment, and a corresponding reduction in the organs of locomotion, sensation, and digestion. The structure and life cycle vary with the type of parasitic existence, which ranges from ectoparasitism on aquatic hosts to extreme endoparasitism in the vascular system of vertebrates.

The species parasitic in man belongs to the DIGENEA, in which sexual reproduction in the adult is followed by asexual multiplication in the larval stages in snails.

Morphology. Adult digenetic trematodes are usually flat, elongated, leaf-shaped worms, but they may be ovoid, conical, or cylindrical, depending upon the state of contraction. They vary in size from less than 1 mm to several centimeters. The worm is enveloped by a noncellular homogeneous tegument, which may be partially or completely covered with spines, tubercles, or ridges. The tegument is shown by electron microscopic studies to be syncytial and without nuclei, to contain many vacuoles, and many small mitochondria, and to be connected by proto-plasmic tubes with an inner layer of cells. There are no microtriches or pore canals as are found in the tegument of cestodes. The tegument plays an important role in the absorption of carbohydrates. It may also serve for secretion of excess meta-bolites and mucus (Fig. 82). The worms are attached to the host by cup-shaped muscular suckers, sometimes bearing spines or hooklets. An oral sucker is situated at the anterior end of the worm, while in most species a larger ventral sucker or acetabulum is located on the ventral surface posterior to the oral sucker. An outer circular, middle oblique, and an inner longitudinal layer of muscles lie beneath the tegument, while bands of muscles traverse the body dorsoventrally. These muscles serve to alter the shape of the worm. There is no body cavity. The intervening space between the various organs is filled with fluid and a network of connective tissue cells and fibers.

A muscular, globular pharynx (Fig. 83) extends from the mouth in the oral sucker to a short narrow esophagus, both receiving the secretions of unicellular salivary glands. Below the esophagus the intestine bifurcates into two straight or branching ceca of variable length that usually end blindly. A system of lymph channels extends along the intestinal ceca with numerous branching canals to the various internal organs. The flow of lymph is maintained by bodily contractions.

The excretory system (Fig. 83) includes diffusely scattered flame cells, capil-laries, collecting tubes, bladder, and an excretory pore. The terminal flame cell is a hollow cell with a tuft of cilia streaming inward toward the capillary end. Through

206

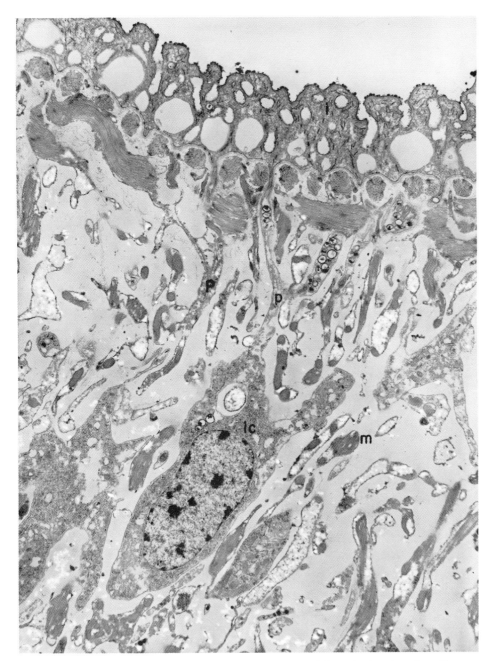

Fig. 82. *Schistosoma mansoni*. Electron micrograph of adult male dorsal surface. P, myo-cytic internuncial process; p, integumental internuncial process; i.c., integumental cytons; m, medullary parenchyma. (*Amer. J. Trop. Med.,* 1969. Courtesy of J. H. Smith, E. S. Reynolds, and F. von Lichtenberg.)

the activity of these cilia the excreted waste products pass into the tubular excretory system and eventually are discharged from the bladder through a pore on the ventral surface at the posterior end of the worm.

The primitive nervous system (Fig. 83) comprises two lateral ganglia in the

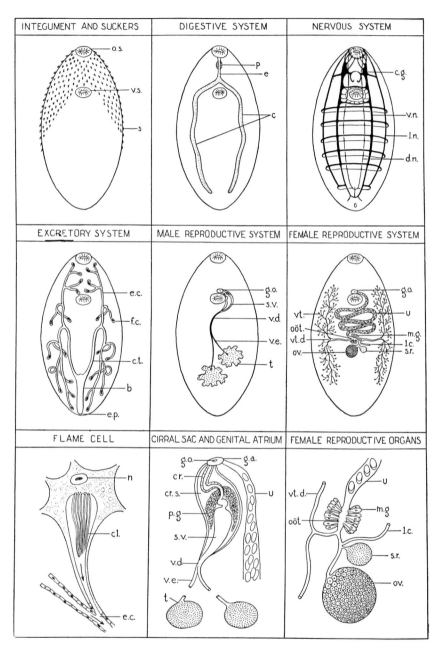

Fig. 83. Schematic representation of morphology of a typical trematode. b, bladder; c, ceca; c.g., cephalic ganglia; cl., cilia; cr., cirrus; cr.s., cirral sac; c.t., collecting tube; d.n., dorsal nerve trunk; e, esophagus; e.c., excretory capillary; e.p., excretory pore; f.c., flame cell; g.a., genital atrium; g.o., genital opening; l.c., Laurer's canal; l.n., lateral nerve trunk; m.g., Mehlis' gland; n, nucleus; oöt, ootype; o.s., oral sucker; ov., ovary; p, pharynx; p.g., prostate gland; s, spines; s.r., seminal receptacle; s.v., seminal vesicle; t, testis; u, uterus; v.d., vas deferens; v.e., vas efferens; v.n., ventral nerve trunk; v.s., ventral sucker; vt., vitellaria; vt.d., vitelline duct.

region of the pharynx connected by dorsal commissures. From each ganglion arise anterior and posterior longitudinal nerve trunks connected by numerous commissures.

Except for the unisexual blood flukes, the parasitic trematodes of man are hermaphroditic (Fig. 83). The conspicuous testes, usually two except in the schistosomes, are located most frequently in the posterior half of the body and may be globular, lobate, tubular, or dendritic, depending upon the species. The vasa efferentia, arising from the testes, unite in the vas deferens that passes anteriorly into the cirral sac, opening into the common genital atrium.

The female reproductive organs comprise a single ovary, an oviduct, a seminal receptacle, vitelline glands and ducts, ootype, Mehlis' gland, and, in many species, Laurer's canal. The rounded, lobed, or dendritic ovary is usually smaller than the testes. A short oviduct leads from the ovary to the ootype, receiving Laurer's canal, the vitelline duct, and a duct from the seminal receptacle. The function of Laurer's canal, which opens on the dorsal surface in some species, is not known. The seminal receptacle is a thin-walled saccular outpocketing of the oviduct for storing spermatozoa. The grape-like vitellaria are usually located in the midlateral part of the body and their tubules converge to form the common vitelline duct. The ootype is a muscular dilation of the oviduct surrounded by Mehlis' gland, of uncertain function. The uterus extends forward from the ootype as a long tortuous tube, often packed with eggs, and terminates in the common genital atrium, which opens to the exterior by the genital pore.

The undeveloped egg (Fig. 84A) consists of the fertilized ovum, vitelline cells, vitelline membrane, and a shell. Its shape, appearance, and size are reasonably constant and diagnostic for each species. The egg shells of most species of digenetic trematodes have a cap-like polar operculum, but the *Schistosoma* eggs are non-operculated.

The adult fluke moves by contraction, elongation, and flexion aided by its cuticular structure. It maintains its position in the host by its suckers. The life span varies with the species, but usually covers several years—up to 30 in the schistosomes.

Nutrition is obtained from the tissues, secretions, or intestinal contents of the host, depending upon the habitat and species of the parasite. Insoluble material is regurgitated through the oral opening while soluble material is distributed throughout the body by the lymph. Waste products are eliminated through the flame cells of the excretory system. Respiration is largely anaerobic, glycogen being split into carbon dioxide and fatty acids. The larval forms, however, require oxygen.

Self-fertilization is the common method of fecundation for the hermaphroditic species. The cirrus is the copulatory organ, and the spermatozoa traverse the uterus and are stored in the seminal receptacle. The ova are fertilized as they pass down the oviduct; yolk and shell material are added from the vitellaria. The assembled eggs in the distended uterus escape to the exterior through the common genital atrium and pore.

Life Cycle. In the definitive host, usually a vertebrate, multiplication takes place sexually with the production of eggs, and in the intermediate molluscan host by asexual generations. In the typical life history of a digenetic trematode, the eggs escape from the definitive host via the intestinal, genitourinary, or pulmonary tracts. When discharged, the eggs may contain fully developed larvae or may require subsequent development outside the body before hatching. At the time of hatching in

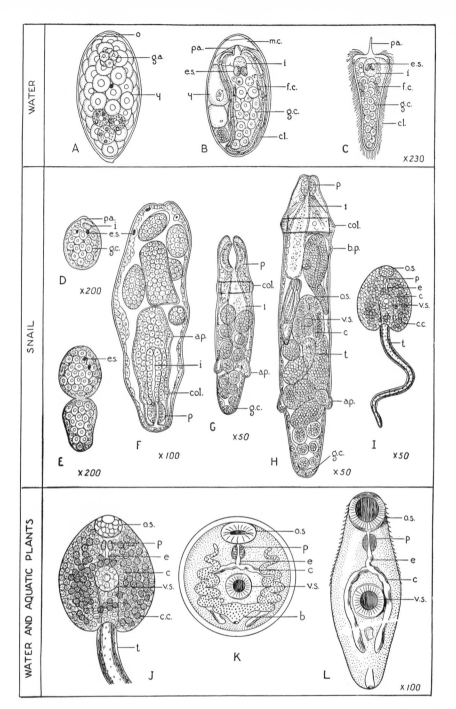

Fig. 84. Larval forms of *Fasciola hepatica*. A, immature egg; B, miracidium in eggshell; C, miracidium ready to enter snail; D, a very young sporocyst, immediately after completion of metamorphosis; E, young sporocyst undergoing transverse fission; F, adult sporocyst with rediae; G, immature redia; H, redia with developing cercariae and one daughter redia; I, cercaria; J, body of cercaria; K, encysted metacercaria; L, excysted metacercaria.

ap, appendages; b, excretory bladder; b.p., birth pore; c, ceca; c.c., cystogenous cells; cl., cilia; col., collar; e, esophagus; e.s., eye spots; f.c., flame cells; g.a., germinal area; g.c., germinal cells; i, digestive tract; m.c., mucoid cap; o, operculum; o.s., oral sucker; p, pharynx; pa., papilla; t, tail; v.s., ventral sucker; y, yolk. (A-J redrawn from Thomas, 1883; K adapted from Hegner, Root, Augustine, and Huff. Parasitology, 1938, courtesy of D. Appleton-Century Company; L redrawn from Leuckart, 1882.)

fresh water, the operculum pops open like a lid to permit the escape of the larval *miracidium,* whereas the nonoperculated shells are split longitudinally by the energetic movements of the larva.

After escaping from the shell, the ciliated pyriform miracidium (Fig. 84C) swims actively in the water. It has anterior secretory glands that discharge enzymes for penetrating the tissues of the snail, a paired excretory system with flame cells, a nervous system with ganglia, and a collection of germinal cells. The miracidium is attracted to an appropriate species of snail by a chemotactic stimulus, probably from the mucus or tissue juices of the snail. It penetrates the exposed portions within a few minutes by a boring motion aided by the glandular secretions and the cilia are shed as the organism enters the snail. Unless the miracidium finds the snail within a few hours, it perishes. In some species, the unhatched eggs are ingested by the snail and hatch in its intestine.

Within the tissues of the snail the miracidium undergoes metamorphosis into an irregular sac-like *sporocyst* (Fig. 84D–F), which serves as a brood sac for the development and production of a generation of daughter sporocysts or *rediae,* which escape through the ruptured wall of the mother sporocyst. The mother sporocyst is usually located near the point of entry, but the sporocysts and rediae migrate along the lymph spaces to the hepatic glands of the snail. The redia (Fig. 84G and H) is equipped with a pharynx and primitive gut, an excretory system with flame cells and collecting tubules, and germinal cells. Within the rediae and daughter sporocyst, cercariae develop and escape into the tissues of the snail and ultimately pass through the integument of the snail into the water. In certain species the rediae may produce an additional intervening generation of daughter rediae.

The mechanism of multiplication in the larval stages of digenetic trematodes involves the production of large numbers of germinal cells and is considered to be a polyembryony of the fertilized ovum. So extensive is the multiplication that thousands of cercariae may develop from one miracidium. The period of intramolluscan development varies with the temperature, snail host, and species of trematode, but usually it extends over 1 month.

The typical cercaria (Fig. 84I and J) has an elliptical body, an elongated tail for swimming, oral and ventral suckers, various spines or stylets, digestive tract, rudimentary reproductive system, an excretory system, and unicellular cephalic glands with ducts opening in the vicinity of the oral sucker. The lytic secretions of the cephalic glands enable the cercaria to penetrate the skin of definitive hosts (*Schistosoma*) or enter the tissues of intermediate hosts. Special cystogenous glands are present in species that encyst in secondary animal hosts or on plants. The liberated cercariae swim with their tails, the body being anterior except in those with forked appendages. The aquatic habits vary with the species, some frequenting the surface and others the lower levels. They may attach themselves to the surface film or settle to the bottom. The life of the cercaria in water is limited unless it finds a suitable plant or animal host on which to encyst or penetrates the skin of a definitive host. In the encysted cercaria, known as the *metacercaria,* the tail and cystogenous and lytic glands of the cercaria have disappeared (Fig. 84K and L).

In order to invade the definitive host, the metacercariae in secondary intermediate hosts (fish, crustacea, and snails) or on aquatic plants must be ingested or the cercariae must penetrate the skin. Within the definitive host the adolescent worm migrates to its normal habitat and grows to maturity.

Snails, mostly fresh-water species, act as primary intermediate hosts for the parasitic trematodes of man. Only certain species serve as hosts, and their identification and control play an important role in the prevention of human infection. Scarcely 70 of the 100,000 or more species of snails are intermediate hosts of helminths of man. The various species and even strains of trematodes have become adapted to a single or, at most, a few species of snails. They either fail to penetrate or else do not complete their larval development in other species. Adaptation to a new host species may occur in nature, but it usually requires a concentration of infected persons and heavy deposits of eggs. Thus, while there is a potential danger, there is little chance of spreading pathogenic trematodes in new areas uninhabited by suitable snail hosts. Effective control measures for a particular species of snails, chiefly drainage and molluscacides, depend upon a knowledge of its ecology.

The designation of a species of snail as an intermediate host requires carefully controlled experimental evidence, difficult to obtain, and should not be based on its mere presence in a locality where the trematode is endemic. The slight differences between species, and even genera, and the great variation within species render classification confusing and subject to constant revision.

Trematodes which infect man may also infect lower mammals and birds. In some instances, although man may be the chief source of infection, the parasite may be of only minor importance because of limitations by climate, presence of suitable intermediate hosts, and the eating habits of the inhabitants. In other instances, man is an incidental host, and mammals are the principal hosts.

Pathology.   The lesions produced by flukes depend upon their location in the host and upon their irritative and toxic actions. The systemic effects are due to the absorption of toxic substances with resultant allergic reactions and to the injury of vital organs. The severity of the infection depends not only upon the number of worms present, but also upon the invasion of the tissues by the eggs, larvae, and adult worms. The flukes that inhabit the intestinal tract are usually less harmful than those that invade the tissues, producing little injury, as a rule, except in heavy infections.

Immunity.   The trematodes that invade the tissues or blood evoke the greatest immunologic response, Hence, studies on immunity are largely confined to those flukes that have a larval or an adult somatic existence. In man, age resistance cannot readily be differentiated from acquired resistance.

Previous infection tends to produce a certain degree of immunity, rarely absolute, as indicated by epidemiologic evidence and by animal and human experimentation with schistosomiasis. The production of complement-fixing antibodies, precipitins, and sensitizing antibodies has been reported in both man and animals. The normal serum of certain vertebrates contains labile antagonistic substances against the cercariae of various trematodes. Partial immunity against *Fasciola* and schistosomes has been produced in experimental animals by injecting suspensions of larval or adult parasites.

12

Intestinal, Hepatic, and Pulmonary Flukes of Man

INTESTINAL FLUKES

Fasciolopsis buski

Disease. Fasciolopsiasis.

Life Cycle. Man, hogs, and, occasionally, dogs are the natural definitive hosts of *F. buski*. The adult fluke (Fig. 85), the largest parasitic trematode of man, is a thick, fleshy, ovate, flesh-colored worm, 2.0 to 7.5 by 0.8 to 2.0 cm. Normally the cuticle is covered with transverse rows of small spines, which are often destroyed by the intestinal juices. The oral sucker is about one-fourth the size of the nearby ventral sucker. The intestinal tract comprises a short prepharynx, a bulbous pharynx, a short esophagus, and a pair of unbranched ceca with two characteristic lateral indentations.

The two dendritic testes lie in tandem formation in the posterior half of the worm. The single branched ovary lies in the middle of the body to the right of the midline. The vitellaria lateral to the ceca extend from the ventral sucker to the posterior end of the body. From the ootype the uterus follows a convoluted course to open into the common genital atrium at the anterior border of the ventral sucker. The yellowish ellipsoidal egg, 130 to 140 by 80 to 85 μ, has a clear, thin shell with a small operculum at one end; it is undeveloped when passed in the feces (Fig. 86).

The fluke inhabits the small intestine, particularly the duodenum and jejunum, but sometimes it may be found in the stomach or in the large intestine. It either is attached to the mucosa by the ventral sucker or lies buried in the mucous secretions. It obtains its nourishment from the intestinal contents and secretions. Its probable life span in man is short. The average daily egg production per fluke is 21,000 to 28,000. In water the eggs at 27° to 32° C hatch in 3 to 7 weeks. The miracidium, covered with cilia, has a spined head, pigmented eye spot, two flame cells, cephalic glands, and germinal cells. Usually within 2 hours after hatching, it penetrates the exposed flesh of a suitable snail host; otherwise it perishes in 5 to 52 hours.

The primary intermediate hosts are species of planorbid snails of the genera *Segmentina, Hippeutis,* and *Gyraulus.* In the snail the miracidium metamorphoses into a mother sporocyst, which, after reaching an average size of 400 μ, migrates to the region of the heart and liver; when ripe it ruptures to liberate mother rediae, which in turn produce daughter rediae. Cercariae, with slender muscular

213

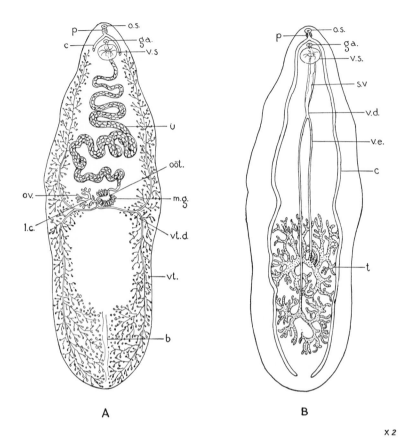

A   B

×2

Fig. 85. Schematic representation of morphology of *Fasciolopsis buski*. A, female reproductive organs, ventral view; B, male reproductive organs and digestive tract, ventral view.
b, bladder; c, ceca; g.a., genital atrium; m.g., Mehlis' gland; l.c., Laurer's canal; oöt, ootype;
o.s., oral sucker; ov., ovary; p, pharynx; s.v., seminal vesicle; t, testes; u, uterus; v.d., vas
deferens; v.e., vas efferens; v.s., ventral sucker; vt., vitellaria; vt.d., vitelline duct. (Adapted from
Odhner, 1902.)

tails 500 μ long, and heavy bodies 195 by 145 μ, are liberated from the daughter
rediae and erupt from the snail in 4 to 7 weeks after its infection. In the water the
cercaria swims by lashing the tail and crawls like a measuring worm using its
suckers. The free-swimming stage is brief, ordinarily of merely sufficient length for
the cercaria to reach a suitable plant for encystment. Cercariae show little selective
specificity and encyst on the surface or in the integument of all sorts of aquatic
vegetation in stagnant waters. The principal plants are the water caltrop *Trapa,*
the water hyacinth *Eichhornia,* the water chestnut *Eliocharis,* and the water bamboo
Zizania. The cercaria, casting off its tail, in 1 to 3 hours becomes a metacercaria
by secreting an outer friable cyst wall, 216 by 187 μ, and a firm inner wall soluble
in the digestive juices. A single plant may harbor a large number of cysts which
are resistant to cold but are susceptible to desiccation at summer temperatures.
When the cysts are swallowed, their inner wall is dissolved in the duodenum, and
the activated larval worm attaches itself to the mucosa of the upper intestine and
becomes an adult worm in 25 to 30 days (Fig. 86).

Epidemiology.   This parasite is found in Central and South China as far

FASCIOLOPSIS BUSKI

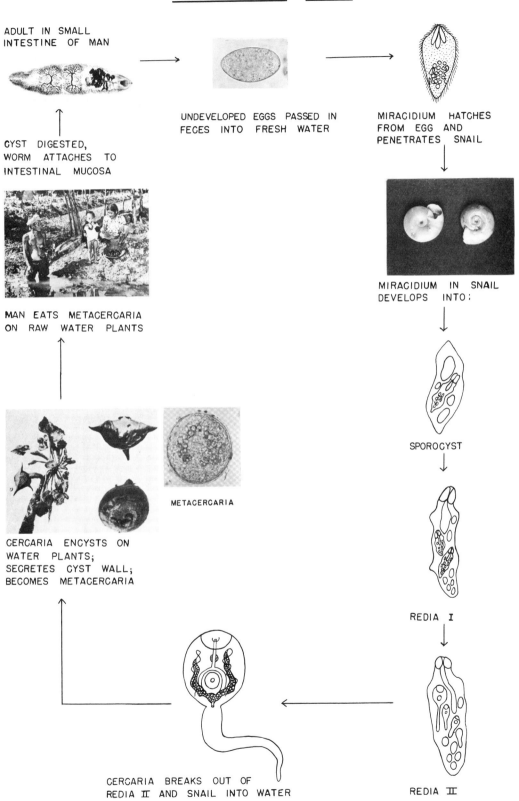

ADULT IN SMALL
INTESTINE OF MAN

UNDEVELOPED EGGS PASSED IN
FECES INTO FRESH WATER

MIRACIDIUM HATCHES
FROM EGG AND
PENETRATES SNAIL

CYST DIGESTED,
WORM ATTACHES TO
INTESTINAL MUCOSA

MIRACIDIUM IN SNAIL
DEVELOPS INTO:

MAN EATS METACERCARIA
ON RAW WATER PLANTS

SPOROCYST

METACERCARIA

CERCARIA ENCYSTS ON
WATER PLANTS;
SECRETES CYST WALL;
BECOMES METACERCARIA

REDIA I

REDIA II

CERCARIA BREAKS OUT OF
REDIA II AND SNAIL INTO WATER

Fig. 86. Life cycle of *Fasciolopsis buski*.

north as the Yangtze valley, Taiwan, Thailand, Laos, Vietnam, Cambodia, and Indonesia. The chief endemic area is in the Kwangtung and Chekiang provinces of China where the incidence of human infection is high. Human infection usually results from the ingestion of metacercariae on fresh edible water plants, which grow in ponds fertilized by night soil rather than in the less severely polluted canals. When eaten raw, the pods of the water caltrop and the bulbs of the water chestnut are peeled with the teeth, thus enabling the detached metacercaria to enter the digestive tract. Dried plants are not dangerous, since desiccation kills the metacercariae.

Pathology and Symptomatology. *Fasciolopsis* attaches to the mucosa of the upper small intestine by means of its ventral sucker. It feeds on the intestinal contents and possibly on the superficial mucosa. Areas of inflammation, ulceration, and abscesses occur at the site of attachment. Epigastric pain, nausea, and diarrhea of varying severity occur, especially in the morning. These are relieved by food, which may be raw water nuts bringing additional infection. In heavy infections, edema, ascites and anasarca are severe. Occasionally, intestinal stasis and obstruction are produced. The clinical manifestations are probably due to toxic products of the worm. There is slight anemia, often a leukocytosis, sometimes a leukopenia or lymphocytosis, and an eosinophilia up to 35 percent. Except in patients with severe anasarca prognosis is good, provided treatment is given. Complete recovery follows the removal of the worms. In advanced cases death may result from exhaustion (Fig. 87).

Diagnosis. The clinical symptoms are sufficiently characteristic to arouse suspicion in an endemic area. Final diagnosis is based on finding the eggs in the feces. The eggs resemble those of *Fasciola hepatica* except for the distribution of the yolk granules, those of *Gastrodiscoides hominis* which are narrower and greenish-brown, and those of *Echinochasmus perfoliatus* which are smaller. Adult flukes are sometimes vomited or passed in the feces.

Treatment. See Page 128, *Treatment* for hookworms. Tetrachlorethylene, hexylresorcinol, and stilbazium iodide are all very effective against *Fasciolopsis*.

Prevention. While treatment will reduce the human sources of infection, it will not diminish porcine sources and will not prevent reinfection, particularly in children, in endemic areas. The infestation of water plants may be reduced by

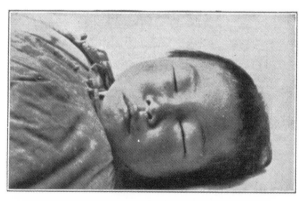

Fig. 87. Patient with fasciolopsiasis, showing edema of cheeks and orbital area. (From Faust. *Human Helminthology,* 2nd ed., 1939. Courtesy of Lea & Febiger, Philadelphia.)

treating night soil containing the eggs by storage or unslaked lime, and by killing the eggs, miracidia, and cercariae in the water with unslaked lime (100 ppm) or copper sulfate (20 ppm). Infected hogs should be restrained from contaminating areas where water plants are growing, a difficult task in the Far East. The intermediate snail hosts may be destroyed in various ways (Page 247). The abolition of eating raw aquatic plants would soon eliminate infection in man, but such a measure would require education of the public and fundamental changes in eating habits. Thorough cooking or steeping the plants in boiling water should afford protection.

Heterophyes heterophyes

Disease. Heterophyiasis.

Life Cycle. The worm is a natural parasite of man and of domesticated and wild fish-eating mammals. The pyriform, grayish fluke (Fig. 88) is identified by: (1) its small size, 1.3 by 0.5 mm; (2) a cuticle covered with fine scale-like spines; (3) a large ventral sucker in the anterior middle third of the body; (4) a protrusible, nonadhesive genital sucker at the left posterior border of the ventral sucker; (5) two ovoid testes side by side in the posterior fifth of the body; (6) absence of cirrus and cirral sac, the seminal vesicle opening within the genital sucker; (7) a subglobose ovary anterior to testes; and (8) vitellaria with large polygonal follicles in the lateral posterior third of the body. The light brown, thick-shelled, operculated eggs, 29 by 16 μ, contain fully developed miracidia at oviposition. The shell has a slight shoulder at the rim of the operculum and sometimes a knob at the posterior pole. They may be differentiated from *Clonorchis* eggs by

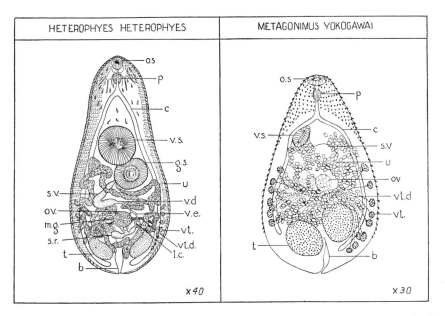

Fig. 88. *Heterophyes heterophyes* and *Metagonimus yokogawai*. b, excretory bladder; c, ceca; g.s., genital sucker; l.c., Laurer's canal; m.g., Mehlis' gland; o.s., oral sucker; ov., ovary; p, pharynx; s.r., seminal receptacle; s.v., seminal vesicle; t, testes; u, uterus; v.d., vas deferens; v.e., vas efferens; v.s., ventral sucker; vt., vitellaria; vt.d., vitelline duct. (*Heterophyes heterophyes* redrawn from Looss, 1894; *Metagonimus yokogawai* redrawn from Leiper, 1913.)

their broad ends with indistinct opercular shoulders and less developed posterior spine, and with greater difficulty from those of *Metagonimus yokogawai,* which have a light-yellow color and a thin shell.

The adult worm inhabits the middle part of the small intestine. It is usually found in the intestinal lumen, but it may be attached to the mucosa between the villi. It apparently obtains its nourishment from the intestinal secretions and contents. The life span is short.

The first intermediate hosts are brackish-water snails, *Pirenella conica* in Egypt and *Cerithidea cingulata microptera* in Japan. The second intermediate hosts are fish, chiefly *Mugil cephalus* (mullet) and *Tilapia nilotica* in Egypt, and *Mugil japonicus* and species of *Acanthogobius* in Japan.

The egg is probably ingested by the snail, in which it develops successively into sporocyst, redia, and cercaria. After leaving the snail the cercaria encysts as a metacercaria in a two-layered cyst on the scales, fins, tail, gills, or, less frequently, in the muscles of susceptible fish. When raw or imperfectly cooked fish is eaten by the definitive host, the metacercaria escapes from the cyst and develops into an adult worm in about a week.

Epidemiology. This parasite is found in Egypt particularly the lower Nile valley, Greece, Israel, Central and South China, Japan, Korea, Taiwan, and the Philippines. There is a high incidence of infection near Port Said, Egypt, where the local fishermen continually pollute the water and a high percentage of mullets are infected. Man acquires the infection by eating raw fresh mullets or fessikh (salted mullets) pickled less than 14 days.

Pathogenicity. Except with heavy infections there is no appreciable mechanical or toxic injury to the intestine, and as a rule no marked symptoms are produced. In heavy infections, irritation of the intestinal mucosa may result in a chronic intermittent mucous diarrhea with colicky pains and abdominal discomfort and tenderness. There is eosinophilia but no anemia. Occasionally, if the worms penetrate the intestinal wall, the eggs may get into the lymphatics or venules and set up granulomatous lesions in such distant foci as heart and brain.

Diagnosis. Diagnosis is made by finding the eggs in the feces. They require differentiation from those of *Clonorchis, Opisthorchis,* and other heterophyid flukes.

Treatment. See Page 128. Tetrachlorethylene, bephenium hydroxynaphthoate, and hexylresorcinol are the drugs of choice.

Prevention. The practical method of preventing human infection is to curtail the practice of eating raw, imperfectly cooked, or recently salted fish in endemic areas. The impossibility of detecting and treating human carriers, the presence of animal reservoir hosts, and the difficulty of enforcing sanitary measures or of destroying the snail hosts renders general control measures impracticable.

Metagonimus yokogawai

Disease. Metagonimiasis.

Life Cycle. The definitive hosts are man, dog, cat, hog, and the pelican and probably other fish-eating birds.

The adult worm (Fig. 88) is identified by: (1) its small size, 1.4 by 0.6 mm; (2) its pyriform shape with a rounded posterior and a tapering anterior end; (3) a cuticle covered with minute scale-like spines more numerous at the anterior end; (4) a large ventral sucker, situated to the right of the midline, with a genital opening at its anterior rim; (5) the two oval testes, obliquely side by side, in the posterior third of the body; (6) the globose ovary at the junction of the middle and lower third of the body; and (7) the coarse vitellaria in a fan-shaped distribution in the posterior lateral fields. The light yellow-brown, thin-shelled operculated eggs, 28 by 17 μ, with nodular thickening on the posterior end, contain at oviposition mature miracidia. They closely resemble the eggs of other heterophyid flukes and differ from those of *Clonorchis sinensis* by having a less distinct opercular groove.

The adult worms inhabit the upper and middle jejunum, rarely the duodenum, ileum, and cecum. They are embedded in the mucus or in the folds of the mucosa. The life span is about 1 year.

The first intermediate snail hosts are species of the genera *Semisulcospira, Thiara,* and *Hua.* The second intermediate hosts are fresh-water salmonoid fishes of the genera *Plecoglossus* and *Salmo,* and the cyprinoids of the genera *Richardsonium (Leuciscus)* and *Odontobutis.*

The egg is probably ingested by the snail, and the miracidium hatches in its intestine. Upon penetration of the tissues the larva develops successively into sporocyst, mother and daughter rediae, and cercariae. The cercaria that emerges from the snail has an elongate, spinous body attenuated anteriorly, and a long tail with dorsoventral flutings. After a short swimming existence, it penetrates an appropriate species of fish, casts off its tail, and encysts in the scales, fins, tail, gills, and, rarely, the muscles. The metacercarial cyst, 140 to 225 μ, has a thin outer hyaline, and a thin inner membranous layer. When ingested by a definitive host, the outer cyst wall is dissolved by the duodenal juices, and the inner membrane is ruptured by the activated larva. The excysted metacercaria becomes an adult worm in 7 to 10 days.

Epidemiology. *M. yokogawai,* the most common heterophyid fluke in the Far East, has been reported in Japan, China, Korea, the Philippines, Taiwan, Siberia, the Balkans, Greece, and Spain.

Since the infection is acquired by man and other mammals by eating raw infected fish, the parasite is common in man in countries where this custom prevails. The waters inhabited by susceptible snails and fish are contaminated by the fecal discharges of man and other mammals.

Pathogenicity. Similar to that of *H. heterophyes.* Occasionally eggs may enter the lymphatics or mesenteric venules and set up granulomatous lesions in such distant foci as the heart and nervous system.

Prognosis. Favorable except in systemic invasion by the eggs.

Diagnosis. Identification of eggs in feces. They are difficult to differentiate from other heterophyid and opisthorchid eggs.

Treatment. See Page 128, *Treatment* for hookworms. The heterophyid flukes are readily expelled by hexylresorcinol, bephenium hydroxynaphthoate, and tetrachlorethylene.

Prevention. Infection may be avoided by eating only thoroughly cooked fish.

Echinostomate Flukes of Man

Species. Some 11 or more echinostomes have been reported in man. A few are natural, and others are incidental human parasites. Most of these species are found in oriental countries. They are discussed here as a group, since they are of minor or only local importance as agents of human disease.

The flukes of the family ECHINOSTOMATIDAE are distinguished from other trematodes by a horse-shoe-shaped collar of spines surrounding the dorsal and lateral sides of the oral sucker. They are elongated, moderate-sized trematodes with slightly tapering rounded extremities. The cuticle bears minute spine-like scales. The more-or-less lobate testes occupy a tandem position in the posterior half of the worm. A cirrus is present. The globular ovary is anterior to the testes. The vitellaria with small follicles usually fill the lateral borders of the posterior two-thirds of the worm. The looped uterus lies anterior to the ovary. At oviposition the large thin-shelled egg contains an undeveloped miracidium.

Life Cycle.   The ovum matures about 3 weeks after leaving the definitive host and the miracidium enters a snail. Apparently the sporocyst stage is abortive, and development takes place directly into mother and daughter rediae and cercariae. The cercariae escape to encyst in snails (even species that serve as first intermediate hosts), fish, or possibly on aquatic vegetation.

Pathogenicity.   It is questionable whether the echinostomes are active pathogens for in spite of the oral circlet of spines, they cause little damage to the intestinal mucosa other than irritation. Heavy infections may produce catarrhal inflammation and even ulceration of the mucosa. Ordinarily, no marked intestinal symptoms are produced. At times children show a clinical syndrome of diarrhea, abdominal pain, anemia, and edema.

Diagnosis.   Diagnosis is made by finding the eggs in the feces. The operculated, ellipsoidal, yellow to yellowish-brown, thin-shelled eggs require differentiation from the undeveloped eggs of other intestinal and biliary flukes. The various echinostome species differ in size of the eggs, although there is some overlapping.

Treatment.   Tetrachlorethylene (See Page 128, *Treatment* for hookworms).

Prevention.   Snails, fish, amphibians, and plants are possible sources of infection. In endemic areas, raw or insufficiently cooked snails or fresh-water fish should not be eaten. Drinking water also should be boiled.

An example of this group is *Euparyphium ilocanum* of the Philippines, Celebes, China, and Java, a fluke 2.5 to 6.5 by 1.1 mm, with 49 to 51 spines on circumoral disc, and eggs 83 to 116 by 53 to 82 μ. Reservoir hosts are the field rat and dog; first intermediate snail host, *Gyraulus;* and second intermediate hosts, snails of the genera *Viviparus* and *Pila,* which are eaten by natives of the Philippines and Java.

Troglotrema salmincola

This is a nonpathogenic incidental parasite of man which is associated with salmon poisoning of dogs in the northwest Pacific Coast of North America and Siberia. The adult fluke has a small pyriform body, 0.9 by 0.4 mm. The suckers are unarmed. The uterus contains usually from 10 to 15 yellowish, broadly oval, operculate, thick-shelled eggs, 70 by 42 μ, with undeveloped miracidia.

The definitive hosts are dogs, cats, and wild fur-bearing mammals; man is an incidental host. The intermediate snail host on the Pacific Coast is *Goniobasis.*

The piscine hosts are species of SALMONIDAE. The eggs hatch 2 to 3 months after leaving the definitive host; the liberated miracidium penetrates a snail, where it develops into sporocyst, rediae, and cercariae, which, when liberated, encyst in the tissues of salmonoid fishes. Man and other mammals are infected by eating raw fish, the excysted metacercaria becoming a mature worm in 5 days or more.

Man manifests no symptoms. The presence of the flukes in dogs, foxes, and coyotes is associated with a local or generalized enteritis due to a rickettsial agent, which can be serially transmitted through the blood. The helminth acts as a reservoir host of *Neorickettsia helmintheca.* Diagnosis is made by finding the eggs in the feces. Thorough cooking of fish will prevent infection.

Gastrodiscoides hominis

G. hominis is found in Assam, Bengal, Malaya, and Vietnam. The natural definitive hosts other than man are hogs and Napu mouse deer.

The reddish, aspinous, dorsally convex worm, 5 to 8 by 3 to 5 mm, is divided into an anterior conical portion and an enlarged posterior disc with a large ventral sucker with a thick overhanging rim. The ceca are relatively short, extending only to the middle of the discoid region. The lobate testes lie in tandem position below the bifurcation of the ceca. There is a tortuous seminal receptacle, a Laurer's canal, and a loosely coiled uterus terminating in the genital cone. The greenish-brown egg, 150 to 170 by 60 to 70 μ, is ovoid with the anterior portion narrow, and the operculum small.

The worm inhabits the cecum and ascending colon. Its life span is unknown.

The egg, unembryonated when passed in the feces, matures in 16 to 17 days at 27° to 34° C. The life cycle is unknown but probably is the same as in other species of GASTRODISCIDAE.

The definitive hosts are mammals; redia, daughter rediae, and cercariae are produced in snails; encystment occurs on aquatic vegetation; and infection takes place by ingestion. The fluke causes mucosal inflammation of the cecum and ascending colon, and may produce diarrhea. Treatment is similar to that for hookworm (Page 128).

Presence of eggs in feces is diagnostic. The eggs resemble those of *Fasciolopsis buski* but are narrower and greenish-brown.

The only known preventive measure in endemic areas is the cooking of vegetables.

A second amphistome fluke has been reported in man. *Watsonius watsoni,* a parasite of monkeys and baboons, has been found once in a West African Negro, who died of a severe diarrhea and toxic inanition. This fluke has a large powerful ventral sucker, the chief cause of trauma to the intestinal mucosa of primates.

LIVER FLUKES

Clonorchis sinensis

The Chinese or oriental liver fluke, *Clonorchis sinensis,* is an important parasite of man in the Far East. The fluke is a parasite of fish-eating mammals and man in Japan, China, South Korea, Formosa, and Vietnam.

Life Cycle (Fig. 89). The natural definitive hosts other than man are the dog, hog, cat, wild cat, martin, badger, mink, and, rarely, ducks. The adult fluke (Fig. 90) is a flat, elongated, aspinous, flabby, opalescent gray worm, tapering anteriorly and somewhat rounded posteriorly. It is identified by: (1) its small variable size, 12 to 20 by 3 to 5 mm; (2) a ventral sucker, smaller than the oral sucker, lying about one-fourth the length of the body from the anterior end; (3) long intestinal ceca extending to the posterior end; (4) deeply lobed testes in tandem formation in the posterior part of the body; (5) a poorly developed

CLONORCHIS SINENSIS

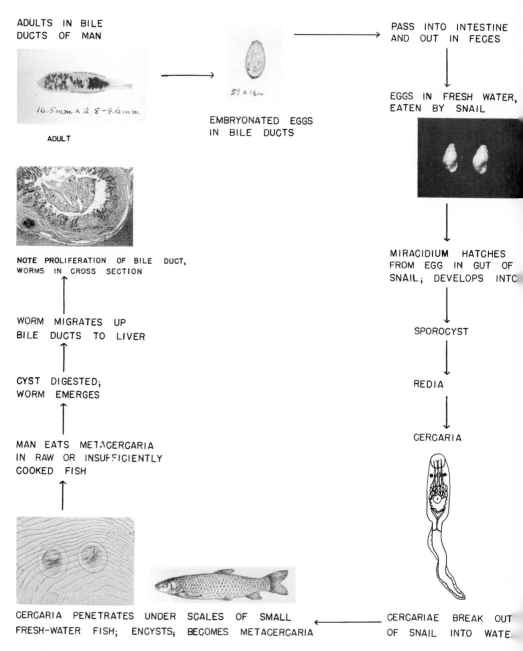

ADULTS IN BILE
DUCTS OF MAN

16.5mm × 2.8-4.6mm

ADULT

29 × 16μ

EMBRYONATED EGGS
IN BILE DUCTS

PASS INTO INTESTINE
AND OUT IN FECES

EGGS IN FRESH WATER,
EATEN BY SNAIL

NOTE PROLIFERATION OF BILE DUCT,
WORMS IN CROSS SECTION

MIRACIDIUM HATCHES
FROM EGG IN GUT OF
SNAIL; DEVELOPS INTO

WORM MIGRATES UP
BILE DUCTS TO LIVER

SPOROCYST

CYST DIGESTED;
WORM EMERGES

REDIA

MAN EATS METACERCARIA
IN RAW OR INSUFFICIENTLY
COOKED FISH

CERCARIA

CERCARIA PENETRATES UNDER SCALES OF SMALL
FRESH-WATER FISH; ENCYSTS, BECOMES METACERCARIA

CERCARIAE BREAK OUT
OF SNAIL INTO WATER

Fig. 89. Life cycle of *Clonorchis sinensis.*

ejaculatory duct without cirrus, cirral sac, or prostatic glands; (6) a small slightly
lobate ovary anterior to the testes in the midline; (7) a loosely coiled uterus end-
ing in the common genital pore; and (8) minutely follicular vitellaria in the
lateral midportion of the body. The light yellowish-brown eggs are 29 by 16 μ.

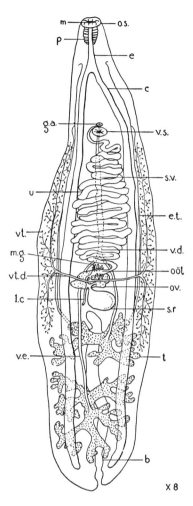

Fig. 90. Schematic representation of morphology of *Clonorchis sinensis*. b, excretory bladder; c, ceca; e, esophagus; e.t., excretory tubules; g.a., genital atrium; l.c., Laurer's canal; m, mouth; m.g., Mehlis' gland; oöt, ootype; o.s., oral sucker; ov., ovary; p, pharynx; s.r., seminal receptacle; s.v., seminal vesicle; t, testes; u, uterus; v.d., vas deferens; v.e., vas efferens; v.s., ventral sucker; vt., vitellaria; vt.d., vitelline duct.

At the smaller end, the operculum rests in a rim with distinct shoulders in such a position that its contour does not follow the curvature of the shell. At the thicker posterior end is a small median protuberance.

The eggs, deposited in the biliary passages of the definitive host, pass from the body in the feces. Although the eggs contain fully developed miracidia, they do not hatch upon reaching water.

The first intermediate hosts are operculate snails of the genera *Alocinma, Bulimus, Parafossarulus, Hua,* and, possibly, *Semisulcospira* and *Thiara.* The miracidium, which has a blunt solid spine on the small head papilla, does not erupt from the shell until the egg is ingested by a suitable snail. In the tissues of the snail it metamorphoses into a sporocyst, rediae, and cercariae. The free-swimming cercaria perishes unless it encounters a fish within 24 to 48 hours. It penetrates beneath the scales and, losing its tail, encysts as an ovoid metaceraria, chiefly in the muscles and subcutaneous tissues, less often in the scales, fins, and gills. The second intermediate hosts are some 40 species of fresh-water fishes belonging to 23 genera of the family CYPRINIDAE. Certain species, especially those cultivated in night-soil-fertilized ponds, are more heavily infected than others; a maximum of 2,900 metacercariae per fish has been reported. The cyst, 138 by 115 μ, has an outer and an inner hyaline wall secreted by the parasite, and a surrounding capsule formed by the tissues of the fish. In the duodenum of man the outer wall is dissolved by trypsin, while the inner layer is ruptured by the activity of the metacercaria. The freed larva migrates to the common bile duct and thence to the distal biliary capillaries, where it becomes a mature worm in 26 to 28 days.

The worm lies unattached in the small branches of the distal portion of the biliary tract. Occasionally in heavy infections, it may be found in the larger bile ducts, the gallbladder, and the pancreatic duct. It is not found in the duodenum, since it can only survive the action of the digestive juices for a few hours. It probably feeds on the secretions of the upper bile ducts. Its life span is 20 to 25 years. The average daily output of eggs per worm in the feces of dogs and cats, though irregular, is 1,100 to 2,400; in guinea pigs 1,600; in rats 330; in man ?

Epidemiology.   Man is usually infected by eating uncooked fish containing infectious metacercariae and, less often, by the ingestion of the cysts in drinking water. The intensity of human infection is dependent upon the eating habits of the population and does not always coincide with the prevalence of the parasite in animal reservoir hosts. In North China, where little or no raw fish is consumed, autochthonous cases comprise only 0.4 percent of the population, although nearly one-third of the dogs and cats are infected. In South China—especially in the Kwangtung Province where raw fish is served in thin slices either with vegetables and condiments or, more often, among the poorer classes by whom it is partially cooked with hot rice congee or gruel—the incidence of human infection is 3 to 36 percent. The rearing of certain fresh-water fish in ponds fertilized by night soil is an important industry in this area, and these fish are largely used in raw-fish food dishes.

We usually associate clonorchiasis with the Oriental race; however, German-Jewish refugees who sojourned in Shanghai for several years before coming to the United States are exhibiting *Clonorchis.* In Shanghai in 1946, some 7,000 of these refugees, whose diet was low in protein, were sold small fish raised on human feces in fresh-water ponds by enterprising Chinese as "herring," a salt-water fish. During the past years we have had several of these patients from the Shanghai epidemic in our medical center, as have others in various parts of the world.

Pathology and Symptomatology.   The distal bile ducts inhabited by *Clonorchis* are irritated mechanically and by its toxic secretions. Early in the infection there is slight leukocytosis and eosinophilia. Depending on the severity of infection, which may run into thousands of worms, the liver may enlarge and become tender. The bile ducts gradually thicken and become dilated and tortuous, and adenomatous proliferation of the biliary epithelium develops. As the disease progresses, fibrosis and destruction of hepatic parenchyma takes place, and liver function is impaired although the SGOT and SGPT are normal.

The relationship between *Clonorchis* infection and the symptoms attributed to it are not entirely clear. Light infections may produce only mild symptoms or go unrecognized. As additional worms are acquired, indigestion, epigastric discomfort unrelated to meals, weakness, and loss of weight become noticeable. In heavy infections anemia, liver enlargement, slight jaundice, edema, ascites, and diarrhea develop. Tachycardia, palpitation, vertigo, and mental depression may ensue. Patients seldom die of clonorchiasis, but because of lowered resistance they may succumb to superimposed diseases. With mild infections the prognosis is usually good even without treatment. With prolonged or heavy infections in highly endemic regions, the outcome is unsatisfactory and depends upon the degree of impairment of the liver.

Diagnosis.   Clinical diagnosis is suggestive in patients with an enlarged liver and symptoms of hepatitis in endemic areas where uncooked fish is eaten. Advanced infections require differentiation from malignancy, cirrhosis of the liver, or other causes of hepatic enlargement. Absolute diagnosis is based on finding the characteristic eggs in the feces or biliary drainage. The eggs require differentiation from those of other opisthorchid and heterophyid flukes.

Treatment.   Treatment is not satisfactory, especially in chronic or heavy infections. Chloroquine (See Page 34, *Treatment* for *Entamoeba histolytica*) after repeated courses has resulted in some cures and has reduced the output of eggs. Various dosages from 0.5 to 1.5 g per day to a total of 21 g have been employed. Gentian violet, given orally, 65 mg three times a day for 30 days, has cured light infections, relieved symptoms, and reduced the number of worms, but the complete destruction of all worms is seldom attained.

Prevention.   The thorough cooking of fish would practically eliminate the disease in man. This depends upon the education of the housewives and those serving raw fish in restaurants—a difficult task. Metacercariae are not killed by refrigeration, salting, or the addition of vinegar or sauce. Reduction of sources of infection is impossible because of animal reservoir hosts. Sterilization of human feces may be effected by storage or by the addition of ammonium sulfate; the curtailment of night soil for fertilizing fish ponds is not economically feasible; and molluscacides capable of destroying the snails may destroy fish and other aquatic life.

Opisthorchis felineus

O. felineus is prevalent in dogs, cats, foxes, and hogs in eastern and southeastern Europe and Asiatic U.S.S.R. In the highly endemic areas of Poland and the Dnieper, Donetz, and Desna Basins, it is also found in man.

O. felineus (Fig. 91), 7 to 12 by 1.5 to 3.0 mm, resembles *Clonorchis sinensis*. The eggs 30 by 12 μ, resemble those of *C. sinensis* but are narrower and have more tapering ends, a pointed terminal knob, and a less conspicuous opercular rim. Its habitat is the distal bile ducts, occasionally the pancreatic duct. The life span is probably several years.

The first intermediate hosts are the snails *Bulimus*. The second intermediate hosts are numerous species of cyprinoid fishes, of which the chub and the tench are infected most frequently. The egg, which contains a miracidium, does not hatch until ingested by a snail, in the digestive gland of which sporocysts and rediae develop. The cercariae leave the snail in about 2 months, encyst in a suitable species of fish, and become infective metacercariae. When ingested by a definitive host, they excyst in the duodenum and pass to the distal bile ducts, where they reach maturity in 3 to 4 weeks.

The infection is acquired by eating raw or insufficiently cooked fish. Cats appear to be the most important reservoir hosts in highly endemic areas. Intermediate snail hosts are infected by feces deposited on sandy shores and washed into streams.

Pathology, prognosis, and treatment are similar to those for *Clonorchis*. Presence of characteristic eggs in feces or duodenal drainage is diagnostic. The infection may be prevented by cooking fish and sanitary excreta disposal.

Opisthorchis viverrini

This fluke is found in Thailand and Laos in southeastern Asia. In general it is similar to *O. felineus* (Fig. 91). The egg is 26 by 13 μ and closely resembles that of *C. sinensis*.

The definitive hosts other than man are the civet cat, cat, dog, and other fish-eating mammals. Intermediate hosts are snails and several species of fish.

The disease is acquired by eating uncooked fish containing the infective metacercariae.

The hepatic lesions are similar to those of *C. sinensis*. At autopsies of patients

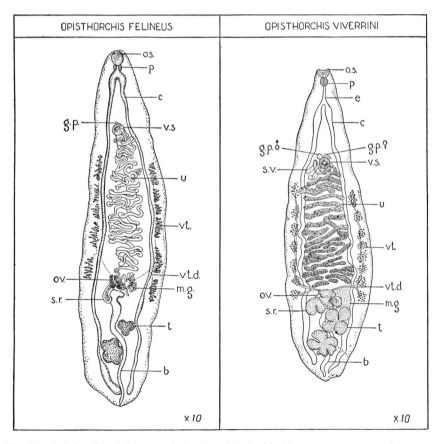

Fig. 91. *Opisthorchis felineus* and *O. viverrini*. b, bladder; c, ceca; e, esophagus; g.p., genital pore; m.g., Mehlis' gland; o.s., oral sucker; ov., ovary; p, pharynx; s.r., seminal receptacle; s.v., seminal vesicle; t, testes; u, uterus; v.s., ventral sucker; vt., vitellaria; vt.d., vitelline duct. (*O. felineus* redrawn from Stiles and Hassall, 1894; *O. viverrini* redrawn from Leiper, 1915.)

infected with 1,000 to 6,000 worms, the findings comprised: enlarged liver, marked dilatation of bile ducts, numerous worms in yellowish fluid in lumens of ducts, thickening of walls of ducts, increase of portal connective tissue, atrophy of liver cells, and, in two cases, papillary adenomatous carcinoma. The early symptoms in these patients included: loss of appetite, dyspepsia and flatulence, anorexia, epigastric discomfort and pain, and, sometimes, leukocytosis and fever. Later there was an enlarged painful liver, transient jaundice and urticaria, watery diarrhea, weakness, and anemia. There was no marked eosinophilia.

Diagnosis is made by finding eggs in feces or duodenal drainage.

Treatment.   See above. Similar to that of *Clonorchis*. The disease may be prevented by eating only cooked fish.

Fasciola hepatica

Disease.   Fascioliasis, "liver rot."

Morphology.   *F. hepatica* (Fig. 92) is identified by: (1) its large size, 20 to 30 by 8 to 13 mm; (2) its flat, leaf shape with characteristic shouldered appearance due to its cephalic cone; (3) oral and ventral suckers of equal size on

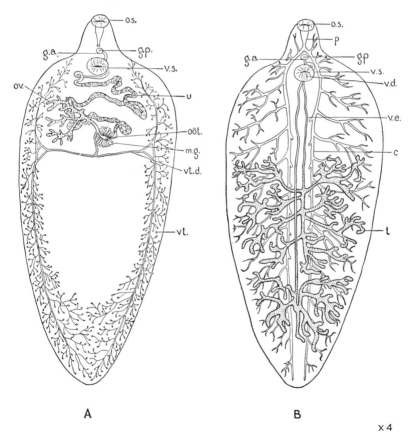

Fig. 92. Schematic representation of morphology of *Fasciola hepatica*. A, female reproductive organs, ventral view; B, male reproductive organs and digestive tract, ventral view.

c, ceca; g.a., genital atrium; g.p., genital pore; m.g., Mehlis' gland; oöt., ootype; o.s., oral sucker; ov., ovary; p, pharynx; t, testes; u, uterus; v.d., vas deferens; v.e., vas efferens; v.s., ventral sucker; vt., vitellaria; vtd., vitelline duct. (Adapted from Sommer, 1880, and from Leuckart, 1863.)

cephalic cone; (4) intestine with numerous diverticula; (5) highly dendritic testes in tandem formation; (6) diffusely branched vitellaria in lateral and posterior portions of body; and (7) short convoluted uterus. The large, oval, yellowish-brown, operculated eggs, 130 to 150 by 63 to 90 μ (Fig. 84A) are unsegmented at oviposition.

The adult inhabits the proximal bile passages, gallbladder, and, occasionally, ectopic sites. It has an anaerobic metabolism and obtains its nourishment from the biliary secretions. The life span is at least 10 years.

Life Cycle. The fluke is a parasite of sheep, cattle, deer, and rabbits, as well as other herbivorous mammals. Its intermediate hosts are some 21 species of lymneid snails, of which *Lymnaea truncatula,* a snail that inhabits transitory bodies of water and sluggish brooks, is the most important. In the snail it metamorphoses into a sporocyst, rediae, at times daughter rediae, and cercariae (Fig. 84D–J). The latter emerge from the snail and encyst on grasses, watercress, bark, or soil (Fig. 84K). When ingested by definitive hosts the metacercariae (Fig. 84L) pass through the intestinal wall, eventually penetrating the liver capsule, and migrate to the biliary tree consuming liver parenchyma en route. They mature in 12 weeks.

Epidemiology. This fluke is cosmopolitan throughout the sheep- and cattle-raising countries of the world. Human infection is frequent in Cuba, southern France, Great Britain, and Algeria. One human infection has been reported from California. An adult worm was found in an intestinal nodule in a woman who had lived in New York State all of her life, except for a visit to Hawaii, where it is common (Fig. 93). It is common in animals in the United States.

Man contracts the disease by ingesting plants such as watercress or possibly water containing the encysted metacercariae. Herbivorous or omnivorous animals acquire the infection in low, damp pastures where the vegetation is infested with metacercariae.

Pathology and Symptomatology. The extent of the damage and symptomatology depend upon the intensity of the infection and the duration of the disease. A single fluke can produce severe symptoms by biliary obstruction. Due to pressure, toxic metabolic products, and feeding habits the worms provoke inflammatory, adenomatous, and fibrotic changes of the biliary tract. Parenchymal atrophy and periportal cirrhosis develop. Severe headache, chills, fever, urticaria, a stabbing substernal pain, and right upper quadrant pains that radiate to the back and shoulders may be the first evidence of infection. As the infection progresses,

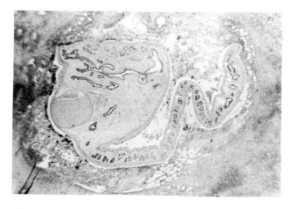

Fig. 93. Section of intestinal nodule showing *Fasciola* adult.

an enlarged tender liver, jaundice, digestive disturbances, diarrhea, and anemia develop. Animal experiments indicate each adult worm consumes 0.2 ml of blood per day. The erythrocyte sedimentation rate may be elevated, and there is usually marked eosinophilia early in the infection with or without leukocytosis.

Young worms migrating to the liver may produce ectopic lesions in the intestinal wall, heart, orbit, lungs, and subcutaneous tissues. In the Near East the laryngopharyngitis, known as halzoun, may be caused by adolescent *F. hepatica* consumed in raw liver, which attach themselves to the pharyngeal mucosa. Recent attempts to produce halzoun (with liver grossly infected with *F. hepatica* or *Dicrocoelium dendriticum*) in 94 volunteers all failed.

Diagnosis.   Clinical diagnosis is difficult because of multiplicity of symptoms, but an enlarged tender liver and a febrile eosinophilic syndrome are suggestive. Laboratory diagnosis is based on finding the characteristic eggs in the feces or bile. Eggs may be found in the stools of patients eating infected liver, leading to false diagnoses. Positive complement-fixation test and intracutaneous reactions have been obtained with *Fasciola* antigens in infected and clinically cured persons, and these tests are useful in extrahepatic infections or when direct examination fails to reveal the eggs.

Treatment.   Several patients infected with *Fasciola* have been treated successfully with dichlorophenol (Bithionol). Emetine (See Page 34, *Treatment* for *Entamoeba histolytica*), 0.030 g (½ grain) daily for 18 days, has given symptomatic relief and caused the disappearance of the eggs from the feces and bile. In animals carbon tetrachloride and oleoresin of aspidium destroy the adult flukes, but do not kill the immature worms in the small bile ducts.

Prevention.   Long-range control is dependent upon the eradication of the disease in herbivorous animals. Treatment is possible for domesticated animals, but not for wild animals. The destruction of snails and the larval parasites is difficult. Infection in man in endemic areas may be prevented by eliminating raw watercress and other uncooked green vegetation from the diet.

Fasciola gigantica

F. gigantica is a parasite of cattle, water buffalo, camels, wild hogs, and other herbivora in Africa, Asia, and Hawaii. The adult worm is distinguished from *F. hepatica* by its greater length, shorter cephalic cone, larger ventral sucker, more anterior position of the reproductive organs, and larger eggs (150 to 190 by 70 to 90 μ). The life cycle is similar to that of *F. hepatica,* with a snail intermediate host and encystment of the cercariae on water plants. The liver is the primary site of the adult worm, and the damage to this organ and the symptoms produced are similar to those of *F. hepatica*. In Hawaii man is infected from eating watercress or other vegetation contaminated with metacercariae or by drinking water from streams containing floating metacercariae. In cattle of Hawaii both species of flukes are present. Raw watercress and other contaminated vegetation should not be eaten in areas where the parasite is endemic.

Dicrocoelium dendriticum

D. dendriticum has a cosmopolitan distribution in sheep and other herbivora in Asia, Africa, Europe, and North and South America. Sporadic cases of human infection, less than 100, have been reported from 12 countries in Europe, Asia, and Africa.

The fluke is identified by: (1) its slender, lancet-shaped, flat, aspinous body, 5 to 15 by 1.5 to 2.5 mm; (2) two large, slightly lobed testes situated obliquely to each other anterior to the small subglobose ovary; and (3) voluminous uterine coils in the posterior two-thirds of the worm. The dark brown, thick-shelled, operculated egg, 38 to 45 by 22 to 30 μ, contains a fully developed miracidium.

The principal definitive host is the sheep. The first intermediate hosts are the land snails of the genera *Abida, Cochlicella, Helicella,* and *Zebrina,* which eat the fluke's eggs.

The egg hatches in the intestine of the snail, and the miracidium metamorphoses into two generations of sporocysts and cercariae. The latter agglomerate in groups of 200 to 300 in slime balls of secreted material in the respiratory chamber of the snail. The crawling snails shed these slime balls on vegetation, where they are ingested by the foraging ant *Formica fusca,* and in which the cercariae encysts, becoming a metacercariae. When the ant is ingested by the definitive host the excysted metacercariae penetrate the intestinal wall and reach the liver and bile ducts probably by the portal system.

The pathology and symptoms are similar to those of *Fasciola hepatica.* In animals the parasite causes enlargement of the bile ducts, hyperplasia of the biliary epithelium, formation of periductal fibrous connective tissue, atrophy of the liver cells, and finally, in heavy infections, portal cirrhosis. The hepatic changes are less pronounced in man, in whom the infection is usually light. The symptoms in man include digestive disturbances, flatulence, vomiting, biliary colic, chronic constipation or diarrhea, and a toxemia less pronounced than in fascioliasis.

Diagnosis is made by finding the eggs consistently in the feces and eliminating spurious infections from eating livers containing the eggs. (See *Clonorchis,* Page 225, for treatment.) There are no effective measures of control.

PULMONARY FLUKES

Paragonimus westermani

Disease. Paragonimiasis, pulmonary distomiasis.

Life Cycle (Fig. 94). The definitive hosts, other than man, are domesticated and wild mammals.

P. westermani is a reddish-brown fluke identified by: (1) its size, 8 to 16 by 4 to 8 mm; (2) its shape when active resembling a spoon with one end contracted and the other elongated, and when contracted or preserved an oval, flattened coffee bean; (3) spinous cuticle; (4) suckers of equal size, the ventral just anterior to the equatorial plane; (5) irregularly lobed testes, oblique to each other, in posterior third of worm; (6) lobed ovary anterior to testes on right side opposite closely coiled uterus; and (7) vitellaria in extreme lateral fields for entire length of body. The oval, yellowish-brown, thick-shelled egg 85 by 55 μ, has a thickened opercular rim and is unembryonated at oviposition.

The first intermediate hosts are operculated snails of the genera *Hua, Semisulcospira, Syncera,* and *Thiara* in the Far East; *Pomatiopsis* in North America; and possibly *Pomacea* in South America. The second intermediate hosts are the fresh-water crabs of the genera *Eriocheir, Potamon, Sesarma,* and *Parathelphusa* in the Far East, and *Pseudothelphusa* in South America; and crayfishes of the genus *Astacus* in the Far East and *Cambarus* in North America and probably elsewhere.

PARAGONIMUS WESTERMANI

ADULT IN LUNGS OF MAN

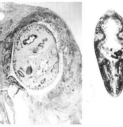

→

UNDEVELOPED EGGS
PASSED IN SPUTUM OR
FECES INTO FRESH WATER

→

MIRACIDIUM HATCHES FROM
EGG; PENETRATES SNAIL

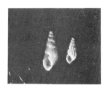

↑

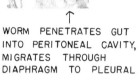

WORM PENETRATES GUT
INTO PERITONEAL CAVITY,
MIGRATES THROUGH
DIAPHRAGM TO PLEURAL
CAVITY AND LUNGS

MIRACIDIUM IN SNAIL
DEVELOPS INTO:

↓

SPOROCYST
↓
REDIA I
↓
REDIA II

↓

CERCARIA BREAKS OUT
OF REDIA AND SNAIL
INTO WATER

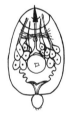

MAN EATS METACERCARIA
IN RAW OR INSUFFICIENTLY
COOKED RIVER CRABS
OR CRAYFISH

↑

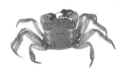

PENETRATES GILLS,
MUSCLES OR VISCERA
OF FRESH-WATER CRUSTACEAN;
ENCYSTS; BECOMES
METACERCARIA

←

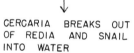

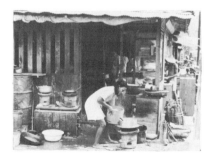

FAR EASTERN STREET RESTAURANT

Fig. 94. Life cycle of *Paragonimus westermani*.

231

The eggs that escape from the ruptured pulmonary cysts leave the host via the sputum or, if swallowed, the feces. Development usually takes place in about 3 weeks at an optimal temperature of 27° C. The free-swimming miracidium cannot survive over 24 hours unless it penetrates a suitable snail, in which it develops into a sporocyst. The first generation rediae, in the snail, migrate to the lymph sinuses near the liver and produce daughter rediae, which in turn yield cercariae that emerge from the snail about 13 weeks after infection. They perish in 24 to 48 hours unless they penetrate a fresh-water crab or crayfish in which they encyst in the gills, legs, body muscles, and viscera as metacercariae, 250 to 500 μ in size. The crustacean also may become infected by eating the snails. One crab may harbor 3,000 metacercariae. After ingestion by the mammalian host the excysted metacercariae pass through the duodenal wall into the abdominal cavity. The adolescent worms burrow through the diaphragm, enter the pleural cavity, and in about 20 days reach the lungs, where in cystic cavities near the bronchi they become adult worms in 5 to 6 weeks. During this prolonged migration, the adolescent worms may remain for long periods in the peritoneum, may enter and leave the liver, and may become lodged in other organs than the lungs—so-called ectopic lesions.

Epidemiology.   *P. westermani* has a cosmopolitan distribution among mammals, but its presence in man is chiefly confined to the Far East. The principal endemic regions are in Japan, South Korea, Thailand, Taiwan, China, and the Philippines. Human infections also have been reported in South and Southeast Asia, Indonesia, islands of the South Pacific, and northern South America. The African *Paragonimus* is possibly a different species. Only one autochthonous case in man has been reported in North America, although *P. kellicotti* has been found in mammals in 10 or more states of the United States.

Man is infected by eating uncooked infected fresh-water crabs and crayfish. It is customary in the Orient to consume these uncooked crustaceans in brine, vinegar, or wine as "drunken crabs," in which the metacercariae may survive several hours. Also, metacercariae, dislodged during food preparation, may contaminate eating and cooking utensils. Crushed crayfish juice, taken orally and used in the treatment of measles in Korea, may be a source of infection in children.

Metacercariae are killed if the crabs are roasted until the muscles turn white or if they are heated in water at 55° C for 5 minutes.

Pathology and Symptomatology.   In the lungs, *Paragonimus* provokes the development by the host of a fibrous tissue capsule. Within this cyst is blood-tinged, purulent material containing eggs. Surrounding the cyst is an infiltrated area. The onset of symptoms is usually insidious: a dry cough at first, and later production of blood-stained, rusty-brown tenacious sputum most pronounced on rising in the morning. Pulmonary pain and pleurisy may be present, and hemoptysis may occur. These signs and symptoms along with a low-grade fever and non-diagnostic x-rays make it difficult to separate this infection from tuberculosis, pneumonia, or bronchiectasis.

Aberrant worms, with cyst formation, may localize in the abdominal wall, abdominal cavity, mesenteric lymph nodes, omentum, and intestinal wall; they may produce abdominal pain, rigidity, and tenderness. Eggs from the worms in the intestinal wall may be found in the stool and be accompanied by diarrhea and blood. In the brain the worms may cause Jacksonian epilepsy, hemiplegia, monoplegia, paresis of various degrees, and visual disturbances. Worms stituated in the subcutaneous tissues cause creeping tumors.

Prognosis is good with light infections, with spontaneous cure and death of the worm in 5 to 6 years. It is unfavorable in heavy pulmonary infections and patients with cerebral involvement. Superimposed tuberculosis and pyogenic infection are especially serious.

Diagnosis. Pulmonary symptoms, blood-tinged sputum, and eosinophilia in patients in endemic regions are suggestive. At times the x-rays aid in diagnosis, although it is difficult to differentiate paragonimiasis from tuberculosis, which is common in areas where *Paragonimus* is endemic. A typical roentgenographic finding is a ring-shadowed opacity, 5 to 10 cm, comprising several small contiguous cavities that give the appearance of a bunch of currants.

Definite diagnosis is established by finding the eggs in the sputum, feces (from swallowed sputum or intestinal lesions), or less frequently in aspirated material from abscesses or pleural effusions. Although eggs are usually present in the sputum, in Taiwan the eggs were found more frequently in the stool. In Korea more than 20 sputum samples of some patients were examined before eggs were detected. At times the adult worm is found at exploratory operation. In ectopic infections, in deep foci with no eggs excreted, complement fixation and intradermal tests with a *Paragonimus* antigen have been used.

Treatment. See Page 34, *Treatment* for *Entamoeba histolytica*. Chloroquine, in adult doses of 0.75 g per day to a total of 40 g is curative in some infections and of clinical value in others. Bithionol, thiobis-dichlorophenol, orally, 40 mg/kg body weight, every other day for 10 to 15 days, gave a cure rate of 90 percent of 1,315 persons treated. Side reactions consisted of diarrhea 30 percent, rash 13 percent and abdominal pain 11 percent.

Prevention. The most practical method of preventing human infection is to avoid eating raw, freshly pickled, or imperfectly cooked fresh-water crustaceans, and to refrain from drinking unfiltered or unboiled river water in endemic districts. The best line of attack is public education, since the elimination of reservoir hosts, crustaceans, and snails is not feasible.

13

Blood Flukes of Man

SCHISTOSOMIASIS, BILHARZIASIS

The blood flukes, the most important digenetic trematodes of man, include three important species: *Schistosoma haematobium,* an inhabitant of the vesical veins; *S. mansoni;* and *S. japonicum* of the intestinal veins.

BIOLOGY OF SCHISTOSOMES OF MAN

Morphology.   The schistosomes differ from the typical trematodes in their narrow elongated shape and separate sexes. The distinctive morphologic characteristics of the three species are given in Figure 95. The larger grayish male has a cylindrical anterior end, and its heavier body is folded to form a long ventral gynecophoric canal in which the darker slender female is embraced during copulation (Fig. 95). The integument is smooth or tuberculated, depending upon the species. The intestine bifurcates into two ceca, which unite in the posterior part of the body in a single blind stem. The number of testes in the male, and the length of the uterus and number of eggs, are distinctive for the species. The excretory system consists of flame cells, collecting tubules, and two long tubules leading into a small bladder with a terminal excretory pore.

Life Cycle (Fig. 96).   The delicate adult worms, which are 0.6 to 2.5 cm in length, reside in pairs, the female lying in the gynecophoric canal of the male. Depending upon the species of worm, from 300 (*S. mansoni*) to 3,500 (*S. japonicum*) eggs are passed daily into the venules. A larval form, miracidium, develops within the egg; its lytic enzymes and the contraction of the venule rupture the wall of the venule, liberating the egg into the perivascular tissues of the intestine or urinary bladder. The eggs effect a passage into the lumens of these organs and are evacuated in the feces or the urine. On contact with fresh water the miracidia hatch from the eggs and swim about until they find an appropriate snail, which they penetrate. After two generations of sporocyst development and multiplication within the snail, the forked-tailed cercariae emerge. During bathing, swimming, working, or washing clothes, the skin of man comes in contact with free-swimming cercariae, which become attached and burrow down to the peripheral capillary bed as the surface film of water drains off. If ingested with water, the cercariae penetrate the mucous membranes of the mouth and throat. The cercariae are transported through the afferent blood to the right heart and lungs. They squeeze through the pulmonary capillaries, are carried into the systemic circulation, and pass through to the portal vessels. Within the intrahepatic portion of the portal system, the blood flukes

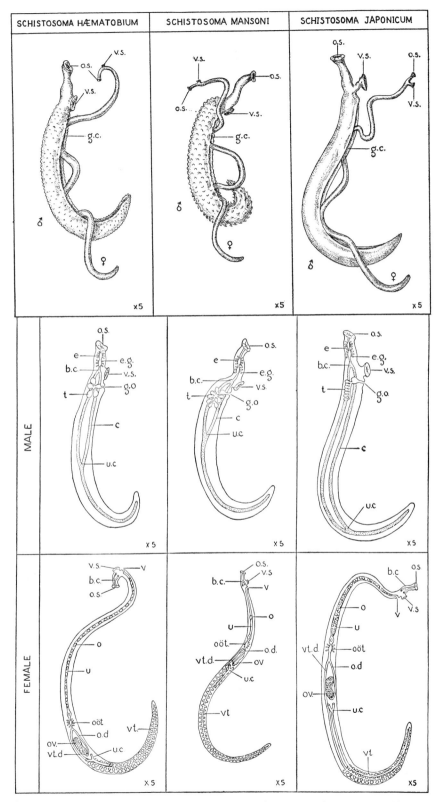

Fig. 95. Schematic representation of important schistosomes of man. b.c., bifurcation of ceca; c., ceca; e., esophagus; e.g., esophageal glands; g.c., gynecophoric canal; g.o., genital orifice; o, eggs; o.d., oviduct oöt., ootype; o.s., oral sucker; ov., ovary; t, testes; u, uterus; u.c., union of ceca; v, vulva; v.s., ventral sucker; vt., vitellaria; vt.d., vitelline duct.

SCHISTOSOMA MANSONI

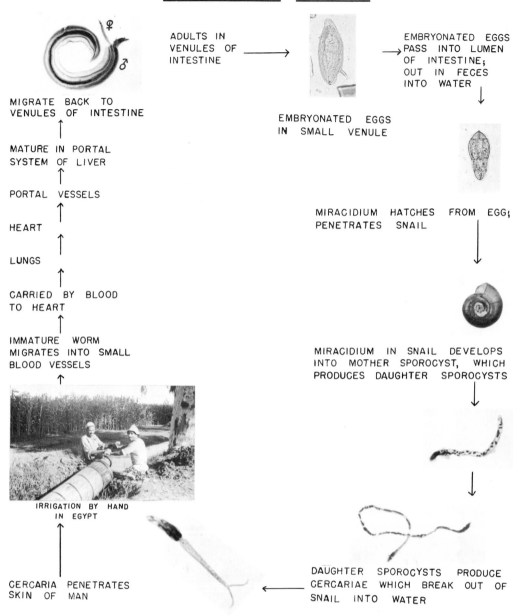

ADULTS IN
VENULES OF
INTESTINE

EMBRYONATED EGGS
PASS INTO LUMEN
OF INTESTINE;
OUT IN FECES
INTO WATER

EMBRYONATED EGGS
IN SMALL VENULE

MIGRATE BACK TO
VENULES OF INTESTINE

MATURE IN PORTAL
SYSTEM OF LIVER

PORTAL VESSELS

HEART

LUNGS

CARRIED BY BLOOD
TO HEART

IMMATURE WORM
MIGRATES INTO SMALL
BLOOD VESSELS

MIRACIDIUM HATCHES FROM EGG;
PENETRATES SNAIL

MIRACIDIUM IN SNAIL DEVELOPS
INTO MOTHER SPOROCYST, WHICH
PRODUCES DAUGHTER SPOROCYSTS

IRRIGATION BY HAND
IN EGYPT

CERCARIA PENETRATES
SKIN OF MAN

DAUGHTER SPOROCYSTS PRODUCE
CERCARIAE WHICH BREAK OUT OF
SNAIL INTO WATER

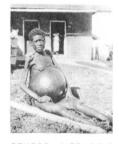

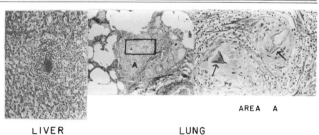

SEVERE CIRRHOSIS
WITH ASCITES

LIVER   LUNG

AREA A

EGGS STIMULATING FORMATION OF PSEUDOTUBERCLES

Fig. 96. Life cycle of *Schistosoma mansoni.*

feed and grow rapidly. Approximately 3 weeks after skin exposure, the adolescent worms migrate against the portal blood flow into the mesenteric, vesical, and pelvic venules. The prepatent period for *S. mansoni* is 7 to 8 weeks, *S. haematobium* 10 to 12 weeks, and *S. japonicum* 5 to 6 weeks. The adult worms live as long as 30 years in man.

Man is the principal host of the three species of human schistosomes, but these flukes differ in their other mammalian hosts. *S. haematobium* and *S. mansoni* have been found in monkeys and baboons, and *S. mansoni* has also been found in rodents and opossums. *S. japonicum* has a wide range of reservoir hosts: natural infections have been reported in dogs, cats, cattle, water buffalo, horses, hogs, sheep, goats, wild rats, and other rodents.

Response of the Host.   Schistosomiasis in man may be divided into 3 stages: (1) developmental, from the penetration of the skin to the mature adult worms; (2) active oviposition and extrusion of eggs; and (3) proliferation and repair. The lesions produced by the three species are similar during the first period, but during the overlapping second and third stages differ chiefly in tissue selectivity and site of oviposition.

The pathologic changes during the developmental period include negligible to mild cutaneous lesions at the site of cercarial entry, tissue reactions to the immature worms inside and outside of the blood vessels, and associated toxic and allergic reactions. The invasion of the tissues by the migrating larval and adolescent worms produces petechial hemorrhages and small foci of eosinophilic and neutrophilic infiltration in the lungs and other organs, and inflammatory reactions in the liver.

The eruption of the eggs through the vascular endothelium is brought about by enzymic secretions, pressure, and an endothelial or subendothelial inflammatory reaction. In the vascular endothelium, perivascular tissues, and parenchyma of the various organs, the eggs produce multiple foci of inflammatory cellular infiltration that develop into granulomas or non-necrotizing pseudotubercles. The fundamental histopathologic unit is the pseudotubercle (Fig. 101), which consists of a layer of epithelioid cells, fibroblasts, and giant cells surrounded by a zone of plasma cells and eosinophils. In addition to the usual selective intestinal and urinary bladder sites, the eggs usually are distributed elsewhere in the body. Often the eggs of *S. mansoni* and *S. japonicum,* when deposited in the larger mesenteric veins, are swept into the intrahepatic portal vessels to evoke pseudotubercle formation in the liver and lungs. The eggs of *S. haematobium* may be carried from the vesical plexus to the inferior vena cava, and ultimately reach the pulmonary arterioles and, occasionally, the liver. At times the eggs of the three species may be distributed to the skin, heart, central nervous system, and other organs. The adult worms may be similarly distributed but the live worms cause only slight inflammation. The dead worms, which are often swept back into the liver, evoke a marked inflammatory reaction that produces complete or partial fibrosis of the walls of the blood vessels.

Diagnosis.   In endemic areas schistosomiasis may be suspected in the developmental stage by a petechial cutaneous eruption, toxic and allergic manifestations, and hepatic and pulmonary disorders. In the advanced ovipositing stage vesical schistosomiasis may be recognized by urinary signs and symptoms, cystoscopic examination, and intravenous pyelography; and intestinal schistosomiasis by diarrheic or dysenteric symptoms and sigmoidoscopic examination. Occasionally, pul-

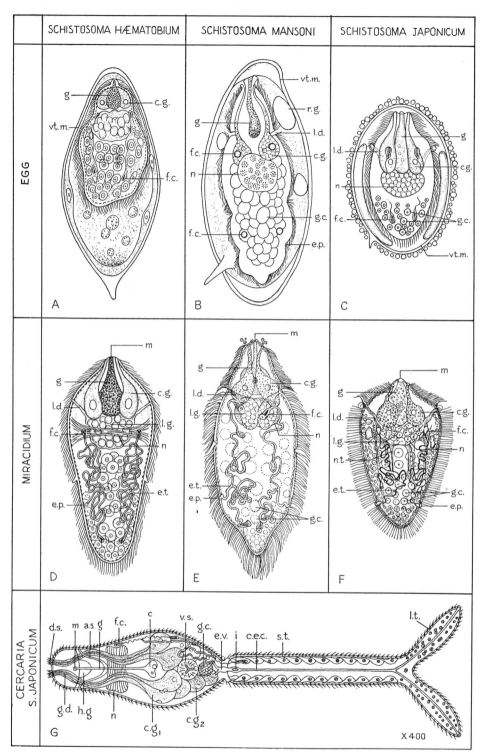

Fig. 97. Egg, miracidium, and cercaria of the schistosomes of man. a.s., anterior sucker; c. cecum; c.e.c., caudal excretory canal; c.g., c.g.1, c.g.2, cephalic glands; d.s., duct spines; e.p., excretory pore; e.t., excretory tubule; e.v., excretory vesicle; f.c., flame cell; g, gut; g.c., germinal cells; g.d., gland ducts; h.g., head gland; i, island of Cort; l.d., lateral duct; l.g., lateral gland; l.t., lobe of tail; m, mouth; n, nervous system; n.t., nerve trunk; r.g., refractile globule; s.t., stem of tail; v.s., ventral sucker; vt.m., vitelline membrane.

238

monary schistosomiasis may be detected by roentgenography. As splenomegaly and cirrhosis of the liver develop, there is evidence of liver cell damage, and some of the liver function tests become significantly positive. Eosinophilia, while helpful, is not consistent.

STOOL EXAMINATION. Eggs may be few in number owing to a light infection, the intermittency of their discharge, or a chronic infection. If a simple smear is negative, concentration by sedimentation should be employed. A whole stool should be thoroughly broken up in 0.5 percent glycerol water and, after sedimentation in a conical glass, the supernatant fluid poured off. Mixing and decanting should be repeated until only a small residue remains, which should be examined microscopically for eggs.

OTHER METHODS. The eggs are identified in the urine by direct examination of the last few drops of urine passed at noon, or in the urine after exercise or prostatic massage. A simple concentration test for diagnosis is sedimentation in a conical urinalysis glass of a day's output of urine. The addition of water, previously heated to $60°$ C to kill any infusoria, to the sediment permits the hatched free-swimming miracidia to be detected by indirect lighting against a black background. The hatching of miracidia furnishes an index of the viable eggs.

AS SCHISTOSOME EGGS MAY BE FEW IN NUMBER, LARGE QUANTITIES OF URINE AND STOOL MUST BE SEDIMENTED. THESE ARE TWO PRODUCTS THAT THE PATIENT CAN SUPPLY ABUNDANTLY AND FREE. THE EXAMINATION OF A SMALL SPECIMEN MAY GIVE INACCURATELY NEGATIVE RESULTS.

Biopsies by sigmoidoscopic or cystoscopic methods or hepatic puncture often yield eggs when the urine and feces examinations are negative. These mucosal snips, unfixed and unstained, should be pressed between two glass microscope slides and examined for eggs under the low power of the microscope. Occasionally, when eggs cannot be found in the feces or rectal mucosa, a liver biopsy may reveal their presence.

All eggs from the feces, urine, or tissues should be examined under high power to determine their viability by the activity of the cilia of the excretory "flame-cell" of the enclosed miracidium. Dead eggs may persist for a long time after successful therapy or natural death of the worms, and their presence should not lead to further therapy.

Various serologic and intradermal tests are useful, and, when positive should stimulate a thorough search for eggs. Various animal schistosomes which temporarily invade man may cause falsely positive results. The complement fixation test remains positive at least 4 years after chemotherapeutic cure.

Treatment. Nutritional therapy and correction of anemia are indicated, and the patient should be brought to a satisfactory physical state before being subjected to the rigors of chemotherapy. Animal experiments and clinical findings in man indicate that good nutrition is protective against the damage of the schistosomes.

Potassium and sodium antimony tartrate, when given in full dosage intravenously on a regular schedule, are highly effective. They are most effective in *S. haematobium* infections and least in *S. japonicum* infections. Their disadvantages are intravenous administration, lengthy treatment causing defaulting on the part of the patient, and high toxicity from long treatment. They inhibit the activity of the phosphofructokinase reaction which controls the rate of glycolysis of the worm.

Potassium antimony tartrate (tartar emetic) is an inexpensive, stable trivalent antimony compound with an antimony content of about 36 percent. It is administered slowly, intravenously, in a freshly prepared 0.5 percent solution in fresh distilled water or 5 percent glucose. In schistosomiasis the initial dose of 0.06 g is increased by the third dose to a maximum of 0.14 g, which is continued every other day to a total of 2.2 g. Nausea, vomiting, diarrhea, abdominal colic, dizziness, fainting, brachycardia, edema, prostration, joint pains, hypotension, electrocardiographic changes, dyspnea, occasional jaundice, and collapse may occur. It is contraindicated in febrile, cardiac, respiratory, renal, and hepatic diseases.

Sodium antimony tartrate (antimonyl sodium tartrate) is a trivalent antimony compound, with an antimony content of about 37 percent. It is used for schistosomiasis in a dosage similar to the potassium compound.

These agents should be given 2 hours after a light meal, and the patient should remain recumbent for an hour.

Stibophen (Fuadin, Neoantimosan, Reprodal, Fantorin) is antimony pyrocatechin sodium disulfonate, a trivalent antimony compound with an antimony content of 14 percent; it is administered intramuscularly. This drug is supplied in ampules of 5 ml of a 6.3 percent solution. The course of treatment for adults consists of 15 injections of 5 ml on alternate days, starting with 1.5 ml and 3.5 ml on the first two injections, a total of 80 ml. Children are given a total dose of 1.0 ml per pound of weight in 17 injections. A high cure rate is achieved in *S. haematobium* and *S. mansoni* infections. Nausea, vomiting, and joint pain are common. This drug is preferred to tartar emetic because of its intramuscular administration and somewhat less severe side effects, although sensitization to it may lead to serious hemolysis.

Antimony dimercaptosuccinate (Astiban) has been introduced recently and has the advantage that the course of intramuscular injections is only 4 or 5 days.

Lucanthone hydrochloride (Miracil D, Nilodin), given orally, is effective against *S. mansoni* and *S. haematobium,* but is of little or no value in *S. japonicum* infections. Various dosage schedules are employed; 20 mg per kilogram of body weight in two divided doses daily for 6 to 8 days is quite satisfactory. Side effects consist of vomiting, abdominal pain, headache, tremor, dizziness, confusion, and yellowing of the skin, and may be especially severe. Severe toxicity is common in adults.

Niridazole (Ambilhar) is a drug upon which recent extensive studies have demonstrated its significant efficacy, usually a 90 percent cure rate in *Schistosoma mansoni* and *S. haematobium* infections and modest efficacy against *S. japonicum.* It is given orally in a daily dose of 25 mg per kilogram of body weight, usually for 7 days. Children rapidly metabolize niridazole to an inactive form which is nontoxic, and they therefore withstand therapy well but with a lower cure rate than treated adults. Vomiting, headache, dizziness, and electrocardiographic changes are frequent, and rare instances of convulsions, psychosis, and loss of consciousness have been encountered. Several patients with severe schistosomal involvement of the liver who were treated with niridazole had a drug-related death, possibly due to the inability of the liver to metabolize the drug, which then accumulated in toxic amounts in the tissues. Niridazole is the active anthelmintic principle and toxic, whereas the metabolic product has neither of these characteristics. The reproductive system of the female worm is damaged by the drug, and carbohydrate metabolism is reduced. Patients should have stool or urine examinations every month or 2 for 6 months and if live eggs are found therapy may be repeated.

Vascular shunts, splenectomy, and other surgical procedures may be indicated when hepatic damage is extensive.

VESICAL SCHISTOSOMIASIS

Schistosoma haematobium

Disease. Schistosomal hematuria, vesical schistosomiasis, urinary bilharziasis.

Epidemiology. The distribution of the schistosomes of man is governed by the range of their molluscan hosts (Fig. 98). *S. haematobium* is highly endemic in the entire Nile valley and has spread over practically all of Africa and the islands of Malagasy and Mauritius. Endemic foci are also found in Israel, Jordan, Syria, Iraq, Iran, Arabia, Yemen, and a small area on the west coast of India. In areas of Egypt and the rest of Africa, 75 to 95 percent of the inhabitants may be infected. Monkeys and baboons are naturally infected, but are probably unimportant in the spread of the infection.

The snail hosts of *S. haematobium* are nonoperculate, reside in fresh water, and belong to the genera *Bulinus, Physopsis,* and *Biomphalaria.*

Pathology and Symptomatology. As *S. haematobium* lives primarily in the pelvic veins, its eggs are mainly deposited in the vesical plexuses, produce lesions in the urinary bladder, genitalia, and, to a lesser extent, in the intestine.

The eggs of *S. haematobium* in the bladder wall are distributed in the submucosa and, to a lesser extent, in the mucosa, while some occlude the blood vessels (Fig. 97A). The resulting inflammatory condition leads to progressive changes in the bladder and neighboring tissues. The early changes are a diffuse hyperemia and minute vesicular or papular elevations of the mucosa. Papillomatous folds and polypoid excrescences develop as the disease progresses. Later inflammatory patches consisting of sloughing tissue, calcium deposits, and eggs give the mucosa a sandy or granular appearance, especially at the trigone of the bladder. Uric acid and oxalate crystals, phosphatic deposits, eggs, blood clots, mucus, pus, and sloughed-off papillomas may be present in the urine. The urethra may be occluded, the ureters obstructed, and occasionally the pelvis of the kidney affected (Fig. 99 and 100).

The mechanical and toxic irritation of the eggs and the chemical deposits evidently predispose to malignancy. In Egypt vesical schistosomiasis is considered the most common cause of malignancy of the bladder in male agricultural workers. The incidence of squamous cell epithelioma of the bladder in patients with vesical schistosomiasis is many times that in uninfected persons. The age incidence is below that of other cancers, most patients being under 40 years of age, some as young as 10 years. The relationship of intestinal schistosomiasis to malignancy is not as definite as that of vesical schistosomiasis.

In the male the seminal vesicles are affected most frequently, sometimes without bladder involvement, and the prostate less frequently. The changes consist of congestion, tissue proliferation, and finally adhesive fibrosis. The external male genitalia may assume an elephantoid appearance with papillomatous growths from obstruction of the scrotal lymphatics. Secondary bacterial infection may produce ulcera-

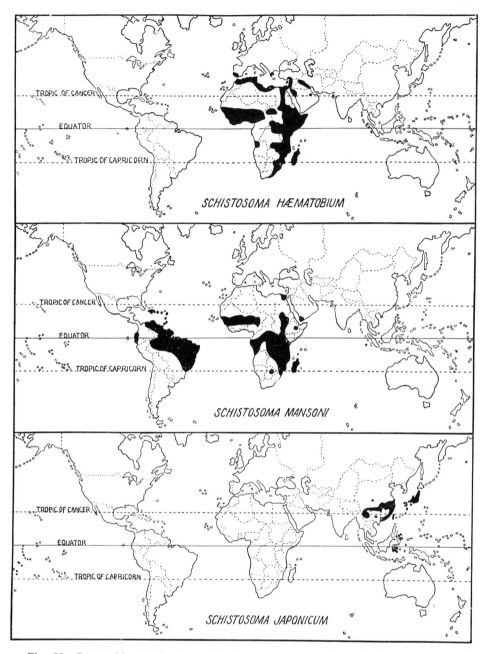

Fig. 98. Geographic distribution of *Schistosoma haematobium, S. japonicum,* and *S. mansoni.* (From Belding. *Textbook of Parasitology,* 3rd ed., New York, 1965, Appleton-Century-Crofts.)

tion, perivesical and periurethral abscesses, and fistulas of the bladder, rectum, scrotum, and penis. The female genitalia are affected in 80 to 90 percent of bladder infections; the vulva may have nodular papillomatous growths that may ulcerate, the cervix and vaginal walls may be thickened, vesicovaginal fistulas may be produced, and the ovaries and tubes may be matted together.

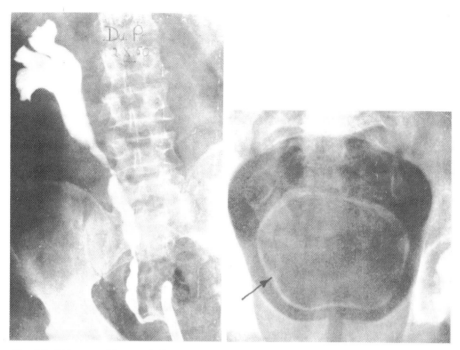

Fig. 99. Urinary schistosomiasis.
A. *Schistosoma Haematobium.* X-ray showing ureteral dilatation and constriction and renal pelvic enlargement.
B. *Schistosoma Haematobium.* X-ray of urinary bladder showing calcification. (From *Urological Aspects of Bilharziasis in Rhodesia,* 1960, E. & S. Livingstone, Ltd., Edinburgh & London. Courtesy of Drs. R. M. Honey, M. Gelfand, and D. M. Blair.)

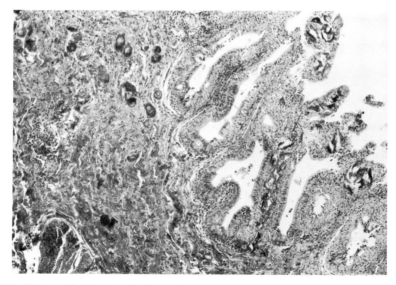

Fig. 100. Urinary bladder heavily invaded with *Schistosoma haematobium* eggs. (X 50)

Symptoms may not develop for years in light infections, but in heavy infections symptoms may be first noticed as early as 1 month after infection. The eggs first appear in the urine in 10 to 12 weeks after infection. The most characteristic symptom is hematuria, usually with blood in the terminal drops of urine, although the whole output may be blood-tinged. As the mucosal surfaces become inflamed, painful micturition and frequency begin, and mucus and pus are found in the urine. The greatly thickened bladder wall loses its elasticity, and there is a constant urinary residual. Daily temperature elevation, sweating, malaise, weakness, and dull pain in the suprapubic region occur. The leukocyte count is increased, and there is usually eosinophilia. There is progressive cystitis with ascending secondary infection of the ureters and kidneys, and hydronephrosis. Urinary fistulas of the scrotum, perineum, and adjacent areas are common. A few patients show intestinal and rectal involvement. Liver involvement, although not less frequent, is much less severe than in *S. japonicum* and *S. mansoni* infection. Pulmonary involvement results early from the migrating immature schistosomes, and later from the embolic eggs, which produce mild parenchymatous pneumonitis around the bronchi and alveoli, but at times cause more serious necrotizing and obliterative arterial lesions with hyperplasia of the endothelium, hyaline thrombosis, and diffuse fibrous thickening of the intima. The endarteritis and periarteritis appear to be allergic responses to substances elaborated by the miracidium in the egg. The condition known as cor pulmonale results from pulmonary hypertension and leads to hypertrophy of the right ventricle and, finally, right heart failure.

Autopsy of a series of patients harboring *S. haematobium* revealed eggs in the following organs (expressed in percents): urinary bladder, 80 percent; ureters, 69; kidney, 46; vagina, 81; cervix, 75; uterus, 79; fallopian tubes, 12; ovaries, 67; prostate, 55; testes, 34; liver, 43; gallbladder, 38; pancreas, 35; stomach, 32; small intestine, 34; cecum, 54; appendix, 60; ascending colon, 66; transverse colon, 73; descending colon, 65; rectum, 75; suprarenal gland, 26; mesenteric lymph nodes, 32; and spleen, 34 percent.

When large numbers of eggs are deposited in these various organs and tissues, symptoms may be produced.

The prognosis of vesical schistosomiasis is good, except in the late ulcerative stages, because *S. haematobium* is relatively susceptible to chemotherapy. Patients with chronic severe infections and superimposed septic infections, especially the old and debilitated, have a poor prognosis. Death usually occurs from exhaustion, pneumonia, or superimposed infections.

INTESTINAL SCHISTOSOMIASIS

Schistosoma mansoni

Disease.   Intestinal bilharziasis, schistosomal dysentery.

Epidemiology.   *S. mansoni* is spread less widely in Africa than *S. haematobium,* occurring intensely in the Nile Delta north of Cairo, and in East Africa from the Upper Nile to Southern Rhodesia, the Republic of the Congo, West Africa east and southeast of Senegal, with several foci in Natal, and on the east coast of Malagasy. Scattered foci are reported in Arabia and Yemen. The parasite, probably introduced into the Western Hemisphere by the slave trade, is established in Brazil, Venezuela, Surinam, Puerto Rico, Vieguez, Antigua, Dominican Republic,

Guadeloupe, Martinique, Montserrat, Nevis, and St. Lucia. It is not in Barbados, Cuba, Haiti, Jamaica, Trinidad, or the Virgin Islands.

The fresh-water snail intermediate hosts are *Biomphalaria* in Africa and *Biomphalaria* (*Australorbis*) and *Tropicorbis* in South America and the West Indies.

Rodents, monkeys, and baboons have been found infected in nature.

Schistosoma japonicum

Disease.   Oriental schistosomiasis, Katayama disease.

S. japonicum is confined to the Far East. It is highly endemic in the Yangtze River valley of Central China and it is present in less abundance on the east coast, south to Hong Kong. There are 5 endemic areas in the coastal river valleys of Japan; numerous foci in the islands of Mindanao, Mindoro, Luzon, Samar, and Leyte in the Philippines; a small focus in Celebes; Thailand; and an animal focus in Taiwan. *Oncomelania* which inhabit canals, ditches and marshes serve as intermediate hosts.

The numerous reservoir hosts include; rats, mice, cats, dogs, horses, cows, water buffalo and swine.

S. mansoni and *S. japonicum*

Pathology and Symptomatology.   The incubation period is initiated by the penetration of the skin by cercariae, which may produce a transient pruritus and rash. During the invasion of the liver and other organs by the immature worms, petechial hemorrhages and foci of eosinophilic and leukocytic infiltration are produced. Toxic and allergic reactions may cause urticaria, subcutaneous edema, asthmatic attacks, leukocytosis, and eosinophilia. Toward the end of the incubation period the liver becomes enlarged and tender, and there are abdominal discomfort, fever, sweating, chilliness, and sometimes diarrhea. The young worms now migrate against the bloodstream—*S. japonicum* to the superior mesenteric and *S. mansoni* to the mesenteric veins—and their eggs invade the walls of the intestine.

With the initiation of egg laying, the acute stage begins. In the normal cycle the eggs work their way through the intestinal wall and escape in the feces; when numerous, they are accompanied by blood and necrotic tissue cells. Many eggs are swept back into the bloodstream to the liver.

Autopsies of 110 persons infected with *S. mansoni* revealed eggs in the following organs (expressed in percents): liver, 20 percent; gallbladder, 4; lungs, 24; pancreas, 5; stomach, 11; small intestine, 16; cecum, 23; appendix, 8; ascending colon, 29; transverse colon, 36; descending colon, 38; rectum, 44; suprarenal gland, 2; mesentric lymph nodes, 2; spleen, 2; urinary bladder, 14; vagina, 19; cervix, 6; uterus, 21; kidney, 2; ureters, 6; prostate, 7; and testes, 6 percent.

The stage of acute symptoms marks the onset of invasion of the intestines, liver, and lungs by the eggs. It is characterized by fever, malaise, urticaria, eosinophilia, abdominal discomfort, diarrhea, weight loss, cough, a slightly enlarged liver, and sometimes an enlarged spleen. In the chronic disease, which begins after 1.5 years in heavy infections and in 4 to 5 years in light infections, there is loss of weight, anemia, symptoms referable to the intestinal tract, and, often, splenomegaly, cirrhosis of the liver, and ascites.

The eggs of *S. mansoni* and *S. japonicum* are deposited in the mesenteric

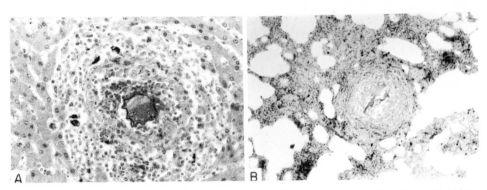

Fig. 101. Pseudo-tubercle formation around eggs of *Schistosoma mansoni*. A, liver (X 200); B, lung (X 50).

lymph nodes and the intestinal wall. The most severe lesions are caused by *S. japonicum,* which produces about 10 times as many eggs as *S. mansoni.* The invading eggs evoke an intense cellular infiltration in the intestinal wall with extensive fibrous tissue proliferation, formation of papillomas, and thrombosis of the small blood vessels (Fig. 101). The early changes are congestion, granular or hypertrophic mucosa, yellowish papillae (diagnostic) and ulcerations; and in the late disease, polyps and strictures. The entire intestinal wall, including the peritoneal surface, may be included in the process and may be bound down by mesenteric and omental adhesions. Fibrous constrictions of the irregularly thickened wall may cause the tearing off of papillomas and polyps, and secondary bacterial infections may produce the discharge of blood, pus, and eggs into the intestinal lumen. In advanced cases, relaxation of the anal sphincter may permit the prolapse of pedunculated papillomatous masses. Fistulas may extend to the ischiorectal fossa, perineum, buttocks, or bladder. Eggs are found in the appendix in 75 percent of intestinal infections, at times accompanied by secondary bacterial invasion, but they rarely are responsible for an appendicitis syndrome.

The embolic eggs are chiefly responsible for the progressive fibroblastic proliferation, periductal fibrosis, and interstitial cirrhosis with rising portal hypertension (Fig. 96). Toxins from the adult worms, pigmentation, and hypoproteinemia from malnutrition may also play a part in the production of the hepatic lesions. Hepatic fibrosis, which leads to cirrhosis, is common in *S. mansoni* and *S. japonicum* infections, but is infrequent in *S. haematobium* disease. It is difficult to correlate cirrhosis and other liver conditions with schistosomal infections, since the diffuse changes of steatosis and fibrosis, other than the reactions around the eggs, are similar to those produced by malnutrition. In late cases, ascites and its attendant complications may develop. The condition of the portal system may be ascertained by roentgenography and venography.

About a year after the initial infection, the spleen shows congestion, medullary hyperplasia, and slight enlargement. Later there is hypertrophy with fibrous tissue formation, atrophy of the malpighian bodies, thickened capsule with patchy adhesive perisplenitis, and tortuous splenic veins. Splenomegaly is caused chiefly by portal obstruction and, to a lesser extent, by the invasion of the eggs and the reticuloendothelial reaction to the toxic products of the worms. Splenomegaly occurs less frequently with *S. haematobium* than with the other two species. Splenectomy may be indicated when there are esophageal varicosities, progressive cirrhosis of the liver with portal hypertension, ascites, and leukopenia.

The uncommon cerebral infections, chiefly caused by *S. japonicum,* are due to embolic eggs, which act mechanically, as foreign proteins and as toxic agents, to set up an intense reaction with edema, neural cellular infiltration, foreign body cells, phlebotic changes, and degeneration of the surrounding tissues.

Abdominal tenderness, hepatitis, anorexia, fever, headache, myalgia, dysentery, and weight loss are characteristic of intestinal schistosomiasis. The acute stage lasts 3 to 4 months, and it is more severe in heavy infections and in *S. japonicum* infections because of the larger number of eggs produced by this species.

The chronic stage of the disease may develop in 18 months with heavy infections and as late as 25 years in light *S. mansoni* infections.

The liver is enlarged in the acute stage of the disease, but as the infection becomes chronic the liver recedes in size and, although usually slightly enlarged, may become subnormal in size. The liver cells are atrophied, and there is a periportal cirrhosis. Although the cirrhosis of the liver may be extreme, especially in *S. japonicum* infections, interference with bile flow rarely occurs. Severe ascites may develop, and dilated abdominal, thoracic, and esophageal veins are often present. The thymol turbidity test is also positive, especially late in the disease, and bromsulfalein is retained. The SGOT and SGPT may be normal or slightly elevated, and antimony therapy may cause both to be elevated. When the patient is placed on an enriched diet, the liver functions revert to normal.

Depending upon the intensity and duration of the chronic infection, the patient may have a colitis of varying degree, with the formation of polyps. Headache, malaise, irregular slight fever, diarrhea, and abdominal pain are common. The appetite becomes poor, and the patient loses weight. As the disease progresses the red blood cells gradually decrease to below 3 million with a corresponding reduction in hemoglobin, producing hypochromic anemia. There is leukocytosis of above 10,000 in 75 percent of patients in the early disease, and leukopenia in the late stages. Eosinophilia, which is usual early in the infection, often disappears in chronic infections. The blood serum shows an increase in globulin and a decrease in albumin. The sedimentation rate is increased. Eggs which pass into the systemic circulation and are filtered out in the brain or spinal cord produce various nervous disorders. The symptoms encountered are headache, disorientation, coma, aphasia, amnesia, confusion, paraplegia, spasticity, altered reflexes, incontinence, cranial nerve involvement, and Jacksonian epilepsy. Eggs carried to the lungs produce an arteriolitis and fibrosis, resulting in a right ventricular failure or cor pulmonale.

The chronic stage may be prolonged for years, and the patient may die of pneumonia or other infections, or rupture of esophageal varices.

Prevention. Prevention of schistosomiasis includes: (1) reduction of sources of infection, (2) protection of snail-bearing waters from contamination with infectious urine or feces, (3) control of snail hosts, and (4) protection of persons from cercaria-infested waters.

Theoretically, the sources of infection of *S. mansoni* and *S. haematobium* may be reduced by the detection and treatment of infected persons, but difficulties in diagnosis, the unsuitability of chemotherapeutic agents to mass therapy, and constant reinfection reduces the effectiveness of this method unless combined with vector control. The presence of animal reservoir hosts renders chemotherapy of less value for the control of *S. japonicum.* Until a cheap, nontoxic, effective, preferably oral, chemotherapeutic agent is developed, mass treatment cannot be attempted with any expectation of success.

The protection of waters from contamination involves sewage disposal and treatment. The sanitary disposal of human feces should eradicate the disease, but its practice runs counter to economic, racial, and religious customs, and to the primitive habit of promiscuous defecation and urination in or near snail-infested waters. The economic need for night soil for fertilizer in the Orient is a complicating factor, although composting of night soil prior to use will kill the eggs. Populations must be educated to use sanitary toilet facilities and to avoid contact with infected water. Safe facilities for bathing and washing of clothes must be provided.

The eradication of snails may be attempted by removal of vegetation, desiccation by drainage, reduction in number by capture with hand nets or palm leaf traps, introduction of natural enemies, and molluscacides. Control of snails is with copper sulfate, sodium pentachlorphenate, dinitro-o-cyclohexylphenol, Bayluscide, and zinc dimethyldithiocarbamate. The cercariae are killed by chlorine, 1 ppm, in 10 to 20 minutes. Migration of snails from nontreated areas into treated areas complicates this method of control.

The avoidance of contact with waters infested with cercariae affords complete protection, but, unfortunately, prohibition of bathing, wading, or working in and the drinking of infested waters cannot be enforced and is nullified by agricultural and other practices. Agricultural workers may be partially protected by clothing, boots, or repellents, but economic considerations, conveniences of working, and ignorance tend to make such measures impracticable.

SCHISTOSOME DERMATITIS

(*Swimmer's Itch, Clam Digger's Itch*)

Schistosome cercariae of several avian and mammalian hosts penetrate the skin of man but can progress no further and are destroyed in the skin, producing a dermatitis. A number of migratory birds, including several species of ducks, harbor the adult worms and, wherever in their travels the suitable snail host is present, the dermatitis may be found in man. Recognition of this clinical entity is gradually expanding the known geographic distribution of the disease (Fig. 102).

Geographic Distribution. Distribution is probably cosmopolitan: At least 25 species of cercariae from fresh-water snail hosts and at least four from marine snails have been reported, and probably many other species exist. The disease was first recognized in Michigan in 1928 and has been reported from the United States, Canada, Europe, Mexico, Central America, Japan, Malaya, Australia, India, Africa, Alaska, South America, Cuba, and New Zealand. Marine forms cause a dermatitis among clam diggers and sea bathers on the east and west coasts of the United States and in Hawaii. The cercariae from the snails either swarm in shallow water or are swept toward the shore by wave action. Their free-swimming existence lasts about 24 hours. The distribution and habits of the snail hosts determine the infestation of bathing beaches.

Pathology and Symptomatology. The cercariae, "strangers in a strange land," are walled off and destroyed in the epithelial layers of the skin, although occasionally some may escape to the lungs. They evoke an acute inflammatory

SCHISTOSOME DERMATITIS

FRESH-WATER   "SWIMMER'S ITCH"   "WATER ITCH"

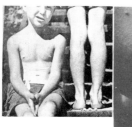
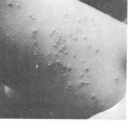

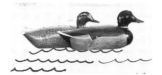

ADULTS IN MESENTERIC VENULES OF
DUCKS, SHORE BIRDS, MICE, MUSKRATS

LESIONS PRODUCED
BY CERCARIAE IN
SKIN OF MAN

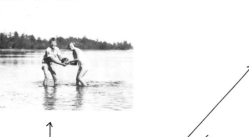

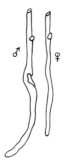
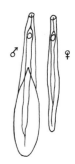

TRICHOBILHARZIA SPP.   SCHISTOSOMATIUM SP.

NORMAL CYCLE

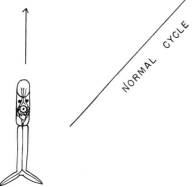

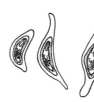

EGG PASSED IN FECES INTO WATER

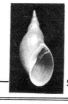

CERCARIA BREAKS OUT
OF SNAIL INTO WATER,
PENETRATES SKIN OF
WARM-BLOODED ANIMALS

MIRACIDIUM HATCHES FROM
EGG, PENETRATES SNAIL

DAUGHTER SPOROCYST ⟵ MOTHER SPOROCYST
IN SNAIL

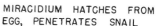

SNAIL HOSTS

MARINE   "CLAM-DIGGER'S ITCH"   "SEA-BATHER'S ERUPTION"

ADULTS, MICROBILHARZIA SP.,
IN DUCKS AND SHORE BIRDS

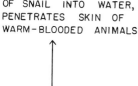

SNAIL
HOST

Fig. 102. Schistosome dermatitis.

response with edema, early infiltration of neutrophils and lymphocytes, and later invasion of eosinophils. Penetration may take place in the water, but usually it occurs as the film of water evaporates on the skin. A prickling sensation is followed by the rapid development of urticarial wheals, which subside in about half an hour leaving a few minute macules. After some hours of severe itching, edema, and the transformation of the macules into papules, occasionally pustules occur, reaching maximal intensity in 2 to 3 days. The papular and sometimes hemorrhagic rash heals in a week or more, but may be complicated by scratching and secondary infection. In heavy infections there may be a general reaction with prostration. There is marked individual variation in the reaction to infection.

The reaction is essentially a sensitization phenomenon. The local skin lesions produced by the schistosomes of man are slight, but with continuous reinfection, sensitized persons may show a definite dermatitis. The dermatitis produced by the animal schistosomes ranges from mild to severe, depending upon the immune response of the individual. Repeated infections tend to become more and more severe.

Diagnosis.   History of contact with water and a cutaneous rash. Serologic and skin tests may be positive, leading to a mistaken diagnosis of human schistosomiasis.

Treatment.   Antipruritic and antihistaminic lotions are of palliative value. Antimicrobial drugs should be used for secondary bacterial infection.

Prevention.   The removal of snails from the neighborhood of bathing beaches is the most practical method of combating "swimmer's itch." The snails may be destroyed by removal of vegetation, and by molluscacides. A mixture of two parts copper sulfate and one part copper carbonate at 3 pounds per 1,000 square feet has proved effective. Sodium pentachlorphenate should also be of value. Vigorous rubbing of the body with a towel immediately after the bather leaves the water tends to prevent the penetration of the skin by cercariae.

ARTHROPODA

14

Arthropods Injurious to Man

The widely distributed and diversified phylum ARTHROPODA contains more species than all the other phyla of the animal kingdom.

Adult and larval arthropods may injure man by venenation, vesication, blood sucking, and tissue invasion; and they transmit bacterial, rickettsial, spirochaetal, viral, and animal parasitic diseases.

Arthropods are characterized by bilateral symmetry, metameric segmentation, jointed appendages, and a hard chitinous exoskeleton. The body comprises head, thorax, and abdomen. The paired appendages are modified into walking legs in the terrestrial species and swimming organs in the aquatic. The appendages of the head are variously adapted as sensory, masticating, or piercing organs. The eyes are compound or simple. Digestive, vascular, excretory, and nervous systems are present. Respiration usually is accomplished in the aquatic forms by gills and in the terrestrial by tracheae, tubular extensions of the outer covering. Usually the sexes are separate, and reproduction is sexual, although parthenogenesis may occur.

The ARTHROPODA are divided into five classes: The ONYCHOPHORA are not injurious, the MYRIAPODA have only the poisonous millipedes and centipedes, and the CRUSTACEA contain a few species that serve as intermediate hosts for animal parasites. The INSECTA and ARACHNIDA include most of the parasitic species or vectors of disease.

CLASS MYRIAPODA

The elongated, terrestrial myriapods have numerous segments bearing legs and tracheal stigmata. The two principal orders are the DIPLOPODA (millipedes) and the CHILOPODA (centipedes). The nonpoisonous, herbivorous millipedes have been incriminated as hosts of the cestode *Hymenolepis diminuta*.

Order CHILOPODA. The poisonous, carnivorous centipedes, 5 to 25 cm in length, have flattened bodies and a single pair of legs on most segments. They live in damp localities under bark, rubbish, or stones, and feed on insects and small animals. The first body segment bears a pair of claws with openings at the tips for the expulsion of a paralyzing venom that is contained in a gland at the base of the claw. The small centipedes of the temperate zones are often incapable of penetrating the skin, and their mild bites seldom produce little more than a sharp pain, erythema, and, sometimes, induration. The larger tropical and subtropical genus *Scolopendra* (Fig. 103) inflicts painful bites and even causes necrotic local lesions. No authenticated deaths from uncomplicated centipede bites have been reported.

The puncture wounds caused by the venomous claws of centipedes may be treated locally with ammonia, alcoholic iodine, or other disinfectants. Necrotic lesions may require surgical dressings. The painful systemic symptoms produced by the larger centipedes may require analgesics and rest in bed.

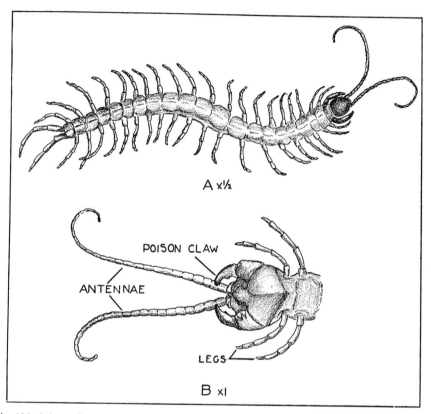

Fig. 103. Schematic representation of centipede (*Scolopendra*). A, Dorsal view of centipede; B, ventral view of head.

CLASS CRUSTACEA

The aquatic CRUSTACEA contain the species which are intermediate hosts of animal parasites of man.

Order COPEPODA. Copepods are small, graceful, symmetrical animals with the head and first two thoracic segments fused into a cephalothorax, and a slender abdomen of 3 to 5 segments. *Cyclops* are intermediate hosts of the Guinea worm *Dracunculus medinensis,* the cestode *Diphyllobothrium latum,* and the nematode *Gnathostoma spinigerum.* Species of *Diaptomus* are hosts of *D. latum.*

Order DECAPODA. The DECAPODA include the large crustaceans such as shrimps, crayfish, lobsters, and crabs. Species of fresh-water crabs and crayfish are second intermediate hosts of the lung fluke *Paragonimus westermani.* Land crabs (*Cardisoma, Birgus*) and the freshwater prawn harbor the infective rat·lungworm larvae (*Angiostrongylus*) that infect man's brain.

15

Class Insecta

The numerous species of insects play an important role in the economic life of man. Relatively few species are parasites of man or act as vectors of human diseases, but these few are intimately concerned with his welfare and have been responsible for the spread of the worst scourges of mankind—malaria, typhus, plague, etc.

Morphology. The primitive insect (Fig. 104) has a 6-segmented head, a 3-segmented thorax bearing three pairs of legs and two pairs of wings, and an 11-segmented abdomen. The segmentation of the ancestral form is evident only in the abdomen of present-day insects. The body is encased in a more-or-less rigid, noncellular integument consisting of hard, chitinized plates or *sclerites* connected by a flexible, slightly chitinous membrane.

The cephalic appendages of the primitive arthropod have been converted into sensory organs such as multijointed antennae, compound and simple eyes, and masticatory organs of varying structure, depending upon the feeding habits. The simplest form of the latter is the chewing or biting mouth (cockroach), but in the highly specialized insects the mouth parts have been modified for piercing-sucking (mosquito) and sponging-lapping (housefly). The thorax is composed of the prothorax, mesothorax, and metathorax, each of which bears a pair of legs. Winged insects theoretically have a pair of wings each on the meso- and metathorax, but there are various modifications, such as the degeneration of the posterior wings

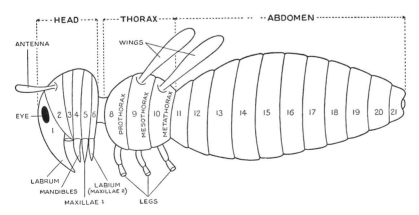

Fig. 104. Diagram of primitive insect, showing segmentation of head, thorax, and abdomen. The numbering includes 20 segments and the neck piece. (Adapted from Patton and Cragg, 1913, after Berlese.)

in the flies to rudimentary *halteres*. The number of abdominal segments is reduced in the more specialized insects.

The abdomen of the adult insect is devoid of appendages. The last segments may
be modified for sexual purposes into the *hypopygium* of the male and the *ovipositor*
of the female.

In the typical insect (Fig. 105), the nervous system is represented by a chain of
ventral ganglia connected by commissures and sub- and supra-esophageal ganglia,
from which nerves pass to the tissues and sensory organs. The respiratory system
comprises branching tracheal tubes communicating with the exterior by *spiracles*.
The poorly developed circulatory system consists of a closed dorsal pulsating organ
and aorta, and an open body cavity (hemocele). The digestive system comprises a
pharynx, a slender esophagus, proventriculus, distensible stomach or midgut, intestine or hindgut, rectum, and anus. In bloodsucking insects the muscular pharynx
acts as a suction pump. Paired salivary glands open into the mouth parts. The excretory system includes several slender malpighian tubules that empty into the
intestinal canal just above the juncture of the mid- and hindgut. The male reproductive organs consist of two testes, a seminal vesicle, accessory glands, and hypopygium. The female reproductive organs include ovaries, oviducts, seminal receptacle
(spermatheca), shell and cement glands, and ovipositor.

Life Cycle.   Insects are both oviparous and viviparous. The types of life cycle,
which afford a basis for classification, are direct development, incomplete metamorphosis, and complete metamorphosis. In the uncommon first type, the newly
hatched insect is a small replica of the adult. Incomplete metamorphosis, in which
the nymphs differ from the adult only in size, proportion, and absence of wings
and external genitalia, occurs in the more primitive insects. Complete metamorphosis is found in the highly specialized insects; the worm-like larva differs from the

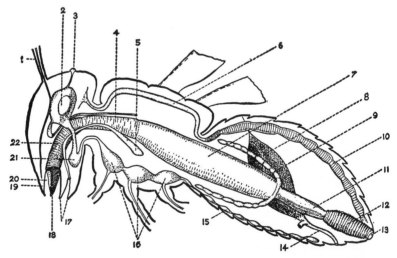

Fig. 105. Internal structure of a typical insect. 1, antennae; 2, supra-esophageal ganglion;
3, ocellus; 4, esophagus; 5, salivary gland; 6, aorta; 7, midgut; 8, gonad; 9, malpighian tubule;
10, dorsal pulsating vessel; 11, intestine; 12, rectum; 13, anus; 14, gonaduct; 15, abdominal
nerve ganglion; 16, thoracic nerve ganglia; 17, maxillae; 18, mandible; 19, labrum; 20, mouth;
21, subesophageal ganglion; 22, pharynx. (From Hegner, Root, Augustine, and Huff. *Parasitology*, 1938, as redrawn from Berlese, "Gli Insetti." Courtesy of D. Appleton-Century Company.)

adult in feeding habits and after several molts passes through a pupal stage, during which the larval structures are transformed into those of the adult. The larva and pupa possess characteristic hairs, bristles, and appendages that aid in the differentiation of species. The duration of life in both the adult and larval stages varies with the species and with the environment.

The insects of special interest as parasites of man belong to four orders, SIPHONAPTERA (fleas), PHTHIRAPTERA (lice), HEMIPTERA (bugs), and DIPTERA (flies, including mosquitoes).

Of less importance are the COLEOPTERA (beetles), HYMENOPTERA (bees, wasps, hornets, ants), LEPIDOPTERA (butterflies and moths), and ORTHOPTERA (cockroaches).

ORDER PHTHIRAPTERA: LICE

Lice are small, degenerate, dorsoventrally flattened, wingless insects, with incomplete metamorphosis. The order includes both biting and sucking lice. Only the sucking lice, of the suborder Anoplura, which have mouth parts modified for piercing and sucking, are ectoparasites of man.

Species. The parasitic lice of man comprise three species or varieties: (1) *Pediculus humanus* var. *capitis,* head louse; (2) *Pediculus humanus* var. *corporis,* body louse; and (3) *Phthirus pubis,* crab louse. The head and body lice are apparently varieties of a single species. They interbreed; their descendants are fertile; and their morphologic differences overlap.

Disease. Pediculosis, crabs. Vectors of epidemic typhus, trench fever, and relapsing fever.

Morphology. The flattened, elongated, grayish-white body has an angular ovoid head, a fused chitinous thorax, and a nine-segmented abdomen (Fig. 106). The head bears a pair of simple lateral eyes, a pair of short five-jointed antennae, and an extensile piercing proboscis. Each of the three fused segments of the thorax bears a pair of strong five-segmented legs that terminate in a single hook-like claw and an opposing tibial process for gripping hairs or fibers. The last abdominal segment in the female bears a median dorsal genital opening and two lateral blunt gonopods, which clasp the hairs during oviposition. The body and head lice differ only in size, the body louse being 2 to 4 mm and the head louse 1 to 2 mm. The crab louse is distinguished by its small size, 0.8 to 1.2 mm, oblong turtle shape, rectangular head, short indistinctly segmented abdomen, and large heavy claws.

Life Cycle. The operculated, white eggs, 0.6 to 0.8 mm, called "nits" are deposited on and firmly attached to the hairs or to the fibers of clothing. They may remain viable on clothing for a month. The eggs hatch in 5 to 11 days at 21 to 36° C. Metamorphosis is incomplete. The nymph develops within the egg case and emerges through the opened operculum. It undergoes three molts within 2 weeks. The average life cycle of the body or head louse covers 18 days, and that of the crab louse 15 days. The life span of the adult is approximately 1 month.

The total number of eggs deposited during the life time has been estimated at 300 for the body louse, 140 for the head louse, and 50 for the crab louse. The daily output for the body louse is 6 to 9 eggs.

Epidemiology. These lice are exclusively human parasites and have worldwide distribution. The favorite locations are the hairs on the back of the head for the head louse, the fibers of clothing and the hairs on the chest and axilla for the

PEDICULUS HUMANUS   HEAD, BODY LOUSE

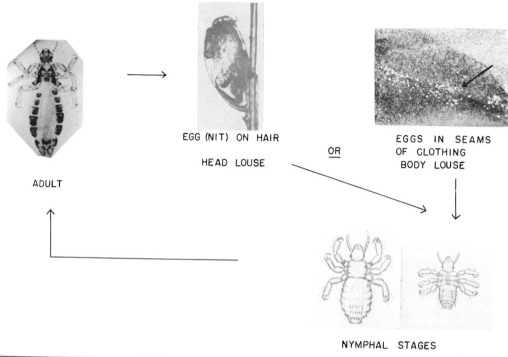

ADULT

EGG (NIT) ON HAIR
HEAD LOUSE

OR

EGGS IN SEAMS
OF CLOTHING
BODY LOUSE

NYMPHAL STAGES

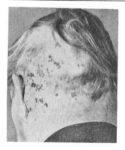

HEAD LOUSE LESIONS
(INFECTED)

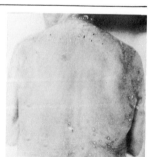

LESIONS CAUSED BY
BODY LOUSE

Fig. 106. Life cycle of head and body louse.

body louse, and the pubic hairs for the crab louse. The body and head lice move fairly rapidly and readily pass from host to host, but the crab louse changes its position infrequently. The body and head lice survive for 10 days at 5° C without food, but the crab louse dies in 2 days. They suck blood for long periods. They exist between 15 and 38° C, but die at over 40° C. Moist heat at 60° C destroys the eggs in 15 to 30 minutes.

Pediculosis is most common in persons of unclean habits in cold climates where heavy clothing is required and bathing is infrequent; in occupants of flophouses, jails, or crowded tenements; and in soldiers during wartime. The head louse, which is easily transmitted by brushes, combs, and hats, is most prevalent in school children, particularly girls. The body louse is transmitted by contact or by clothing or personal effects infested with "nits." The crab louse is usually transmitted during coitus by the transfer of adults or "nits" on broken hairs and less frequently through toilet seats, clothing, or bedding (Fig. 107).

Pathogenicity. The irritating saliva, injected during feeding, produces a roseate elevated papule accompanied by severe itching. The head louse bites most frequently on the back of the head and neck, the body louse on the parts of the body in contact with clothing, and the crab louse chiefly in the pubic region. Individuals vary in sensitivity. Scratching increases the inflammation and secondary bacterial infection results in pustules, crusts, and suppurative processes. Severe infestations may produce scarring, induration, pigmentation, and even ulceration of the skin. Infestation of the eyelashes with secondary infection may lead to phlyctenular conjunctivitis and keratitis. The symptoms are the result of cutaneous irritation, loss of sleep, and mental depression. Itching is the earliest and most prominent symptom, and the sequelae of scratching are the most characteristic signs.

Vectors of Diseases. The body louse is the vector of epidemic typhus, European relapsing fever, and trench fever. The head louse is a less important vector, while the crab louse has never been incriminated. Typhus fever occurs in epidemics in crowded jails, in armies, and during famines. Lice become infected with the causative organism, *Rickettsia prowazeki,* by ingesting the blood of a diseased person. The parasites multiply in the epithelium of the midgut of the louse and are passed in the feces. The louse remains infective throughout its shortened life. Man usually acquires the infection by the contamination of a bite wound, abraded skin, or mucous membranes with the infected feces or crushed bodies of the lice, or, more rarely, from the contaminated proboscis. The spirochaete *Borrelia recurrentis,* the causative agent of European epidemic relapsing fever, when ingested with the blood of the patient, multiplies rapidly throughout the body of the louse, which remains infective throughout its life. The various strains of tick-borne relapsing fever do not survive in the louse. Man is infected by the contaminative method, the crushed body of the louse coming in contact with the bite wound or abraded

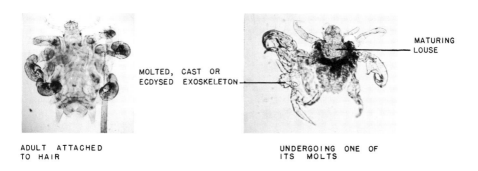

PHTHIRUS PUBIS   CRAB LOUSE

MATURING LOUSE

MOLTED, CAST OR ECDYSED EXOSKELETON

ADULT ATTACHED TO HAIR

UNDERGOING ONE OF ITS MOLTS

LIFE CYCLE SIMILAR TO THAT OF HEAD AND BODY LOUSE

Fig. 107. Crab louse.

skin. Trench fever, an incapacitating but nonfatal disease of rickettsial origin, which was present in epidemic form in World War I and later in endemic form in Europe and Mexico, is transmitted by the bite of the infected louse or by the contamination of abraded skin by its feces.

Diagnosis. Diagnosis, suspected from itching and the sequelae of scratching, depends upon finding the adult louse or the "nits" of the head and crab louse. The eggs of the body louse are usually hidden in the seams of the clothing.

Treatment. Topical applications of soothing lotions relieve the itching and thus, by preventing scratching, allow the lesions to heal.

BODY LICE. The elimination of body lice is effected by thorough cleansing of the body, application of insecticides, and sterilization of clothing and bedding. Dusting of the body and clothing with 10 percent DDT in pyrophyllite or powdered talcum, which is blown beneath the clothing, kills all lice, and prevents reinfestation for 3 to 4 weeks. Strains of lice resistant to DDT have been reported in Egypt, Japan, and North China. In such instances "benzene hexachloride" BHC (Lindane) in a 1 percent dust with treatments every other week, or 1 percent Malathion powder, which is lethal to both adults and eggs, may be used. The disinfection of infested clothing by boiling or autoclaving at 60° C for 15 minutes is necessary to destroy the resistant eggs. Chemical fumigation with methyl bromide is as effective and is less damaging to woolen and leather goods.

HEAD LICE. The head may be rubbed with Lindane ointment (1 percent BHC) or dusted with 10 percent DDT or 1 percent BHC in pyrophyllite or talc, using 3 to 5 g of the mixture for one application. The powder is left in the hair for a week, then the hair is washed and combed to remove the nits. An emulsion of benzyl benzoate has also proved effective.

CRAB LICE. (Fig. 107). The infested areas may be shaved and treated with (Lindane) ointment, followed 12 hours later by a soap and water bath. The hairy parts may also be dusted with 10 percent DDT powder followed by a bath in 2 days; the treatment is repeated in a week because of hatching of the eggs. Lice and nits on the eyebrows may be removed by forceps, or yellow oxide of mercury may be applied.

Control. Mass delousing methods are designed not only to exterminate the lice but also to control the epidemic diseases that are transmitted by lice. Various types of delousing plants for handling large numbers of persons have been devised for military personnel and civilian populations. For the mass delousing of civilians, it is much simpler to administer insecticidal powders such as DDT simultaneously to the body and clothing. Persons coming in contact with lice-infested individuals in typhus epidemics may be protected by wearing silk or rubber outer garments fastened tightly at the wrist, ankles, and neck, and by impregnating their clothing with repellents.

ORDER SIPHONAPTERA: FLEAS

Fleas are bloodsucking ectoparasites that, for feeding purposes, temporarily infest mammals and birds.

Morphology. Fleas are small brown wingless insects, 2.0 to 2.5 mm, with laterally compressed bodies (Fig. 108). The males are smaller than the females. The small chitinous head may bear eyes and combs; all have antennae and suc-

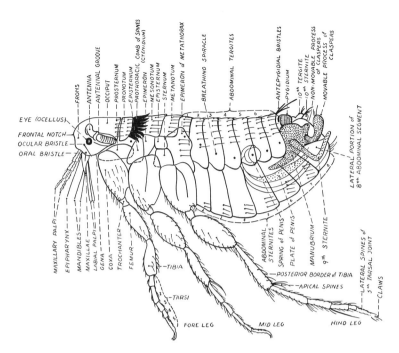

Fig. 108. External anatomy of a male flea. (*Nosopsyllus fasciatus*). (Adapted from Stitt, Clough, and Clough. *Practical Bacteriology, Hematology and Animal Parasitology,* 1938. Courtesy of The Blakiston Company.)

torial mouth parts. Each segment of the three-segmented thorax bears a pair of powerful legs terminating in two curved claws.

Life Cycle. The hosts of fleas are domesticated and wild animals, especially wild rodents. The various species tend to be host specific, but their activities permit the infestation of animals other than their preferred hosts. The life span is about a year under favorable conditions of cool, moist temperature, but the maximal survival period apart from the host is 38 to 125 days, depending upon the species. The larvae die at 36° C, but the adults can withstand 38° C for 24 hours.

The adult fleas feed on their hosts, while the larvae live on any nutritive debris, particularly dried blood and the feces of the adults. Both sexes are able to suck blood. Fleas have unusual leaping powers, which enable them to transfer readily from host to host.

In order to produce a large number of eggs, the female must copulate more than once and take frequent blood meals. The small, ovoid, white or cream-colored eggs (Fig. 109), about 0.5 mm in length, are laid in the hairs or in the habitat of the host. In houses they are deposited in small batches under rugs, in floor cracks, or on the ground near and under buildings. Those deposited on the host usually drop off before hatching.

Fleas develop by complete metamorphosis, passing through a larval and a pupal stage in the host's environment (Fig. 109). In 2 to 12 days the larva emerges from the egg as an active worm-like, white, eyeless, legless, bristled creature of 14 segments, approximately 4.5 mm in length. It has a chewing mouth. It avoids light

XENOPSYLLA CHEOPIS

RAT FLEA

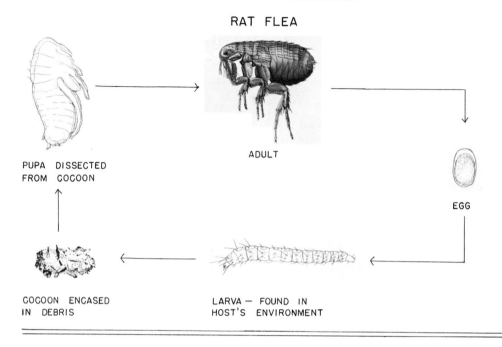

PUPA DISSECTED
FROM COCOON

ADULT

EGG

COCOON ENCASED
IN DEBRIS

LARVA — FOUND IN
HOST'S ENVIRONMENT

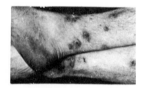

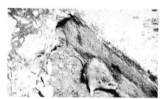

FLEA BITES ON ANKLE

RAT FLEAS ARE
VECTORS OF DISEASE

Fig. 109. Life cycle of *Xenopsylla cheopis.*

and seeks crevices. The larval period usually lasts 7 to 30 days, but may be prolonged for months, during which time it undergoes two or three molts, the last being within the silky pupal cocoon. The pupal stage lasts 14 to 21 days, but at low temperatures may extend over a year. When the development of the pupa is completed, the adult flea breaks out of the cocoon.

Epidemiology. The incidence of human infestation varies with hygienic standards and the association of man with animals. The jumping ability of the flea facilitates access to new hosts. Some of the differential morphologic characteristics of the more common species associated with the diseases of man are shown in Figure 110. Classification is based chiefly on the presence, size, and position of the eyes; the location of the ocular bristles; presence, arrangement, and spines of combs; structure and appendages of the head; and the genitalia. Man is an important host of *Pulex irritans* and *Tunga penetrans,* and an incidental host of several species parasitic on other animals.

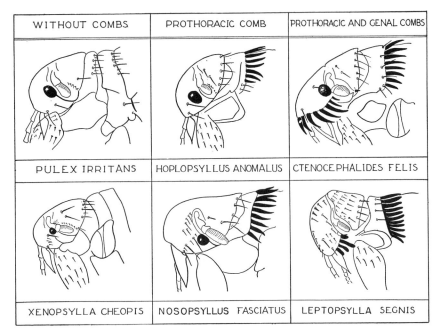

WITHOUT COMBS	PROTHORACIC COMB	PROTHORACIC AND GENAL COMBS
PULEX IRRITANS	HOPLOPSYLLUS ANOMALUS	CTENOCEPHALIDES FELIS
XENOPSYLLA CHEOPIS	NOSOPSYLLUS FASCIATUS	LEPTOPSYLLA SEGNIS

Fig. 110. Schematic representation of heads of various fleas, showing differential characteristics of shape, combs, eyes, and antennae.

Vectors of Disease. Fleas are of medical interest chiefly in connection with the transmission of plague and endemic typhus. They also may act as intermediate hosts of animal parasites.

PLAGUE. Man acquires plague from the fleas that transmit the infection from rat to rat, although human infection may be derived from wild rodents by contact. On the death of the rat near human habitations, the infected fleas seek new hosts, either man or other rats. *Xenopsylla cheopis* is the most important and efficient vector. It is readily infected, remains infectious for a long time, and has a wide distribution. Other species of fleas are prominent locally in various parts of the world. *Pulex irritans* has been found infected on persons dying of plague and is a plague vector in the Chilean Andes, above the "rat-line." *Pasteurella pestis* may be transferred from flea to man by infected mouth parts; the regurgitation of organisms that have multiplied in the gut, particularly if the proventriculus has been blocked; and, infrequently, the contamination of the wound by the feces. Most successful transmissions are from blocked fleas, which are persistent in their efforts to feed. Sylvatic plague in Asia, Africa, and North America is spread by the fleas of wild rodents. *Diamanus montanus* is an important vector among ground squirrels in the United States for both plague and tularemia.

TYPHUS. Endemic or murine typhus is transmitted from rat to rat and from rat to man by fleas. *X. cheopis* and *Nosopsyllus fasciatus* are considered the common vectors, but any species frequenting rats may be incriminated. A single feeding renders the flea infectious for life. The causative agent, *Rickettsia prowazeki* var. *typhi,* is excreted in the feces. Infection is transmitted by the contamination of the bite wound or abraded skin with the infectious feces or the crushed bodies of the fleas.

MISCELLANEOUS DISEASES.   Fleas may act as mechanical vectors of a number of bacterial and viral diseases, chiefly through contaminated feces. *Ctenocephalides canis, Ct. felis,* and *P. irritans* act as intermediate hosts of the dog tapeworm, *Dipylidium caninum,* and together with *Nosopsyllus fasciatus, X. cheopis,* and *Leptopsylla segnis* of the rat tapeworm *Hymenolepis diminuta.* Both of these tapeworms are incidental parasites of man.

Pathogenicity.   The cutaneous irritation caused by the salivary secretions of the flea in different persons varies from no reaction to a raised, roseate, slightly edematous lesion, and in sensitive individuals to a more extensive inflammation or papular rash.

TUNGA PENETRANS.   The chigoe, jigger, nigua, sand flea, or burrowing flea is a parasite of man, hogs, and dogs in tropical America and parts of Africa. The flea is differentiated from the other fleas by its small size (1 mm), its large pointed double-curved head with its sharp upper angling, and its shortened thorax. In addition to sucking blood, the female flea burrows into the skin of mammals and man for oviposition—usually in man on the feet and hands. Man is infected by contact with soil infested with immature fleas. The burrow is usually located about the toes, soles of the feet, fingernails, or interdigital spaces. The lesion, at first characterized by a central black spot in a tense, pale area, becomes a festering painful sore. Secondary bacterial infection may produce an extensive, painful ulcer, sometimes crippling and even causing the death of the host (Fig. 111). The burrowing *Tunga penetrans* may be removed surgically. A 10 percent DDT powder dusted into shoes will prevent infection.

PULEX IRRITANS.   The human flea is the most common flea found on man in Europe and western United States. It also infests hogs, calves, dogs, rats, mice, and small wild rodents.

FLEAS OF LOWER ANIMALS.   The Indian rat flea, *Xenopsylla cheopis,* is the most abundant rat flea in tropical and subtropical regions. It is the most important flea associated with the transmission of plague. It attacks man and other mammals, as well as its natural host, and has cosmopolitan distribution. *Hoplopsyllus anomalus* and *Diamanus montanus* are common fleas of ground squirrels and other rodents in western United States. *Ctenocephalides canis* and *Ct. felis* infest dogs and cats, but may attack man and other animals. These cosmopolitan fleas are the most common species in house infestations in eastern and southern

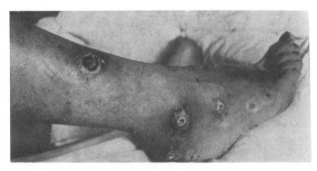

Fig. 111. Lesions caused by *Tunga penetrans.* (Courtesy Dr. P. H. Manson-Bahr, from Andrews and Domonkos. *Diseases of the Skin,* 5th ed., 1963. W. B. Saunders Co.)

United States. The mouse flea, *Leptopsylla segnis,* is a common parasite of the house mouse, rat, and other small rodents. The stick-tight or southern chicken flea, *Echidnophaga gallinacea,* infests birds, dogs, cats, rats, and man.

The bites of fleas may cause an itching dermatitis in some persons. The local irritation may be relieved by calamine lotion or menthol-phenol paste.

Control. Environmental control of fleas consists of spraying rat runways, harborage areas, floors, and other areas with one of the following solutions in kerosene, fuel oil, or in emulsion concentrates: chlordane 2 percent, DDT 5 percent, Diazinon 1 percent, Lindane 1 percent, Malathion 3 percent, Methoxychlor 5 percent, Ronnel 1 percent, Trichlorfon 1 percent. The oil sprays are applied at a rate of 1 gallon per 1,000 square feet. Powders in inert dust of 10 percent DDT, 1 percent Ronnel, and 1 percent Trichlorfon may be used. Before an anti-rat campaign is initiated, their environment should be thoroughly sprayed to kill all fleas, otherwise as the rats die and the fleas seek new hosts, man may be the only one available to receive their attentions. Dogs and cats may be dusted with 4 percent Malathion powder, 1 percent Rotenone dust, 10 percent Methoxychlor, or a 10 percent DDT powder. Cats groom themselves with their tongue, hence care must be exercised in applying these potentially toxic products to them. Their sleeping areas should also be dusted or sprayed.

ORDER HEMIPTERA: TRUE BUGS

Cimex, Bedbugs

The genus *Cimex* contains important bloodsucking species, of which *Cimex lectularius,* the common bedbug, and *C. hemipterus,* the oriental bedbug, are parasites of man.

Morphology. The bedbugs have oval, dorsoventrally flattened, chestnut-brown bodies covered with short, stout, simple or serrated hairs (Fig. 112). The female, slightly larger than the male, has a length of 5.5 mm. Its flattened, pyramidal head bears prominent compound eyes, slender antennae, and specialized mouth parts in a long proboscis flexed backward beneath the head and thorax when not in use. The large conspicuous prothorax has a concave border and rounded lateral horns that give the head a shrunken appearance. Each of the three thoracic segments bears a pair of legs that terminate in a pair of simple claws. The hind wings are absent, and the forewings are reduced to small pads.

Habits. Bedbugs feed at night on man and small mammals, they conceal themselves during the day in the crevices of wooden bedsteads, in wainscoting, or under loose wallpaper. They pass readily from house to house and are easily transported in clothing and baggage. In cold weather they remain inactive in their hiding places. They can survive starvation for over a year. They emit a characteristic odor from stink glands. A blood meal seems essential to the production of a normal quota of eggs.

Life Cycle. The common bedbug may deposit as many as 200 eggs at the rate of about two per day. The white ovoid eggs, about 1 mm in length, have an oblique, projecting, collar-like ring with an operculum at the anterior end and are coated with an adhesive gelatinous substance (Fig. 112). Hatching takes place in 4 to 10 days. Development is by incomplete metamorphosis. The yellowish-white

CIMEX LECTULARIUS

BEDBUG

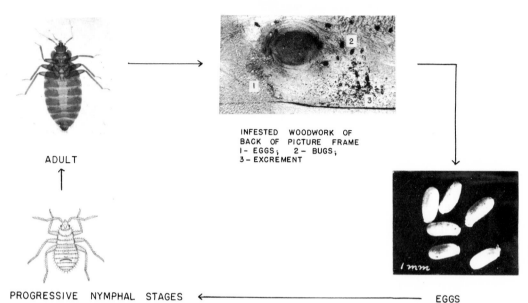

INFESTED   WOODWORK   OF
BACK   OF   PICTURE   FRAME
1- EGGS;   2 - BUGS;
3 - EXCREMENT

ADULT

PROGRESSIVE   NYMPHAL   STAGES   ←——————————————   EGGS

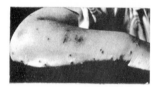

BITES   IN   TYPICAL   GROUPS   OF   2

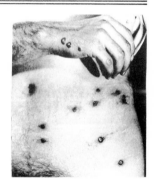

HEMORRHAGIC   BULLAE

Fig. 112. Life cycle of *Cimex lectularius.*

to brown larval bedbug passes through five or six molts at intervals of about a week to become a sexually mature adult. The life span of the adult is 6 to 12 months.

Pathogenicity.   The bite of the bedbug produces red itching wheals. Some persons show little or no reaction; others, particularly children, have local urticaria; and still others may manifest allergic symptoms with generalized urticaria and even asthma.

The role of the bedbug in the transmission of human disease is problematic. It may act as a mechanical carrier, but it is not a proved vector of human diseases. Although capable of harboring pathogenic organisms in the digestive tract, there is no regurgitation of infected blood on biting a second host, and the feces rarely contaminate the bite wound.

Treatment.   The irritation and itching of the bites of bedbugs may be relieved by ammonia, spirits of camphor, menthol-phenol paste, or calamine lotion.

Control.   In infested houses the repair of cracked plaster and wallpaper, and the substitution of iron for wooden bedsteads, is recommended. A 5 percent DDT solution in kerosene, a 0.1 percent Lindane oil solution, or a 1 percent Malathion solution is applied to floors, walls, furniture, and mattresses. It may be supplemented by the dusting of DDT powder into the crevices of the floors and walls. Care must be exercised in using these compounds on bedding used by infants.

Cone-nosed Bugs

The reduviid bugs are called "cone-nosed" bugs because of the pointed head; "barbers" or "kissing bugs" because they bite the face; "assassin" bugs, and "flying bedbugs." They are found in North and South America. The species acting as vectors of disease usually have a limited tropical distribution.

Morphology.   The triatomid bugs (Fig. 113) have long narrow heads with prominent compound eyes; usually two ocelli; four-jointed antennae; a three-segmented, ventrally folded, slender proboscis; and an obvious neck. The long, rather narrow, flattened body has functional wings and elongated legs with three-jointed tarsi. The color is dark brown with red and yellow markings on the thorax, wings, and sides of the abdomen.

Life Cycle.   The female lays, in batches of 8 to 12, about 20 white or yellowish-pink, smooth, barrel-shaped eggs, which hatch in 10 to 30 days. Development is by incomplete metamorphosis. The young bug obtains its first blood meal within 5 days and undergoes a lengthy metamorphosis of over a year with blood meals between each molt.

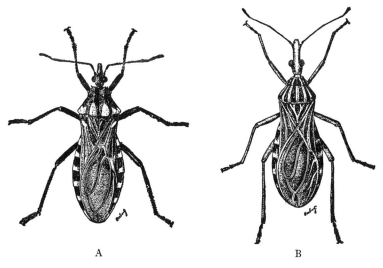

A   B

Fig. 113. A, adult male *Panstrongylus megistus;* B, adult male *Rhodnius prolixus.* (After Brumpt, from Hegner, Root, Augustine, and Huff. *Parasitology,* 1938. Courtesy of D. Appleton-Century Company.)

Pathogenicity.   Both sexes bite. Some species have a painless bite, while in others the salivary toxin produces a painful wound with oozing blood and pronounced swelling, itching, cellulitis, lymphangitis, and lymphadenitis. Some persons react severely to the bites.

Vectors of Disease.   Several species of reduviid bugs are important vectors of *Trypanosoma cruzi,* the causative agent of Chagas' disease, and *T. rangeli,* which appears to be nonpathogenic for man. Most reduviid bugs are capable of transmitting this pathogenic organism, but only certain species are efficient vectors. The most important vectors are *Triatoma infestans, Panstrongylus megistus* and *Rhodnius prolixus.*

Several species frequent houses, especially native huts, while others infest the burrows of rodents and armadillos. They move rapidly both in flight and on foot. They hide during the day in crevices and dark recesses. They feed about every third night. Natural and experimental vectors have numbered as high as 14 in Brazil and 19 in southwestern United States, where, strange to say, there have been only two cases of Chagas' disease in man. From 3 to 44 percent of the reduviid bugs are naturally infected, having acquired *T. cruzi* chiefly from wild and domesticated animals. The trypanosome undergoes a cyclic development in the mid- and hindgut of the bug over a period of 20 days. Infection is usually transmitted by fecal contamination of the bite, though occasionally directly by regurgitated blood.

Treatment.   The irritation and itching of the bites of reduviid bugs may be relieved by ammonia, spirits of camphor, menthol-phenol paste, or calamine lotion.

Control.   The control of reduviid bugs is difficult because of their activity and tendency to infest the burrows of rodents and armadillos. Lindane, hexachlorocyclohexane, is the most effective insecticide. It may be applied as an emulsion of 5 percent gamma isomer in kerosene with 0.3 percent Triton X-45 as an emulsifier, to the walls, roofs, and elsewhere in the huts, at 0.5 to 0.7 g of isomer per square meter. It may be applied also as a dusting powder on beds, cracks and holes in the walls on thatched roofs, and other possible hiding places of the bugs. An application lasts for 3 to 6 months. It has no effect on the egg, necessitating repeated applications. Dieldrin spray at a rate of 1.2 g per square meter is highly effective. Improved housing also prevents access of bugs to man.

ORDER DIPTERA: FLIES

From a medical standpoint the DIPTERA is the most important order of arthropods. It embraces many species of bloodsucking and nonbloodsucking flies, some of which are intermediate hosts or mechanical vectors of bacterial, viral, protozoan, and helminthic agents of disease.

Morphology.   The general morphology is that of insects. The relatively large head bears two compound eyes that meet in the midline (*holoptic*) or are separated by a frontal space (*dichoptic*), and usually three ocelli or simple eyes (Fig. 114).

The chitinous box-like thorax is chiefly a base of attachment for the powerful muscles of flight. The enlarged mesothorax (second segment) comprises most of the thorax and bears the large membranous wings, the prothorax (first segment) and the metathorax (third segment) being reduced to small rings that unite the thorax with the head and abdomen, respectively. Each thoracic segment carries a pair of variously colored legs adorned with spines and hairs.

The jointed legs may terminate in a pair of toothed claws and elongated hairy

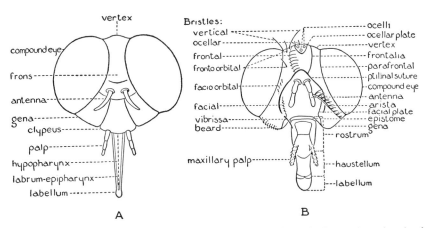

Fig. 114. Diagrammatic representation of heads of flies (frontal view). A, orthorrhaphous fly; B, cyclorrhaphous fly.

pads, the pulvilli, that secrete a sticky substance. The first two segments of the abdomen are atrophied, and the remaining segments are not always distinguishable.

The antennae, equipped with sensory organs, are composed of a series of similar and dissimilar joints, the number, shape, and hirsute adornment of which are characteristic for the various genera (Fig. 115). The more primitive flies have long antennae with numerous joints, while the more highly developed species have short antennae with fewer and heavier joints.

Various adaptations of the mouth parts enable flies to feed upon the blood and tissue juices of animals, the nectar of flowers, liquids, or food that may be liquefied by their digestive secretions. The various modifications of the mouth parts are important in distinguishing genera and species (Fig. 116). The penetration of the skin is accomplished by the saw-like mandibles and the file-like maxillae; the food channel is formed by the labrum-epipharynx and hypopharynx (Fig. 116A and B). In the bloodsucking muscid flies, the cutting organs are highly developed prestomal teeth at the labellar tip of the labium (Fig. 116D). In the nonbloodsucking species, the fly absorbs its food in liquid state through its labella (Fig. 116C).

Flies have paired true wings arising from the mesothorax and small club-like

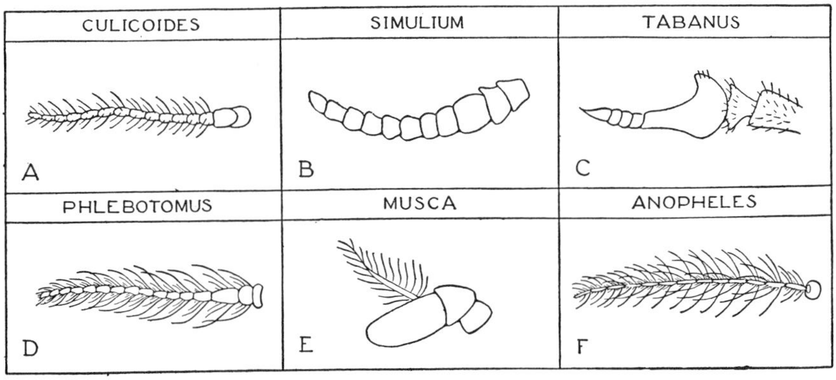

CULICOIDES	SIMULIUM	TABANUS
A	B	C
PHLEBOTOMUS	MUSCA	ANOPHELES
D	E	F

Fig. 115. Antennae of various genera of DIPTERA. (A, B, C, and E redrawn from Hegner, Root, Augustine, and Huff. *Parasitology*, 1938. Courtesy of D. Appleton-Century Company.)

halteres, considered homologous with the metathoracic wings of other insects. The true wings are thin, membranous extensions of the tergal integument, supported by longitudinal, chitinous, tracheal tubes or "veins" that radiate from the base of the wing and are connected at intervals by cross veins. They may be transparent or covered with spines, scales, or hairs that give an iridescent or mottled appearance. The spaces between the veins are called cells. The number and position of the veins and enclosed cells, and the distribution of hairs and scales, are of value in identifying genera and species (Fig. 117).

Life Cycle.   Most species of flies are oviparous, but a few deposit larvae in various stages of development. The eggs or larvae are deposited in water, on the ground, in excreta, or in the bodies of vertebrates. Metamorphosis is complete. The elongated, legless, wormlike larva (Fig. 124) leads an aquatic or terrestrial existence. It feeds voraciously with its chewing mouth parts on organic material or becomes adapted to a parasitic existence. After three to four molts, it becomes a nonfeeding pupa that eventually develops into an adult fly.

Mosquitoes

Mosquitoes are slender, delicate flies of evil reputation. The bloodsucking mosquitoes of the family CULICIDAE include important vectors of viral, protozoan, and helminthic diseases of man and lower animals.

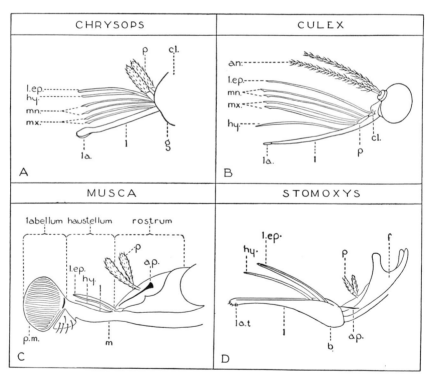

Fig. 116. Schematic representation of mouth parts of various genera of DIPTERA. Orthorrhaphous flies: A, *Chrysops* (bloodsucking); B, *Culex* (bloodsucking). Cyclorrhaphous flies; C, *Musca* (non-bloodsucking); D, *Stomoxys* (bloodsucking).

an., antennae; ap., apodeme of labrum; b, bulb; cl., clypeus; f, fulcrum; g, gena; hy., hypopharynx; l, labium; la., labella; la.t., labellar teeth; l.ep., labrum-epipharynx; m, mentum; mn., mandibles; mx., maxillae; p, palps; p.m., pseudotracheal membrane.

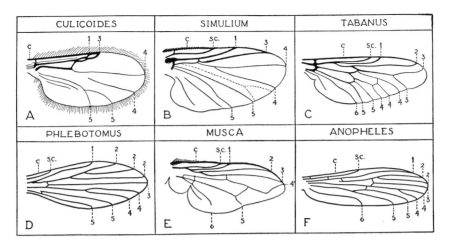

Fig. 117. Wing venation of certain genera of diptera of medical importance. c, costal vein; sc., subcostal vein; 1-6, longitudinal veins. (A, B, C, and E redrawn with modifications and D and F redrawn from Hegner, Root, Augustine, and Huff. *Parasitology,* 1938. Courtesy of D. Appleton-Century Company.)

Morphology. Mosquitoes (Fig. 118) are distinguished from other flies by: (1) the elongated mouth parts of the females, adapted with few exceptions for piercing and sucking blood; (2) the long 15-jointed antennae, plumose in the males and pilose in the females; and (3) the charactersitic wing venation and scales. The roughly spherical head is almost covered by a pair of compound eyes that nearly meet. The rigid thorax, covered by a dorsal scutum, bears three pairs of long, slender legs. The coloration and pattern of the thoracic scales and bristles are useful in differentiating genera and species.

The mouth parts of the bloodsucking female consist of the grooved lower labium, the upper labrum-epipharynx, the hypopharynx, the stylet-like paired mandibles, and the serrated maxillae (Fig. 116B). The maxillary palps of the female are slender and hairy, while those of the males are long and ornamented like the antennae with tufts of hair, giving a plumed appearance (Fig. 119). The salivary glands are located in the prothorax. The male mosquito with its weak mouthparts is unable to penetrate human skin and is therefore relegated to a vegetarian diet— plant juices. "It's the female of the species that's more deadly than the male."

A pair of strong wings is attached to the mesothorax, and a pair of vestigial wings to the metathorax. The venation, especially the anterior and posterior forked cells, and the structure, size, and distribution of the flat squamous and long plume scales distinguish the mosquito from other flies and differentiate genera and species.

Habits. Each species has an effective flight range between the breeding grounds and the sources of the blood meal, as well as a maximal range—1 to 3 miles for *Anopheles;* up to 10 miles for *Culex;* and 50 to 100 miles for some *Aedes.*

Mosquitoes are attracted by bright light, dark-colored clothing, and the presence of man and animals. Long-distance attraction is due to the olfactory stimulus of animal emanations, especially CO_2 and certain amino acids, and immediate localization to warmth and moisture. Certain species in their bloodsucking preferences are pre-eminently anthropophilic (man), and others are essentially zoophilic (animals). Host preference of the different species may be determined by precipitin tests on the blood meals. Predilection for man determines the importance of

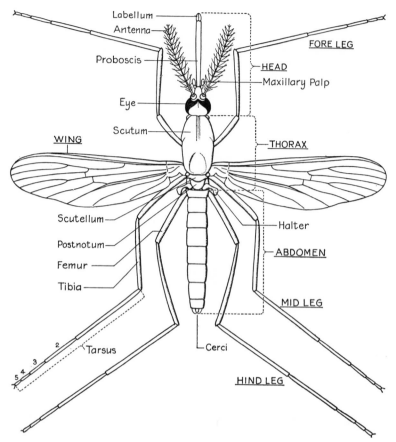

Fig. 118. Diagram of mosquito (female). Dorsal view, showing nomenclature of parts. (Adapted from MacGregor, 1927, and Marshall, 1938.)

an anopheline species as a vector of malaria. With the exception of a few species, the females are the bloodsuckers. As a rule females cannot produce fertile eggs without ingesting blood, which is required to produce the gonadotropic hormone necessary for ovulation. This hormone from the corpora allata, "pituitary" of the insect brain, may be activated by serotonin and adrenaline of the victim's blood. The biting activities of the different species vary with age, time of day, and environment. Likewise, the daily rhythm of attack varies with the season and temperature. Certain species frequent houses for feeding and resting, while other species enter houses only for feeding and spend their resting periods elsewhere. The former are readily destroyed by residual spraying of the houses with insecticides.

Mating is preceded by the prenuptial swarming of the males. Cross-matings between species are rarely successful. The anopheline and culicine mosquitoes deposit their eggs in water, but many *Aëdes* mosquitoes select shaded ground subject to intermittent flooding. The maximal number of eggs deposited at one time is 100 to 400. Many anopheline species lay over 1,000 eggs in a lifetime. The average life span of the adult female mosquito is about 30 days, rarely reaching 8 weeks.

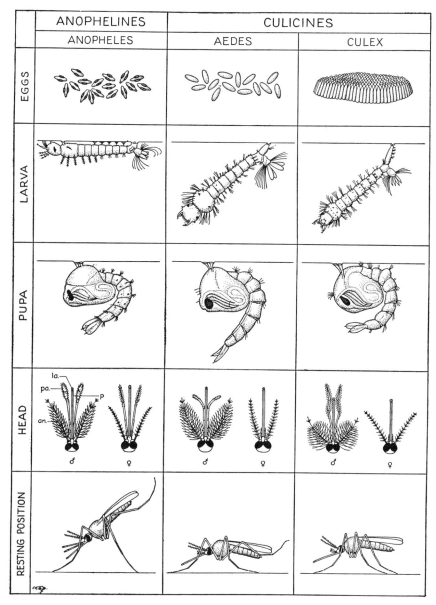

	ANOPHELINES	CULICINES	
	ANOPHELES	AEDES	CULEX
EGGS			
LARVA			
PUPA			
HEAD			
RESTING POSITION			

Fig. 119. Schematic representation of differential characteristics of anopheline and culicine mosquitoes. an., antennae; la., labella; p, proboscis; pa., palp.

The females of species frequenting houses may hibernate as adults during winter, and a few species pass the winter in the larval stage. Species vary in their natural susceptibility to environmental conditions and, possibly, in their ability to develop resistance against insecticides. Birds and bats are natural enemies of the adults; and waterfowl, fish, and insects prey on the larvae.

Life Cycle. The larval development of the diverse species occurs under extremely varied environmental conditions, moisture being the chief essential. Most species use fresh water for their aquatic stages, but some, chiefly culicines, breed in brackish or salt water. Domesticated mosquitoes, such as *Culex quinquefasciatus* and *Aëdes aegypti,* breed in small pools of water in the vicinity of human habitations.

The egg, about 0.7 mm in length, is encased in a three-layered shell that has a funnel-shaped passage for the entry of the spermatozoa. The eggs of *Anopheles* resemble boats with lateral, ribbed, exchorionic floats; the tapering eggs of *Culex,* with cup-shaped corona, are cemented in raft-like masses; and the elliptical eggs of *Aëdes* are polygonally sculptured. The eggs that are laid in water hatch in 1 to 3 days at 30° C, but may require 7 days at 16° C, while those of *Aëdes* do not hatch until the ground is flooded with water. The eggs of different species vary in their resistance to desiccation and to high and low temperatures. Anopheline eggs usually perish above 40° C and below 0° C, and do not develop below 12° C.

The elongate, limbless larva (Fig. 119), with simple or transversely branched tufted hairs symmetrically arranged along its body, passes through four instars to attain a length of about 10 mm. The head bears compound eyes, hirsute antennae, and chewing mouth parts. The eighth abdominal segment carries two spiracles. The anal aperture is surrounded by four flexible papillary processes, the anal gills. Their function is probably the absorption of water rather than respiration. The resting anopheline larvae are suspended horizontally at the surface of the water and the culicine hang at an angle (Fig. 119). The larvae feed on algae, bacteria, and forms of particulate matter, 20 to 100 μ in size. The anopheline larvae obtain their food at the surface, and the culicine larvae beneath the surface, by sweeping particles with their mouth brushes or by nibbling decaying matter at the bottom. They swim with a jerky motion, rising to the surface to breathe. They are able to withstand moderately cold temperatures. The length of the larval cycle, under optimal conditions, averages a little over 3 weeks, but may range from 2 weeks to 6 months, depending upon the food supply and temperature.

The fourth instar larva becomes a megalocephalic curved pupa that resembles a question mark (Fig. 119). The pupa has respiratory trumpets on the thorax, an air vesicle situated between the future wings of the adult, and a pair of overlapping paddles with terminal hairs on the last abdominal segment. These paddles enable the pupa to dive rapidly in a succession of jerky somersaults in response to stimuli. Pupae are readily destroyed by freezing or drying. The nonfeeding pupal stage lasts 2 to 5 days, but may be prolonged to 10 days at low temperatures; no development takes place below 10° C. In hatching, the pupal skin is ruptured by the air vesicle and the activity of the escaping adult insect.

Classification.   The family CULICIDAE is divided into three subfamilies, of which only the ANOPHELINAE (the large genus *Anopheles*) and the CULICINAE (containing the *Theobaldia-Mansonia,* the *Aëdes,* and the *Culex* groups) have species that are vectors of human diseases. The principal genera thus associated are *Anopheles, Culex, Aëdes,* and *Mansonia,* and, to a lesser extent, *Haemagogus* and *Psorophora.*

Species are differentiated by the coloration and pattern of scales and bristles, wing venation and scales, male hypopygium, and the type of distribution of hairs, bristles, and appendages of the fourth-instar larva. The main differences between anopheline and culicine mosquitoes are given in Figure 119.

The numerous species of *Anopheles* vary greatly as to habitat, being found in open country, wooded areas, urban or rural communities and at various altitudes.

The different species have a wide range of preferential breeding grounds, from shaded to sunny places, from fresh to strongly brackish water, and from puddles of water to moderately swift streams, with a wide range in free-oxygen content. Anopheline mosquitoes are the only vectors of human malaria, and certain species transmit Bancroft's and Malayan filariasis.

The genus *Aëdes* includes many species of mosquitoes of cosmopolitan distribution. They breed in tree holes and in temporary pools of fresh or tidal waters. Many North American species are troublesome biters. Certain species may act as vectors of yellow fever, dengue, filariasis, and the viral encephalitides.

A large number of species of the genus *Culex* with its many subgenera are distributed throughout the world, mostly in warm regions. These small- to medium-sized mosquitoes breed for the most part in permanent bodies of water and have both an urban and a rural distribution. Certain species transmit filariasis and the viral encephalitides.

Adults of the genus *Mansonia* have white-banded legs and usually a mixture of black and white scales on the wings. Their distribution is cosmopolitan but largely tropical. The eggs are deposited in clumps on aquatic plants (*Pistia*) from which the larvae obtain oxygen and food. Certain species are vectors of Malayan filariasis.

Pathogenicity. In biting, the piercing apparatus probes beneath the skin until a blood supply is tapped, at which time feeding may take place from the blood vessel or from the extravasated blood. The intermittently injected saliva may contain substances that stimulate capillary dilation or slow coagulation. Some bites cause little irritation, and others a considerable amount. The ordinary bite is followed by erythema, swelling, and itching. Vesicular bullae may appear, and secondary infections may result from scratching. Occasionally, persons manifest severe local symptoms of the urticarial, tuberculoid, and eczematous types. An immediate allergic response is due to sensitization to the multiple antigens of the saliva and a delayed response to a slow-acting toxin.

Vectors of Disease. Mosquitoes serve as cyclic or mechanical vectors of bacterial, helminthic, protozoan, and viral diseases of man and lower animals. Also, day-flying and day-biting mosquitoes of the genera *Psorophora* and *Janthinosoma* carry the eggs of the myiasis-producing warble fly, *Dermatobia hominis,* to the skin of man and other mammals. The species that are important vectors are listed under the respective diseases.

MALARIA. The only cyclic vectors of human and simian malaria are anopheline mosquitoes, while both anopheline and culicine mosquitoes carry avian malaria.

Practically every species of *Anopheles* may be infected experimentally, but many species are not natural vectors. Some 110 species have been associated with the transmission of malaria, of which 50 are of general or local importance. The aptitude of a species for transmitting malaria is determined by: (1) its presence in or near human habitations; (2) its preference for human rather than animal blood, although when animals are scarce, zoophilic species may feed on man; (3) an environment that favors its propagation and provides a life span sufficiently long for the plasmodia to complete their life cycles; and (4) physiologic susceptibility to infection.

The suitability of a species as a potential vector may be determined by recording the percentage of infected mosquitoes after feeding on a malarial patient, but its importance as a vector is ascertained by obtaining the index of natural infections, usually 1 to 5 percent, in female mosquitoes collected in houses in a malarial district.

The following species are among the more important vectors of malaria:

Americas
A. albimanus	Central and South America, West Indies, Mexico
A. albitarsis	South America
A. aquasalis	South America, West Indies
A. darlingi	South and Central America
A. freeborni	Western U.S.A., Mexico
A. pseudopunctipennis	Central and South America, Mexico, southwestern U.S.A.
A. punctimacula	Central and South America
A. quadrimaculatus	East, Central and South U.S.A.

Europe and Mediterranean Area
A. atroparvus	Europe
A. claviger	Eastern Mediterranean, Near East
A. labranchiae	Southern Europe, North Africa
A. maculipennis	Southeastern Europe
A. sacharovi	Southeastern Europe, Near East, Asia
A. sergenti	Egypt, Near East
A. superpictus	Eastern Mediterranean, Near East

Asia
A. culicifacies	Southern Asia
A. hyrcanus sinensis	Southeast Asia, Pacific Islands
A. fluviatilis	India
A. maculatus	Southeast and East Asia, Taiwan
A. minimus	Southeast and East Asia, Taiwan
A. stephensi	South Asia
A. sundaicus	South and Southeast Asia, Indonesia
A. umbrosus	Southeast Asia, Indonesia

Africa
A. funestus	East, West, Central, and South Africa; Malagasy; Mauritius
A. gambiae	East, West, Central, and South Africa; Malagasy; Mauritius, Reunion, and Cape Verde Islands
A. melas	West African coast, Mauritius

Pacific Islands
A. farauti	Solomons, Hebrides, New Guinea, New Britain to eastern Celebes, Australia
A. punctulatus	New Guinea, Solomons, other islands

FILARIASIS. Mosquitoes are vectors of *Wuchereria bancrofti* and *Brugia malayi*. Numerous species of *Anopheles, Aëdes, Culex,* and *Mansonia* have shown complete development of *W. bancrofti,* but most of these species are unimportant as natural vectors. In the tropics and subtropics *Culex quinquefasciatus* (= *fatigans*), a night-biting mosquito of domesticated and urban habits that breeds in partially polluted water near human habitations, is the common vector of the nocturnal periodic form of Bancroftian filariasis. *Aëdes polynesiensis* is the common vector of the nonperiodic type of Bancroftian filariasis in certain South Pacific islands. This rural mosquito, which rests in bushes (never in houses) and breeds in coconut shells and cavities of trees, feeds on domesticated mammals and chickens, but prefers man.

YELLOW FEVER. Yellow fever, a viral disease of high mortality, has spread from its original West African focus over the tropical and subtropical regions of the world. The mosquito, which acquires the infection by biting the patient during the first 3 days of the disease, becomes infective for life, after the incubation of the virus for 12 days. Some 38 species of mosquitoes, chiefly of the genus *Aëdes,* and *Haemagogus* are vectors. During 1853 to 1854 New Orleans (U.S.) reported 11,500 yellow fever deaths.

Aëdes aegypti, the principal vector of epidemic yellow fever, is an anthropophilic species that frequents the vicinity of houses. It breeds in all manner of domestic water receptacles, the larvae thriving as bottom feeders in clean or foul water containing organic material. Consequently, it can be readily controlled by the destruction of its breeding places and larvae. Persons may be protected against epidemic yellow fever by screening and by control of *A. aegypti,* and against the endemic jungle disease by vaccination.

Dengue is an endemic viral disease of the tropics and subtropics that at times becomes epidemic. The virus, which requires an incubational period of 8 to 10 days before the mosquito becomes infective, is transmitted chiefly by species of *Aëdes,* especially *A. aegypti.*

VIRAL ENCEPHALITIDES.   The various encephalitides are transmitted by species of *Culex* and *Aëdes* and occasionally by *Anopheles* and *Mansonia.* Japanese B encephalitis, which has its natural reservoir in domestic mammals and occurs in epidemics at times with high mortality, is transmitted by *Culex pipiens* var. *pallens, C. tritaeniorhynchus,* and *Aëdes togoi.* In central and western United States, St. Louis encephalitis, which has its reservoir mostly in domesticated birds, is transmitted chiefly by *Culex tarsalis* and *C. pipiens,* while species of *Aëdes, Culex,* and *Anopheles* have been found infected in nature. Equine encephalomyelitis, a highly fatal disease of horses and at times of man, the virus of which is found in wild and domesticated birds, is capable of being transmitted by *Aëdes, Culex, Anopheles,* and *Mansonia* mosquitoes. *Culex tarsalis* is probably the most important vector of the western type, and *Culiseta melanura* of the eastern type. The Venezuelan type is carried by *Aëdes taeniorhynchus, Anopheles neomaculipalpis,* and *Mansonia titillans.* West Nile encephalitis is transmitted by several species of *Culex* and *Aëdes. Aëdes aegypti* is an experimental vector of lymphocytic choriomeningitis. Numerous other viruses have been isolated from mosquitoes.

In Norway, tularemia has been spread among sheep and rodents by species of *Anopheles, Aëdes,* and *Mansonia.*

Control.   Mosquito control requires a knowledge of the habits of the particular species, the topography and climate of the country, and the racial and socioeconomic status of the population. Mosquitoes may be controlled by: (1) elimination or reduction of their breeding grounds, (2) destruction of the larvae, and (3) destruction of adult mosquitoes. More than one method may be required. The effectiveness of control measures may be determined by the local reduction in mosquitoes and the decline in the incidence of the transmitted diseases.

The destruction of breeding grounds, essentially an engineering problem, gives permanent results, but involves high initial and maintenance costs. Drainage is applicable to species of limited flight range that breed in quiet bodies of waters, but it must be supplemented by the filling of depressions. Extensive drainage operations are seldom practicable, but they are of value at selected sites. Water level management, and the removal of vegetation from the banks and surfaces of streams and ponds, reduces the breeding grounds of many species. Changing the water level by intermittent flushing has proved useful for controlling species that breed in impounded waters and flowing streams. Tide gates have been installed for the control of brackish water breeding mosquitoes.

Destruction of the larvae may be accomplished by the introduction of larva-eating fish such as *Gambusia,* by oiling the waters with toxic and suffocating films that affect the surface-inhabiting larvae, and/or by the use of such larvicides as DDT, DDD, BHC, Chlordane, Dieldrin, Malathion, or Paris green.

Adult mosquitoes may be caught by hand, trapped, or killed by insecticides. Pyrethrum insecticidal sprays may be used for immediate killing both inside and outside of houses and for residual killing inside buildings.

The residual spraying of the interior walls of houses or outbuildings with DDT has proved particularly effective in reducing the number of the anopheline vectors of malaria that frequent buildings for their blood meals and resting periods. An application of an aqueous suspension at a concentration of 50 to 200 mg per square foot of surface is effective for nearly 4 months. Halogenated hydrocarbons may owe their activity to the formation of a protein complex with charge-transfer properties that interfere with the normal conductivity of the nerve axon. BHC, Chlordane, Malathion, and Dieldrin may also be used.

The protection of man against mosquitoes comprises mosquito-proofing of buildings with 18-mesh wire screening; mosquito nets over beds; protective clothing such as head nets, gloves, and high boots; and repellents applied to skin and clothing. Effective repellents such as indalone, dimethyl phthalate, and Rutgers 612, diethyltoluamide, "Off," are effective for several hours.

Culicoides, Midges

The genus *Culicoides* includes several hundred species of aggressive biters and contains species that are vectors of human parasites. They are cosmopolitan, except Patagonia and New Zealand.

Common Names.   Midges, gnats, punkies, and no-see-ums.

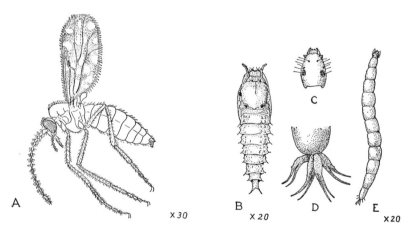

Fig. 120. The genus *Culicoides*. A, *Culicoides austeni*, adult female; B, pupa of *C. kiefferi;* C, head of larva of *C. kiefferi;* D, last segment of larva of *C. kiefferi* showing tracheal gills extruded; E, larva of *C. kiefferi*. (A redrawn from Sharp, 1928; B-E redrawn from Patton, 1913.)

Morphology. These delicate brown or black flies (Fig. 120) are chiefly identified by their small size, 1.0 to 1.5 mm; slightly humped thorax that projects over the head; and the venation of, and spots on, the wings.

Habits. The midges swarm during the day near ponds and swamps. They breed in forest, jungle, and swampland, in fresh and brackish water, but may be found far from these breeding places. Only the bloodsucking female has blade-like cutting mouth parts.

Life Cycle. The small oval eggs are deposited on plants or vegetable material in such shallow water as margins of ponds, puddles, and tree holes. In about 3 days the smooth, elongated, 12-segmented larvae wriggle into the bottom mud, where they feed on vegetable debris with their toothed mandibles. In 1 to 12 months they become elongated pupae with terminal spines and respiratory trumpets. The adult fly emerges from the pupa in 3 to 5 days.

Pathogenicity. The bite of the fly causes considerable irritation, and sensitive persons may experience severe local pruritus and fever.

Vectors of Disease. Certain species are hosts of filarial parasites which infect man—in Africa, *C. austeni* and *C. grahami* of *Acanthocheilonema perstans* and *C. grahami* of *Dipetalonema streptocerca;* and in the Western Hemisphere, *C. furens* and *C. paraensis* of *Mansonella ozzardi.* Other species are intermediate hosts of filarial parasites of lower animals. A number of viruses have been isolated from *Culicoides.*

Control. Control measures are unsatisfactory. Local breeding grounds may be reduced by drainage and filling operations. Ordinary screens do not exclude these small flies. The residual spraying of the door and window screens and interiors of houses with DDT or other insecticides may prevent their entrance. Individuals may be protected by repellents.

Phlebotomus, Sandflies

Members of the genus *Phlebotomus* are called sandflies, humpbacked sandflies, moth flies, and owl midges.

Geographic Distribution. Cosmopolitan in tropical and subtropical countries.

Morphology. The slender, humpbacked, yellowish or buff-colored sandflies (Fig. 121) are characterized by their small size (3 mm), extreme hairyness of bodies and wings, and erect V-shaped position of the wings at rest. The hairy, oval, or lanceolate wings are devoid of scales, and the second longitudinal vein forks near its middle with a second fork in the anterior branch before reaching the margin. The 16-jointed antennae are long and hairy. The mouth parts have blade-like cutting organs.

Habits. Most species feed on mammals, a few on reptiles. As a rule, the females are the bloodsuckers, but in some species the males have piercing mouth parts. Most species are active nocturnal feeders, especially on warm humid nights. During the daytime the flies rest in crevices in stone, concrete, or earth constructions, or in rodent burrows. Inability to fly against slight winds limits their flight range to less than a mile from their breeding places. They enter houses in a series of short intermittent flights and rest on the walls before biting man.

Life Cycle. In 30 to 36 hours after the blood meal, the female fly deposits, in

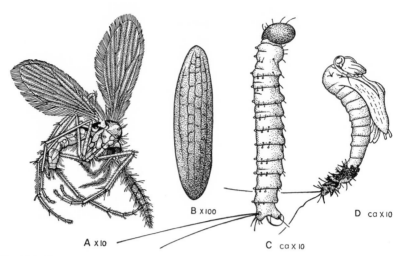

Fig. 121. The genus *Phlebotomus*. A, adult fly; B, egg of *P. papatasii;* C, larva of *P. papatasii;* D, pupa of *P. papatasii.* (A redrawn from Hegner, Root, Augustine, and Huff. *Parasitology,* 1938. Courtesy of D. Appleton-Century Company; B-D redrawn from Newstead, 1911.)

dark, moist crevices near nitrogenous waste, 30 to 50 elongated eggs (Fig. 121). After 6 to 12 days the egg develops into a sluggish, segmented, caterpillar-like larva with long caudal bristles, which feeds on dead leaves and nitrogenous wastes. The larva undergoes four molts in 25 to 35 days before it becomes a buff-colored pupa with a triangular head and curved abdomen. The adult fly, which emerges from the pupa in 6 to 14 days, has a life span of about 14 days. The entire period from egg to adult is 5 to 9 weeks.

Pathogenicity. The bite of the fly produces a rose-colored papule surrounded by an erythematous area 10 to 20 mm in diameter. There is a stinging pain and an itching that persists for some time. In sensitive persons the local lesions are more pronounced and may be accompanied by nausea, fever, and malaise.

Vectors of Disease. Sandflies are the vectors of leishmaniasis, pappataci fever, and bartonellosis. *Leishmania donovani,* the cause of kala-azar; *L. tropica,* the agent of oriental sore; and *L. braziliensis,* the etiologic agent of American leishmaniasis, are transmitted by *Phlebotomus.*

Pappataci or phlebotomus fever, a viral disease prevalent in Mediterranean countries and southern Asia, is chiefly transmitted by *P. papatasii,* which becomes infectious after a developmental period of 7 to 10 days for the virus.

Bartonellosis occurs in northwestern South America as the acute febrile Carrión's disease and as a chronic granulomatous verrucous condition. The causative bacillus, *Bartonella bacilliformis,* is transmitted by the Andean sandflies.

Control. The reduction of breeding grounds by filling, drainage, and the elimination of cracks and crevices is a satisfactory method of control because of the short flight range of the insect. Residual spraying of the interiors of houses with DDT has proved highly successful in freeing dwelling houses of sandflies and reducing leishmaniasis, although the flies remain abundant outdoors. Persons may be protected by repellents such as diethyltoluamide (Off).

Simulium, Black Fly

Common Names. Black flies, buffalo gnats, turkey gnats, and Kolumbtz flies.
Geographic Distribution. Cosmopolitan.
Morphology. Black flies (Fig. 122) are identified by their small size (2 to 3 mm), stout hump-backed forms, short legs, conspicuous compound eyes, short smooth antennae, and venation of the unspotted wings. The short proboscis has blade-like cutting organs. The body is covered with short golden or silver hairs that give it a longitudinally striped appearance.
Habits. Black flies breed in moderately swift woodland streams in upland regions. They remain near, or move along, these shaded watercourses. Their migratory range is usually 2 to 3 miles, rarely over 8. The females bite during the daytime, particularly in the morning and toward evening in open places at the edge of thick vegetation. They may enter darkened houses, and they bite men in the vicinity of buildings. They are a particular scourge to fishermen at certain seasons.
Life Cycle. The triangular-shaped eggs are laid in batches of 300 to 500 and are attached by a gelatinous secretion to stones, leaves, submerged plants, stakes, and branches. In 3 to 5 days a yellowish-green, cylindrical larva with hairy mouth parts and finger-like anal gills emerges and attaches itself in an upright position to rocks, aquatic vegetation, and other debris. In Africa the larva and pupa of *S. neavei* are found on the surface of fresh-water crabs (*Potamon*). It molts seven times in 13 days before spinning a cocoon with an open pocket, in which the dark brown pupa with posterior hooklets and long respiratory filaments is attached. The adult emerges in about 3 days; the females live only a few weeks.

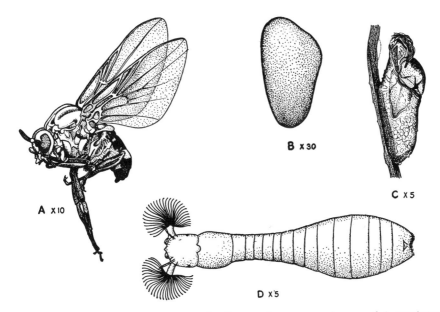

Fig. 122. The genus *Simulium*. A, adult fly; B, egg; C, cocoon and pupa of *S. mexicanum*, lateral view; D, larva, dorsal view. (A and D redrawn from Hegner, Root, Augustine, and Huff. *Parasitology*, 1938. Courtesy of D. Appleton-Century Company; C redrawn from Bequaert, 1934.)

Pathogenicity. The bite, painless at first, often bleeds profusely. Later, swelling, pruritis, and pain develop, which may continue for some days. In susceptible individuals even a few bites may cause marked local inflammation and general incapacity.

Vectors of Disease. In Africa *S. damnosum* and *S. neavei,* and in the Americas *S. metallicum, S. ochraceum,* and *S. callidum,* are vectors of onchocerciasis. Other species are probably minor vectors, and still others transmit onchocerciasis of cattle and protozoan diseases of birds.

Treatment. The painful, itching, slow-healing bites of black flies may be partially relieved by antiseptic and soothing lotions.

Control. Black flies are difficult to control. The adult flies may be reduced in number by spraying their bushy resting places with 20 mg DDT or 4 mg γ isomer BHC per square meter. Better results are obtained by using DDT as a larvicide in the form of a wettable powder or in solution for streams, usually by the drip method. An initial concentration of 0.1 ppm applied for 3 minutes for streams with a flow below 5,000 gallons per minute and 2 ppm for streams with over 5,000 gallons, is effective for 2 miles. The reduction of onchocerciasis has been most promising, but complete extermination of the flies except in limited areas is not worth attempting. Mechanical destruction of breeding places is effective but expensive. Travellers in black fly districts may be protected by fine head nets, tight sleeves and trouser bottoms, and repellents.

Chrysops, Deer Fly

Of the 60 genera of the family TABANIDAE, only the genus *Chrysops* contains vectors of human diseases, although other species are vicious biters.

Common Names. Species of *Chrysops* are known as deer flies; other tabanids as horse flies, mangrove flies, breeze flies, green-headed flies, clegs, and seroots.

Geographic Distribution. *Chrysops* flies are cosmopolitan, but are more abundant in the Americas.

Morphology. The tabanid flies are recognized by their robust shape and brilliant color. *Chrysops* flies are small tabanids with conspicuous markings, slender antennae, brilliantly colored eyes, yellow-banded abdomens with dark stripes, and clear wings with one dark band along the anterior margin and a broad crossband at the level of the discal cell. The bloodsucking female has an awl-shaped epipharynx, bladelike mandibles, and serrated maxillae (Fig. 116A).

Habits. *Chrysops* flies are found in shady woodlands. In Africa their main habitat is the woodlands and savanna grass lands, and the rain forest species have probably been derived from this source. The bloodsucking females attack man most actively in the early morning and late afternoon. This midday diminution probably is associated with light intensity, since at ground and canopy level there is no marked bimodal activity.

Life Cycle. The female deposits 200 to 800 elongated, spindle-shaped eggs in adhesive masses on aquatic plants, grasses, or rocks overhanging water. The carnivorous larvae, which hatch in 4 to 5 days, pass through six molts in mud and water before they pupate in dry ground. The adult emerges from the pupa in 10 to 18 days. The life cycle may be completed in the tropics in 4 or more months, but in the temperate zones it may extend over 2 years.

Pathogenicity. The fly usually makes several thrusts of the cutting mouth parts before it starts drawing about 30 cu mm of blood from the hemorrhagic pool. The ugly puncture wound is not immediately painful. Within a few hours there is considerable irritation and, often, swelling that may persist for days.

Vectors of Disease. Species of *Chrysops* are associated with the transmission of the filarial parasite *Loa loa* and of *Pasteurella tularensis,* the cause of tularemia. The western deer fly *C. discalis* has transmitted tularemia to both man and animals. The chief cyclic vectors of human loasis are the numerous *C. silacea* and *C. dimidiata,* both of which have close contact with man.

Treatment. Soothing lotions.

Control. Control measures are unsatisfactory. The adult flies may be killed by DDT. Larvicidal measures are effective only for certain species. Domestic animals may be given some protection by smudges, sprays, and repellent dips. Man may be protected by nets and repellents.

BLOODSUCKING FLIES OF THE FAMILY MUSCIDAE

The bloodsucking flies of the family MUSCIDAE comprise relatively few genera: *Stomoxys* (stable flies) and *Glossina* (tsetse flies) that attack man and animals, and *Haematobia* and *Philaematomyia* that prey on domesticated animals.

Stomoxys, Stable Flies

The cosmopolitan stable fly, *S. calcitrans,* is a typical representative of the genus *Stomoxys,* which includes 10 or more similar species. It is an annoying pest of man and animals, and a mechanical vector of animal diseases.

Common Names. Stable fly, storm fly, and stinging fly.

Morphology. The oval, grayish fly resembles, but is slightly larger than, the house fly. It may be distinguished by its bayonet-shaped proboscis, robust appearance, dark color, thorax with four dark longitudinal stripes, and banded abdomen. The labium, which in other flies usually forms a sheath for the mouth parts, is itself a piercing organ (Fig. 116D).

Life Cycle. The flies usually frequent stables and farmyards, attracted by animals and decaying vegetation. Both males and females attack domesticated animals and man during the day. They invade houses during or after rain storms. The life span of the adult is about 17 days. The female deposits up to 275 eggs during her lifetime, in batches of 20 to 50, on moist decaying vegetation in barnyards, marshy ground, or on the banks of streams. The elongated, creamy-white, banana-shaped egg produces in 1 to 3 days, a creamy-white, translucent, footless larva that becomes a pupa in 1 to 3 weeks. Under favorable conditions, the life cycle is completed in 3 to 4 weeks.

Pathogenicity. The bite causes a sharp initial, and subsequent prickling, pains, but after the extraction of blood there is little discomfort. A drop of blood collects at the site of the puncture and a small roseola with a scarlet center persists for some time. Cattle and horses, subjected to frequent and heavy attacks, lose flesh and are unable to work.

Vectors of Disease. The habit stable flies have of leaving one animal to feed on another makes them ideal mechanical vectors of disease. *S. calcitrans* is the natural mechanical vector of *Trypanosoma evansi* (surra) in cattle and horses.

Several human diseases have been experimentally transmitted by the stable fly, such as African sleeping sickness, oriental sore, and poliomyelitis. Stable flies have also been accused of spreading anthrax and the infectious anemia of horses among animals.

Treatment.　Soothing lotions.

Control.　Control is best achieved by destroying the breeding places through the removal of decaying vegetable material. Chemical treatment of manure, without impairing its value as fertilizer, will kill the larvae. Stables may be screened and their walls sprayed with DDT to destroy the adult flies.

Glossina, Tsetse Flies

The genus *Glossina* includes some 20 or more African species of tsetse flies, several of which are intermediate hosts of the trypanosomes of man and animals.

Geographic Distribution.　Equatorial Africa from 18° N to 31° S latitude. *G. tachinoides* is also found in southern Arabia.

Morphology.　The yellow, brown, or black flies (Fig. 123), 6 to 13 mm, are distinguished by: (1) the resting position of the wings, which fold over each other like the blades of scissors; (2) the slender, horizontal proboscis with its bulbous base; (3) the branched, curved bristles on the arista of the three-jointed antennae; and (4) the distinctive venation of the light brown wings. *G. palpalis* is a blackish-brown fly with pale lateral markings on its abdomen. *G. morsitans* is a gray fly with brown transverse bands on its yellowish-orange third to sixth abdominal segments. The mouth parts are the labium-piercing type, the whole proboscis entering the wound.

Habits.　The various species occupy a wide range of habitats, each species having preferred climate, vegetation, and fauna, but all requiring warmth and moisture.

There are two general classes: (1) the riverine species as *G. palpalis,* which frequent hot damp areas on the borders of streams, rivers, and lakes in West and Central Africa; and (2) the bush species such as *G. morsitans,* which are found in wooded and bush country that provides moderate shade in East Africa. The fly belts are irregular zones of varying dimensions surrounded by localities that are practically fly-free. For the bush species, ridge-top glades and thickets in valleys or along the slopes of hills are good habitats, but species vary in preference.

The life span of the male is half that of the female, which in the case of *G. palpalis* is about 13 weeks (in captivity). Both male and female flies are day biters of animals and man. Vision and, to a lesser extent, smell are the primary factors in directing the flies to their hosts. *G. palpalis* is attracted by black or blue cloth, particularly if flapping in the wind. The effective flight range is short; it is probably less than one-half mile for *G. morsitans,* but *G. palpalis* is capable of crossing barriers over 3 miles wide.

Life Cycle.　The breeding grounds of the riverine species are sandy beaches and loose soil near water; those of the bush species loose soil near fallen trees or low-branching limbs. The female produces single, large, mature, third-stage larvae at intervals of about 10 days. *G. palpalis* yields a total of nine larvae. The yellow, knobbed larva (Fig. 123E), nearly as long as the abdomen of the fly, has a pair of dark protuberances, tumid lips, on the last segment. It burrows to a depth of

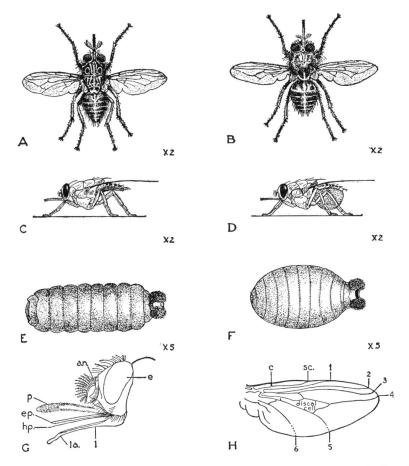

Fig. 123. Tsetse flies. A, *Glossina palpalis,* male; B, *G. morsitans,* female; C, *G. palpalis,* lateral view, before feeding; D, *G. palpalis,* lateral view, after blood meal; E, larva of *G. palpalis;* F, puparium of *G. pallidipes;* G, head and mouth parts of *G. palpalis;* H, wing of *G. palpalis,* showing venation.

an., antenna; c, costal vein; sc., subcostal vein; e, eye; ep., epipharynx; hp., hypopharynx; l, labium; la., labella; p, palps; 1-6, longitudinal veins. (A-D and F redrawn from Austen, 1911; G redrawn from Surcouf and González-Rincones; H adapted from Hegner, Root, Augustine, and Huff. *Parasitology,* 1938. Courtesy of D. Appleton-Century Company.)

2 inches in the ground and immediately pupates. The adult fly emerges in about 5 weeks.

Pathogenicity. The bite of the fly is of minor consequence. Persons may become sensitive to the saliva.

Vectors of Disease. Tsetse flies are important vectors of trypanosomiasis of man and domesticated animals. At least seven species are vectors of trypanosomal infections of domesticated animals. The vectors of *Trypanosoma rhodesiense,* the causative agent of Rhodesian trypanosomiasis are *G. morsitans, G. swynnertoni,* and *G. pallidipes.* The chief vectors of *T. gambiense,* the agent of Gambian sleeping sickness, are the riverine *G. palpalis, G. palpalis fuscipes,* and in certain districts *G. tachinoides.*

Control. The control of the riverine species comprises reduction of their habitats and breeding places in areas frequented by man, and the destruction of the adult flies. An unsuitable environment may be created by: (1) clearing trees and bush from stretches of river bank at least 800 yards in length by 50 to 150 yards in width in the vicinity of water holes and crossings, (2) the erection of barrier clearings to prevent the passage of flies along the river courses, and (3) more extensive clearance of river systems by selective removal of shrubs and trees, starting upstream. The number of flies may be reduced by hand-catching, by trapping, and by insecticides in the lightly foliated small rivers and waterholes.

The woodland tsetse flies are more difficult to eradicate. Methods of control are: (1) barrier clearance to isolate blocks of infested country by removing the upper canopy of trees; (2) clearance of tracts for agricultural purposes; (3) selective bush clearance in crucial areas; (4) trapping of flies; (5) the use of insecticides such as Dieldrin, BHC, and DDT to eliminate residual flies by aerial spraying or by herding cattle, sprayed twice a week with DDT, in infested bush areas; and (6) the destruction of the wild game animals upon which the flies feed. The destruction of game, a controversial subject, is only suitable to isolated fly belts of manageable size. It is less effective in reducing the versatile *G. pallidipes* than *G. morsitans* and *G. swynnertoni;* the areas are susceptible to reinfestation; and discriminative clearance, especially if it is accompanied by human settlements, is preferable because of its permanence.

NONBLOODSUCKING FLIES

The nonbloodsucking flies have mouth parts adapted for sucking liquids or minute particles. They live under filthy conditions, the larval stage usually being passed in decaying material. They affect the health of man by the mechanical transmission of disease-producing organisms and by the parasitic activities of their larvae. The invasion of mammalian tissues by dipterous larvae is known as myiasis.

Myiasis. Clinically myiasis may be classified as cutaneous, atrial, wound, intestinal, and urinary. Larvae are able to burrow through either necrotic or healthy tissue with their chitinous mandibular hooks, aided by secondary bacterial infection and possibly by their proteolytic secretions. Some migrate in tortuous channels, producing a type of larva migrans creeping eruption (*Hypoderma*). When the larvae mature they migrate out of the host in an effort to reach soil and to pupate. The larvae deposited in the atria either remain there or migrate to the sinuses and adjacent tissues. The larvae of several species of flies have been found in the urine. Urethral infections with dysuria, hematuria, and pyuria are presumed to be due to the invasion of larvae deposited upon the genitalia. Intestinal myiasis is largely accidental through ingestion in food. Larvae that are able to live in the intestinal tract may cause nausea, vomiting, and diarrhea.

Classification of Myiasis-Producing Flies. A satisfactory classification is to group the myiasis-producing flies by their ovi- or larvipositing habits as: (1) specific, (2) semispecific, and (3) accidental. The specific flies deposit their eggs or larvae in or near the tissues of obligate hosts, and the larvae inevitably become parasites by invading the skin or atria. These flies may deposit their eggs or larvae in the habitat, on the hairs or body, or in the wounds and diseased tissues of the host. The semispecific flies usually deposit their eggs or larvae in decaying flesh or vegetable matter and, less frequently, as facultative parasites in diseased tissues or neglected wounds, although a few species have acquired a purely parasitic habit.

The accidental myiasis-producing flies of diverse genera and habits deposit their larvae in excrement or decaying organic material and, at times, in food. Man becomes infested by the accidental ingestion of the eggs or larvae or by the contamination of external wounds or atria. Human infection with flesh fly larvae is largely confined to infants and small children, particularly those with nasal discharges sleeping unscreened out of doors. The deposited larvae are able to penetrate the tender skin of infants and to produce furunculous lesions. Extensive superficial lesions of the cheek, neck, arms, and chest of infants have been reported. The genera and families of myiasis-producing flies of medical and veterinary importance are listed below with their clinical types. They are designated as: (1) specific and (2) semispecific; the location of deposition of eggs or larvae as: (A) hairs and body of host, (B) external habitat of host, and (C) wounds of host. In addition, flies of the families ANTHOMYIDAE, MUSCIDAE, and SYRPHIDAE occasionally produce an accidental myiasis. Also the adult nonmyiasis-producing flies of the family OSCINIDAE attack the eyes of man.

Family CALLIPHORIDAE
  Genus *Auchmeromyia*   (1 B) bloodsucking (Congo floor maggot)
    Calliphora   (2 C) wounds
    Chrysomyia   (1 C) atrial, wounds
    Cochliomyia   (2 C) atrial, cutaneous, wounds
    Cordylobia   (1 B) cutaneous
    Phormia   (2 C) wounds

Family OESTRIDAE
  Genus *Dermatobia*   (1 B) cutaneous (arthropod transmitted)
    Gasterophilus   (1 A) atrial, intestinal, cutaneous
    Hypoderma   (1 A) cutaneous
    Oestrus   (1 A) atrial
    Rhinoestrus   (1 A) atrial

Family SARCOPHAGIDAE
  Genus *Sarcophaga*   (2 C) wounds
    Wohlfahrtia   (1 C) atrial, cutaneous, wounds

Morphology of Larva. The mature third-stage larva (Fig. 124) of the nonbloodsucking fly usually has a broad truncated posterior, a narrow anterior with hooklike processes and paired papillae, and a spinose area on each segment. Certain structures are useful for identifying genera and species: (1) shape and ornamentation; (2) structure of the anterior end; (3) the small fan-like, branched anterior

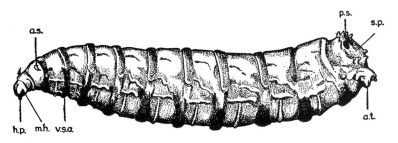

Fig. 124. Mature larva of a muscid fly.
  a.s., anterior spiracles; a.t., anal tubercle; h.p., head papillae; m.h., mouth hooks; p.s., posterior spiracles; s.p., stigmal plate; v.s.a., ventral spinose area. (Redrawn from Hegner, Root, Augustine, and Huff. *Parasitology,* 1938. Courtesy of D. Appleton-Century Company.)

spiracles on the second segment; and (4) most important of all, the posterior spiracles with their depressed or invaginated stigmal plates on the dorsal surface of the posterior segment. Also, identification of certain species may be made by rearing the adult fly from the larva.

Treatment.   Cutaneous and subcutaneous myiasis may require the surgical removal of the larvae after local anesthesia. The maggot is removed from the incision with forceps, and the wound is dressed. The eggs and maggots may be washed from hair, skin, and wounds with soap and water. Urinary myiasis usually terminates spontaneously, although cystoscopic treatment is sometimes necessary. Purgation with sodium sulfate or anthelmintics may be used for gastrointestinal myiasis.

Control.   Diverse methods are employed to reduce the number of myiasis-producing flies. Prevention in man necessitates the control of infestations in animals by larvicides and other measures. Destruction of carcasses and the disposal of offal reduces the breeding grounds of certain species. Fly traps are effective. The screening of susceptible domesticated animals, treatment of wounds, and repellents are useful. Persons, especially infants, with catarrhal or suppurative lesions should not sleep in the open. Control of the African floor maggot consists of the application of insecticides and raising sleeping mats to platforms off the floor.

Vectors of Disease.   Filth flies are mechanical vectors of pathogenic organisms, especially those of enteric diseases. Pathogenic viruses, bacteria, protozoa, and helminthic eggs may be carried on their bodies, legs, and mouth parts, or even may pass unharmed through their intestinal tracts. Several species, especially the common house fly, have been incriminated on experimental and epidemiologic evidence as vectors of typhoid, salmonellosis, cholera, bacillary and amebic dysenteries, tuberculosis, plague, tularemia, anthrax, yaws, conjunctivitis, undulant fever, trypanosomiasis, leishmaniasis, and spirochetal diseases.

Musca domestica, House Fly

The common house fly, *Musca domestica,* infests human habitations throughout the world. The eggs are laid in lots of about 100 in manure or refuse. The entire life cycle occupies 10 to 14 days, and the adult fly lives about a month (Fig. 125). Its larvae are responsible for an occasional intestinal and genitourinary myiasis. The fly, however, is a mechanical vector of pathogenic bacteria, protozoa, and helminthic eggs and larvae, especially of enteric disease organisms. The extent of disease transmission by flies under natural conditions is difficult to determine. Control is a community measure, since flies travel considerable distances, but screening and trapping protect the individual home. Adequate control involves the elimination of breeding places by the disposal, or chemical treatment, of animal excrement, garbage, and decaying vegetation, and residual spraying of the interiors of houses and barns with DDT, Chlordane, or Malathion.

ORDER ORTHOPTERA: COCKROACHES

Cockroaches of the family BLATTIDAE are important household pests and may be mechanical vectors of pathogenic organisms as well as intermediate hosts of helminthic parasites. They are large, swift-running, omnivorous, terrestrial insects

MUSCA DOMESTICA

HOUSE FLY

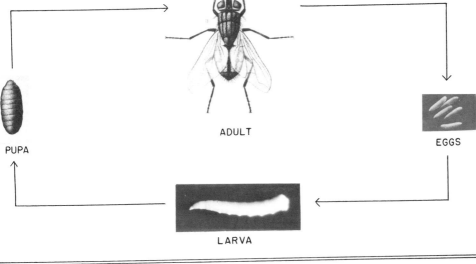

PUPA   ADULT   EGGS

LARVA

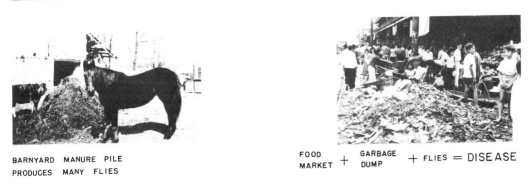

BARNYARD MANURE PILE
PRODUCES MANY FLIES

FOOD MARKET + GARBAGE DUMP + FLIES = DISEASE

Fig. 125. Life cycle of *Musca domestica.*

with long antennae, biting mouth parts, narrow hardened forewings, membranous hindwings, and legs approximately equal in length.

In North America, north of Mexico, there are several species of cockroaches of economic importance which infest buildings (Fig. 126). The oriental cockroach, *Blatta orientalis,* a dark brown insect about 2.5 cm in length has spread from the Far East throughout the world. The smaller, light brown German cockroach or Croton bug, *Blattella germanica,* about 1.3 cm in length, and the large reddish-brown American cockroaches, *Periplaneta americana,* about 3.8 cm in length, have well-developed wings. *Periplaneta fuligniosa* is common in southern United States. The brown-banded *Supella supellectilium,* the common household cockroach of Hawaii, has become, in the last 10 years, increasingly prevalent in the United

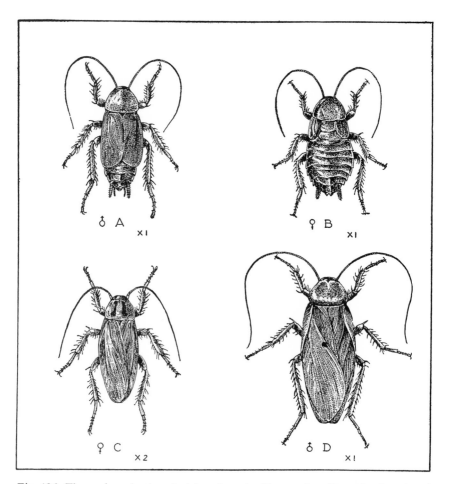

Fig. 126. The cockroach. A, oriental cockroach, *Blatta orientalis,* male; B, oriental cockroach, *Blatta orientalis,* female; C, German cockroach, *Blattella germanica,* female; D, American cockroach, *Periplaneta americana,* male. (Redrawn from Laing, 1938.)

States. *Parcoblatta pennsylvanica* occasionally becomes established in a house, if the dwelling is situated near woods.

Habits.   The oriental and German cockroaches frequent homes and food-handling establishments, while the American and Australian species prefer ships, warehouses, sugar refineries, sewage systems, and hothouses. Cockroaches are nocturnal, shun bright sunlight, and seek concealment during the day in crevices and basements. They are omnivorous with a partiality for starchy foods. They may infest buildings through their introduction in food supplies or by migrating along plumbing installations. *B. germanica,* the most resistant species, has been used for testing insecticides.

Life Cycle.   The eggs are deposited in oothecas, so-called egg cases, in crevices. The incubation period at 25° C varies from 26 to 69 days for the several species. Development is by incomplete metamorphosis. The nymph passes through 13 molts to reach the adult stage. The length of the life cycle is 2 to 21 months according to the species. The life span of the adult is slightly over 40 days (Fig. 127).

BLATELLA GERMANICA

COCKROACH

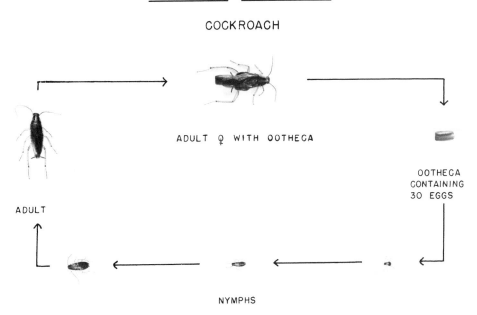

ADULT ♀ WITH OOTHECA

OOTHECA
CONTAINING
30 EGGS

ADULT

NYMPHS

Fig. 127. Life cycle of the cockroach.

Pathogenicity.   The omnivorous habits of these pests cause damage to books, leathers, and woolen goods, while the roachy odor from the glandular secretions spoils food. Its dual contact with filth and food suggests the mechanical transmission of pathogenic organisms. The oriental, German, and American cockroaches have been incriminated as intermediate hosts of the cestode *Hymenolepis diminuta;* the German of the nematode *Gongylonema pulchrum;* and the American of the acanthocephalid, *Moniliformis moniliformis.*

Control.   Their wary habits make methods of control difficult. Cleanliness in kitchens and the protection of stored foods are primary essentials. Repair of cracks and tight-fitting plumbing installations in the walls are preventive measures. Kerosene sprays of 2 percent Chlordane, 3 percent Malathion, or 0.5 percent Diazinon are effective against roaches. Dusts containing 5 percent Chlordane or Malathion are usually more effective than sprays and are spread in cracks and across lines of traffic of the insects.

ORDER COLEOPTERA: BEETLES

A few families of beetles contain species that are injurious to man by the action of vesicating or blistering fluids, or by being intermediate hosts of helminthic parasites. The blister beetles of the family MELOIDAE produce cantharidin, a volatile vesicating substance. The commercial preparation, obtained from the Spanish fly, *Lytta vesicatoria,* is used as a rubefacient, diuretic, and aphrodisiac. When cantharidin comes in contact with the skin, mucous membranes, or conjunctiva by crushing the beetle or by the discharge of its body fluids, it causes a painful, burning blister. Species of rove beetles of the family STAPHYLINIDAE produce another vesicating substance. Rare instances of the canthariasis of the digestive tract, urinary system, and nasal passages, due to the incidental invasion of vesicating beetles, have been reported.

Larval and adult beetles serve as intermediate hosts for rare helminthic parasites of man.

Treatment.   The skin lesions are treated by soothing lotions and at times by antiseptics. Purgation with sodium sulfate is recommended for intestinal canthariasis.

ORDER HYMENOPTERA: BEES, WASPS, ANTS

Bees, wasps, ants, the venenating insects, possess membranous wings; mouth parts adapted for chewing, licking, or sucking plants; and an ovipositor modified for piercing, sawing, or stinging. The stinger has a barbed sheath, a pair of serrated lancets, and a pair of lateral palps. The venom, secreted by paired glands, is forced down the canal formed by the sheath and lancets. During the act of stinging the ovipositor is cast off by the honeybee and some wasps, but it is retained by other species. The exact nature of the venom is unknown, but the active principle is believed to be a complex protein poison.

The sting of bees, wasps, and hornets causes pain, edema, and local inflammation. Ordinarily, the symptoms disappear after a few hours, but at times there may be marked swelling and inflammation, depending upon the location and number of the stings. Supersensitive persons manifest mild to severe systemic reactions, depending upon the degree of sensitiveness and the rapidity of absorption of the venom. A number of cases of severe systemic manifestations, in some instances with fatal terminations, have been reported in medical literature. Such individuals manifest symptoms of anaphylactic shock with respiratory and cardiac impairment, general edema, and urticaria. Among 50 patients who died of stings, death was attributed to respiratory tract angioedema in 35, anaphylactic shock in 6, vascular reactions in 6, and nervous system reactions in 3. Thirteen were known to be allergic. Twenty-nine patients died within 6 hours from one sting; in a small number, death was delayed for more than 96 hours; 38 died of only one or two stings. Supersensitive persons should avoid, as far as possible, exposure to these insects, although accidental stings are unavoidable.

The stinging ants of the temperate zones cause little injury, but the large tropical species give rise to considerable pain and inflammation, and if the stings are numerous, may even endanger life. The foraging ants of India and Africa bite viciously with their mandibles. The small fire ant of the genus *Solenopsis,* which is spreading in southern United States, causes a fiery sting and pruritic vesicles (Fig. 128).

Treatment.   The stings of bees, wasps, and ants are treated locally with soothing lotions. The stingers of bees should be removed from the wound. Hypersensitive persons who experience severe reactions from a bee sting and manifest symptoms of anaphylactic shock with respiratory and cardiac impairment, edema, and urticaria should be treated with epinephrine and 30 mg Prednisone along with a quick-acting anthistaminic, to be repeated in 15 to 30 minutes if necessary. Allergic persons may be hyposensitized by injections of extracts of bee venom or of whole bees, which are group specific for bees and wasps. Polyvalent, whole-body extract antigens of honeybee, bumblebee, wasp, yellow jacket, hornet, red

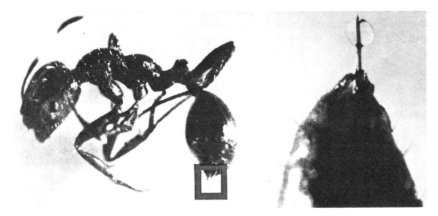

Fig. 128. Fire ant (*Solenopsis saevissima richteri*). Note posterior stinging apparatus with drop of venom. (Courtesy Medical World News.)

ant, and fire ant are reported to produce comprehensive protection against the stings of HYMENOPTERA.

Control. Yards infested with the fire ant should be treated with an emulsion spray of Heptachlor or Dieldrin at a rate of 2 pounds per acre.

ORDER LEPIDOPTERA: CATERPILLARS, MOTHS, BUTTERFLIES

In the United States the common form of caterpillar dermatitis is caused in the eastern part by the brown-tail tussock moth, *Nygmia phaeorrhoea,* and in the eastern and central sections by the silkworm moth, *Automeris io.*

The poisonous hairs are of two types, the venom being secreted: (1) by a single gland cell at the base of the hair (tussock moth and puss caterpillar), and (2) by cells lining the lower part of the sharp chitinized spines (flannel moths). The exact composition of the poison is unknown, but it is probably proteic or linked with a protein. Poisoning is acquired by contact with caterpillars or their nests, or by windblown hairs settling upon the exposed body or upon drying underclothing. The severity of the dermatitis depends upon the species of caterpillar, the site and extent of the exposure and the sensitiveness of the victim. There is an early burning or prickling sensation with numbness and pronounced itching, followed by a vesicular edematous erythema. Windblown hairs may produce an irritating ophthalmia and a serious inflammation of the respiratory tract. Allergic reactions may occur in sensitive persons. Prevention requires the avoidance of localities frequented by poisonous caterpillars and the destruction, where possible, of the caterpillars and their nests by insecticidal sprays of DDT or Chlordane, or the application of creosote to the egg masses.

Several species of moth larvae serve as intermediate hosts of the tapeworm *Hymenolepis diminuta.*

Treatment. Calamine lotion, lime water, or zinc oxide may be applied to the cutaneous lesions. Systemic reactions in supersensitive persons are treated with epinephrine.

16

Class Arachnida: Ticks, Mites, Spiders, Scorpions

The arachnids differ from the insects in the absence of wings, the presence of four pairs of legs in the adult stage, and the fusion of the head and thorax into a cephalothorax. The ARANEIDA (spiders) and SCORPIONIDA (scorpions) are injurious to man by their bites and stings, the degenerate worm-like PENTASTOMIDA are rare parasites of man, and the ACARINA (ticks and mites) are of special importance as vectors of human diseases.

ORDER ACARINA: TICKS, MITES

The order ACARINA, ticks and mites, includes many parasites and vectors of diseases of man and lower animals. The head, thorax, and abdomen of these arachnids are fused into an unsegmented body. The mouth parts and their base, the capitulum, are attached to the anterior portion of the body by a movable hinge. The sexes are separate.

Parasitic Ticks

The tick differs from the mite in its larger size, hairless or short-haired leathery body, exposed armed hypostome, and the presence of a pair of spiracles near the coxae of the fourth pair of legs. About 300 species are bloodsucking ectoparasites of mammals, birds, reptiles, and amphibians, and nearly all are capable of biting man.

Classification. Ticks are divided into the ARGASIDAE or soft ticks and the IXODIDAE or hard ticks. The argasid ticks are more primitive, are less constantly parasitic, produce less progeny, and infest the habitat of the host. The ixodid ticks are more specialized, are more highly parasitic, produce more progeny, and infest the host itself.

FAMILY IXODIDAE. The hard ticks, so-called because of the horny scutum, have a cosmopolitan distribution. The sexes are usually dissimilar; there is a hard dorsal scutum; the capitulum is visible dorsally at the anterior end.

Morphology. The reddish or mahogany-brown cephalothorax and abdomen are fused into an oval or elliptical body with four pairs of six-jointed legs that arise from the plates of the basal coxae (Fig. 129). The false head or capitulum projects from the anterior end in the hard ticks and is concealed in the soft ticks. In the hard ticks it consists of a basal plate or basis capituli of taxonomic value,

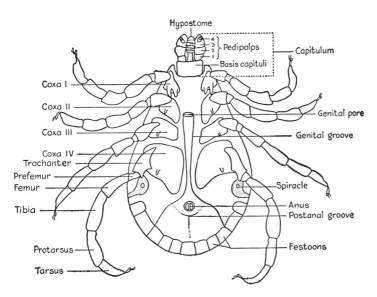

Fig. 129. Ventral view of male *Dermacentor andersoni* showing anatomic structures.

and the mouth parts comprising hypostome, chelicerae, and pedipalps. The median hypostome with its transverse rows of recurrent file-like teeth anchors the parasite to the host. The lateral, paired, chitinous, shaft-like chelicerae act as cutting organs to permit the insertion of the hypostome. The paired four-jointed pedipalps do not penetrate the tissues, but serve as supports. In the hard ticks a chitinous shield, the scutum, covers the entire dorsal surface in the male and the anterior part in the female. The eyes, when present, are on or near the anterior lateral margin of the scutum. Coxal glands between the first two coxae, secrete a tenacious fluid during feeding and copulation, by the soft ticks.

Life Cycle. Both sexes are bloodsuckers. The female hard tick *Dermacentor* increases greatly in size after an engorgement of blood for 5 to 13 days; then drops off the host to deposit, in 14 to 41 days, 2,000 to 8,000 small, oval, brown eggs; and then dies in 3 to 36 days after oviposition (Fig. 130). The soft ticks lay 100 to 200 eggs in several batches following successive blood meals. After 2 to 7 weeks, larvae with three pairs of legs emerge from the eggs. These active "seed" ticks attach themselves to small animals for a blood meal, then drop off and molt into nymphs with four pairs of legs, but without a genital pore. Hard ticks have a single nymphal stage, but soft ticks may have several. Nymphs may hibernate unfed over the winter, and then, after one or more blood meals, molt into adults on the ground. The life cycle is usually completed in 1 or 2 years, occasionally in 3. The adults may hibernate unfed and then the fertilized female, after a blood meal, deposits her eggs. The same or different species of mammals may serve as hosts for the various stages. Various modifications of the cycle such as change of host, length of time on the host, number of molts, and frequency of oviposition occur in different species.

During their larval, nymphal, and adult stages, ticks are intermittent parasites of animals and spend most of their existence on the ground. Some species (*Boo-*

DERMACENTOR ANDERSONI

HARD TICK

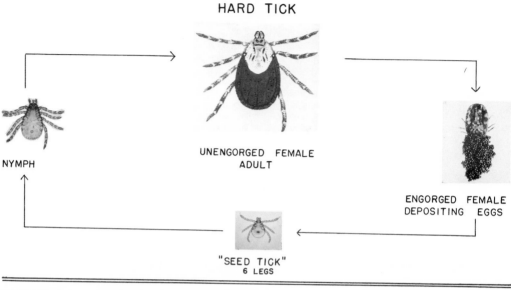

UNENGORGED FEMALE
ADULT

NYMPH

ENGORGED FEMALE
DEPOSITING EGGS

"SEED TICK"
6 LEGS

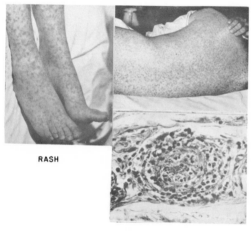

RASH

RASH

ARTERIOLAR THROMBOSIS
AND NECROSIS OF SKIN

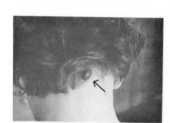

TICK ATTACHED AT
BACK OF NECK

TICK PARALYSIS

ROCKY MOUNTAIN SPOTTED FEVER

Fig. 130. Life cycle of *Dermacentor andersoni.*

philus), however, spend most of their lives on animals. Favorable environmental conditions include abundant vegetation, moisture, and numerous animal hosts. Ticks are susceptible to sunlight, desiccation, and excessive rainfall, but are resistant to cold. Ticks are long-lived, the soft tick, *Ornithodoros turicata,* surviving over 25 years and undergoing starvation for 5 years. The larval and nymphal ticks feed on small animals, and the adult ticks on medium to large ones, attaching themselves when the animals come in contact with infested vegetation.

Pathogenicity. Ticks harm man and lower animals by: (1) the mechanical injury of their bites, (2) the production of tick paralysis, and (3) the transmission of bacterial, viral, rickettsial, and protozoan diseases.

After the chelicerae have cut the skin, the toothed capitulum anchors the tick during the blood meal. Its insertion produces an inflammatory reaction of the perivascular tissues of the corium with local hyperemia, edema, hemorrhage, and thickening of the stratum corneum. The wound may become necrotic or secondarily infected. If the capitulum is broken off in the skin during removal, it may cause a festering wound.

Tick paralysis occurs in sheep, cattle, dogs, and, occasionally, in man and cats. About 12 ixodid ticks, and even soft ticks of the genus *Ornithodoros,* have been implicated. The disease is usually associated with species of *Dermacentor* and *Amblyomma* in North America, and of *Ixodes* in Australia and South Africa. The paralysis is sometimes severe in domesticated animals. The disease manifests itself as a progressive, ascending, flaccid motor paralysis which is due to a failure in the liberation of acetylcholine at the neuromuscular junction because of a block in the somatic motor fibers produced by the tick toxin. The toxin is elaborated by the tick's ovaries and secreted by the salivary glands. The pathology comprises small hemorrhagic foci, diffuse hyperemia, and focal agranulocytic infiltration around the nerve cells in the brain and cord. The lower motor neurons of the spinal cord and cranial nerves are chiefly involved. There is destruction of the myelin sheath and perivascular infiltration.

The disease has a rapid onset with malaise, vague body pains, lassitude, cephalgia, irritability, and slight or no fever. In a few hours an ascending flaccid paralysis ensues with muscular incoordination and, less frequently, sensory changes. There is ataxia, dysphagia, and muscular paralysis, usually bilateral but sometimes localized. Death occurs from respiratory paralysis, although most affected persons recover. Children are affected usually, occasionally aged adults. Children under 2 years of age succumb rapidly. The paralysis subsides after the removal of the tick.

Vectors of Disease. Ticks have been recognized as vectors of disease ever since 1893, when Smith and Kilbourne discovered that *Boophilus annulatus* was the transmitting agent of Texas fever in cattle. In some species the causative organisms pass not only through the metamorphic stages of the tick, but also through the eggs, to succeeding generations. The diseases transmitted among domesticated animals cause heavy financial loss. An incomplete list of the vector ticks for the various human diseases is given below.

A. Rickettsial Diseases
1. American spotted fever (*Rickettsia rickettsii*)
   Amblyomma (*americanum, cajennense, striatum, ovale, brasiliensis*); *Dermacentor* (*andersoni, occidentalis, variabilis*); *Ixodes dentatus; Ornithodoros* (*hermsi, nicollei, parkeri, rudis, turicata*); *Rhipicephalus sanguineus*

2. Boutonneuse fever (*R. conorii*)
   Amblyomma hebraeum
   Rhipicephalus sanguineus
3. African tick fever (*R. conorii*)
   Amblyomma hebraeum; Haemaphysalis leachi; Hyalomma aegyptium;
   Rhipicephalus (*sanguineus, appendiculatus*)
4. Russian tick typhus
   Dermacentor nuttalli
5. Q fever (*R. burneti*)
   Dermacentor (*andersoni, occidentalis*); *Amblyomma americanum;*
   Haemaphysalis humerosa; Ixodes (*dentatus, holocyclus*); *Ornithodoros*
   (*moubata, hermsi*)—experimentally; *Rhipicephalus sanguineus*

B. Viral Diseases
   1. Colorado tick fever
      Dermacentor andersoni
   2. Hemorrhagic Fevers
      Hyalomma marginatum; H. anatolicum; Dermacentor pictus
   3. Louping ill
      Ixodes ricinus; Rhipicephalus appendiculatus
   4. Kyasanur Forest Disease
      Haemaphysalis spinigera
   5. Powasson Virus
      Dermacentor andersoni; Ixodes marxi; I. cooki
   6. Russian spring and summer encephalitis
      Dermacentor silvarum; Haemaphysalis concinna; Ixodes (*persulcatus,*
      ricinus)

C. Bacterial and Spirochetal Diseases
   1. Relapsing fever (*Borrelia duttoni*, etc.)
      Ornithodoros (*erraticus, hermsi, marocanus, moubata, parkeri, papil-*
      lipes, savignyi, talaje, turicata, venezuelensis); *Rhipicephalus sanguineus*
   2. Tularemia
      Amblyomma americanum; Dermacentor (*albipictus, andersoni, occi-*
      dentalis, silvarum, variabilis); *Ixodes ricinus* and other species; *Rhipi-*
      cephalus sanguineus

FAMILY ARGASIDAE.   The soft ticks are primarily ectoparasites of birds, less commonly of mammals and man. They have a cosmopolitan distribution but are more abundant in warm climates. The sexes are similar; there is no dorsal plate; the capitulum is not visible dorsally; the spiracles lie in front of the third pair of unspurred coxae; and the tarsi bear no pads or pulvilli. They are nocturnal feeders and seldom travel far from their local habitat. *Argus persicus*, a natural parasite of fowl and a vector of avian disease in many tropical and semitropical countries, occasionally bites man, producing painful wounds that are subject to secondary infection. *Ornithodoros moubata* (Fig. 131) of Africa, an oval, yellowish-brown, tuberculated, leathery tick, 8 to 9 mm, is the best known parasitic species of this genus. This tick inhabits the cracks in the floors of native huts, and bites its victims at night. The bites of both nymphs and adults produce hard red wheals that remain painful for 24 hours. It is an important vector of endemic relapsing fever. Several

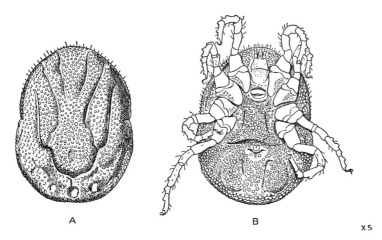

Fig. 131. *Ornithodoros moubata*. A, dorsal view, female; B, ventral view, female.

other species of *Ornithodoros* are vectors of local types of relapsing fever throughout the world.

Treatment. The painless bite of the tick seldom calls for treatment. The ticks may be removed from the skin by gentle traction after applying chloroform, ether, alcohol, gasoline, kerosene, glycerol, ethyl chloride, or a glowing match or cigarette to the tick. Care should be taken not to break off the capitulum in the wound. Early removal is indicated in order to prevent tick paralysis. Paralysis, if present, soon subsides after the removal of the tick. In endemic areas of rickettsial and spirochetal diseases, careful search for ticks should be made on persons exposed to tick-infested areas, and care should be taken not to contaminate the hands with the fluid secretions of the tick during its removal.

Control. Argasid ticks are best combated by destroying their nests or lairs. Infested native huts should be burned, or the floors and walls should be plastered to eliminate the crevices and then sprayed with BHC or the less effective DDT. More than one application is required, since these insecticides are ineffective against the eggs. Rodent proofing of buildings is desirable. Inmates should avoid sleeping on the floor.

Ixodid ticks may be eliminated by exterminating their rodent hosts and destroying their habitats. The infested grounds, houses, and animals may be sprayed with DDT, Chlordane, Dieldrin, or BHC. BHC has the most rapid immobilizing action, but has less residual toxicity than the others, which give good control within a few days and prevent reinfestation for a month or more. Sprays and 5 to 10 percent dusts are equally effective. Suspensions and emulsions are preferable to oil solutions. Effectiveness depends upon the amount and the thoroughness of distribution. It is advisable to start spraying in the spring, but a subsequent treatment at the peak of population in the summer is necessary. Ticks may be brought into houses on clothing or animals, and the dog tick *R. sanguineus* may pass its entire life cycle indoors. It is difficult to eliminate ticks from houses. Both DDT and Chlordane, when applied as liquid sprays to floors and walls, are effective for several weeks; more than one application may be required. It is preferable to prevent house infestation by the removal of infested clothing and the treatment of dogs with DDT or BHC. Men traversing tick-infested areas should use tick-proof clothing and, after removing the clothing, a search should be made for ticks on their bodies. Repellents applied to the skin provide little protection, but clothing treated with diethyltoluamide gives protection for from several days to a week. Indalone is a better tick repellent than dimethyl phthalate and Rutgers 612, but all give fairly good protection.

PARASITIC MITES

The term "mite" is usually applied to members of the order ACARINA other than the ticks. Mites are much smaller than ticks and do not have a leathery covering; spiracles are present on the cephalothorax of some mites; and the hypostome may be unarmed. The parasitic species infest plants and animals, and some cause direct injury to man or transmit human diseases. The parasitic mites are chiefly ecto-parasites, but a few are endoparasites. Most species have a cosmopolitan distribution. Some species use insects as a means of transportation and a source of food. General rather than specific host specificity seems to be the rule.

Life Cycle.   The eggs are deposited in the soil or on the skin of the host. The 6-legged larvae, which feed on blood or plant juices, metamorphose into 8-legged nymphs, and finally into 8-legged adults.

Family TROMBIDIIDAE: Red Bugs, Chiggers

The larvae of the trombiculid mites, known as harvest mites, red bugs, or chiggers, are annoying pests to picnickers, sportsmen, berry pickers, and campers.

Morphology.   The orange-red or brilliantly spotted adult mites are usually scavengers. The body is partly covered with minute hairs and has four pairs of legs (Fig. 132).

Habits.   Chiggers inhabit moist grassy or bushy terrain frequented by domesticated animals or wild rodents. As larvae they feed on blood and tissues of mammals, birds, reptiles, and amphibians.

Life Cycle.   The eggs are laid in clusters on the moist ground rich in humus. The hatched larvae (Fig. 132) feed on animals and then drop to the ground to become nymphs and, finally, adults. The life cycle covers 50 to 70 days, and the adult females live over a year.

Pathogenicity.   The North American chigger or redbug, *Trombicula alfred-dugèsi,* infests grasses and bushes, whence it attacks animals and man. The larva crawls actively up the legs and attaches itself to the skin by the capitulum. Its bite, typical of other chiggers, causes itching increasing to a maximum on the second day. Then the swelling subsides, and a light pinkish color, which gradually turns to a deep red on the third day, surrounds the puncture. The patient suffers severe discomfort with attendant loss of sleep. Severe infestations may produce fever and secondary infection from scratching.

Trombicula autumnalis, the harvest mite of Europe, and allied species in other parts of the world are also annoying pests.

Vectors of Disease.   Tsutsugamushi disease or scrub typhus is characterized by an initial ulcer at the site of the bite, remittent fever, lymphadenitis, spleno-megaly, and a bright red eruption. Chloramphenicol and the tetracyclines give rapid and dramatic cure. The chief vectors are *Trombicula akamushi* and *T. deli-ensis,* while several other species of *Trombicula* have been incriminated epidemi-

TROMBICULA ALFREDDUGESI

CHIGGER

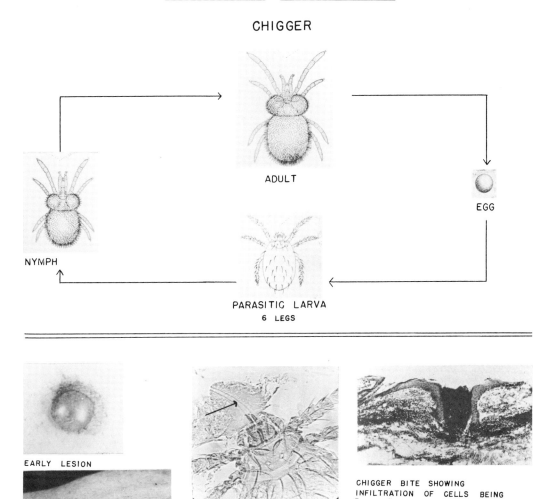

Fig. 132. Life cycle of *Trombicula alfreddugesi.*

ologically. The larval mites are parasites of the vole in Japan and of various house and field rats in Taiwan and Indonesia. Man is an incidental host, the larvae attaching themselves to field workers. The organism, *Rickettsia tsutsugamushi,* has been isolated from the salivary glands of the larval mites. It can be transmitted from generation to generation, so that the larvae of the second generation are capable of infecting man.

Treatment.   For the irritating dermatitis caused by chiggers, a hot soap and water bath is followed by the application to the affected skin of a 10 percent sulfur ointment containing 1 percent phenol. Palliative treatment includes the application of alcohol, ammonia, baking soda, alcoholic iodine, camphor, or a saturated solution of salicylic acid in alcohol with a little sweet oil. Pyogenic infections are treated with 30 percent ammoniated mercury ointment.

Control.   Control of mites in their habitats is difficult: (1) The breeding grounds may be destroyed by burning and clearing the tall grasses and underbrush, by cultivation, and by sheep grazing; and (2) the rodent hosts may be destroyed. Diesel oil, 40 gallons per acre, causes a temporary reduction in the mites and is useful for camp sites. Chlordane sprays, 1 g per 4 square meters, are effective for a month. Lindane sprays are also effective. Persons may be protected by boots and closely woven clothing with tight-fitting edges or, better, by clothing impregnated with repellents such as a mixture of equal parts of diethyltoluamide and benzyl benzoate with an emulsifier.

Family SARCOPTIDAE: Scabies

The itch and mange mites of the family SARCOPTIDAE are of medical and veterinary importance. Species of the genus *Sarcoptes* cause itch or mange by burrowing into the skins of mammals; *Sarcoptes scabiei* is the only species that commonly produces human disease, although domestic animal species occasionally infest man temporarily. This mite has a cosmopolitan distribution, especially among the poorer classes.

Morphology.   *S. scabiei* is a small, oval, dorsally convex, ventrally flattened, eyeless mite, the male measuring 200 to 250 μ, and the female 330 to 450 μ (Fig. 133). The anterior notothorax bears the first two pairs of legs, and the posterior notogaster the second two pairs. The first pairs of legs terminate in long tubular processes each with a bell-shaped sucker and claws. The posterior legs end in long bristles, except the fourth pair in the male which have suckers. The dorsal surface is ridged transversely and bears spines, scales, and bristles. The mouth parts consist of toothed chelicerae, three-jointed conical pedipalps, and labial palps fused to the hypostome.

Life Cycle. (Fig. 133).   The mites live in slightly serpiginous cutaneous burrows. When activated by warmth from the skin the female, usually at night, burrows into the skin, progressing at the rate of about 2 to 3 mm per day. The burrow is confined to the corneous layer of the skin. The male excavates lateral pockets or branches in the burrows. The female, during her life span of 4 to 5 weeks, deposits up to 40 to 50 eggs, 2 to 4 at a time, in the burrow. Larvae emerge from the eggs usually in 3 days, but sometimes not for 10 days. The hexapod larva either forms a lateral branch or a new tunnel, in which it becomes an eight-legged nymph. The female has two nymphal stages, the male only a single one. The life cycle is completed in 8 to 15 days. The female may survive off the host for 2 to 3 days at room temperature. Scabies is transmitted by personal contact, especially by persons sleeping together, and less frequently by towels, clothing, and bed linen. Infectivity is low, and the infection tends to run a limited course in healthy persons of cleanly habits. Infection is common in slum sections, jails, and armies.

SARCOPTES SCABIEI

SCABIES OR ITCH MITE

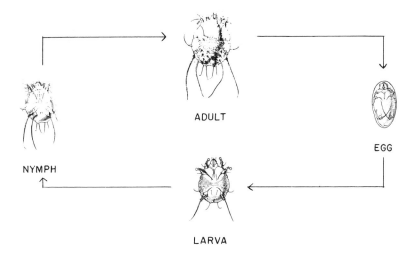

ADULT

EGG

NYMPH

LARVA

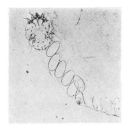

SKIN BURROW CONTAINING
ADULT FEMALE AND EGGS

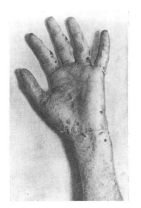

LESIONS ON HAND AND WRIST

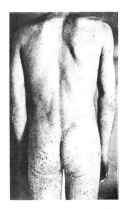

TYPICAL SCABIES RASH

Fig. 133. Life cycle of *Sarcoptes scabiei*.

Pathogenicity.   The preferential sites are the interdigital spaces, the flexor surfaces of the wrists and forearms, elbows, axillae, back, inguinal region, and genitalia. The lesions appear as slightly reddish elevated tracts in the skin. Minute vesicular swellings, possibly produced by the irritating fecal deposits or excretions, form beneath the gallery a short distance behind the mite. The intense itching, aggravated by warmth and perspiration, causes scratching, which spreads the infestation, irritates the lesions, and induces secondary bacterial infection. As a result, multiple papular, vesicular, and pustular lesions may be produced. At first, clinical manifestations may be mild, but after some weeks the skin becomes sensitized, resulting in an itching, widespread, erythematous eruption.

Diagnois.   The type of lesion and an itching rash are suggestive. Conclusive evidence is obtained by removing the mite from its burrow with a needle. The mites are not always easy to find, since the number of females, in spite of the high rate of reproduction, is small.

Treatment.   The most satisfactory treatment of scabies is the application of Kwell, a 1 percent Lindane (hexachlorocyclohexane) ointment, after a hot soapy bath. A second application is seldom necessary, since the ointment kills both mites and eggs. Benzyl benzoate and DDT lotion may also be used, but a second application is necessary, since these agents do not destroy the eggs.

Control.   Prevention of scabies requires the treatment of infected individuals, the sterilization of garments and bedding, and personal cleanliness.

Family DEMODICIDAE

Species of the genus *Demodex* (Fig. 134) are parasites of the sebaceous glands and hair follicles of mammals. They produce mange in dogs and tubercles in the skin of hogs and cattle. *D. folliculorum* is a cosmopolitan parasite of the hair follicles and sebaceous glands of man. It is a worm-like mite with a short capitulum and long tapering abdomen. It rarely causes discomfort. Its presence may manifest itself in acne, blackheads, or localized keratitis, particularly in women using facial cream instead of soap and water. Treatment is rarely required.

MITES OF INCIDENTAL IMPORTANCE TO MAN

The chicken mite, *Dermanyssus gallinae,* a serious pest of poultry, sometimes attacks man. Its bite causes an itching dermatitis in poultrymen, usually on the backs of the hands and on the forearms. The virus of St. Louis encephalitis and

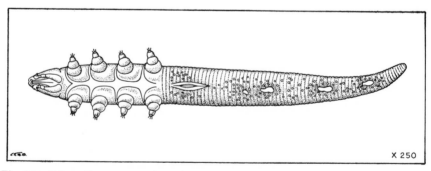

X 250

Fig. 134. Schematic representation of female *Demodex folliculorum.*

western equine encephalomyelitis has been isolated from naturally infected chicken mites.

The rat mite, *Ornithonyssus bacoti,* is prevalent in warm countries, including the United States and Canada. Its bite produces a papulovesicular dermatitis with urticaria in workers in stores, factories, warehouses, and stockyards. It serves as a vector of *Rickettsia typhi,* the agent of endemic typhus, from rat to rat, and is a suspected vector of Q fever. *Allodermanyssus sanguineus,* an ectoparasite of mice, causes a dermatitis by its bite and is the vector of *R. akari,* the agent of rickettsialpox. These mites may be controlled by destruction of their hosts and the use of Malathion or other insecticides.

Species of the genus *Pediculoides* produce dermatitis among workers in the grain-producing countries of the world. The North American grain-itch mite, *P. ventricosus,* feeds upon the larvae of insects that infest grains, straw, or hay. Threshers, grain handlers, and persons sleeping on straw mattresses are subject to infestation. The mites do not penetrate, but burrow superficially in the skin over the entire body, producing petechiae and erythema followed by wheals, vesicles, and pustules.

The food mites of the family TYROGLYPHIDAE feed on cheeses, cereals, on dried vegetable products, and a few on hairs, feathers, and insects. Although not blood-suckers, they produce a temporary pruritus by penetrating the superficial epidermis. Species of *Glyciphagus* that infest sugar, and species of *Tyroglyphus* that infest cheese, cereals, flour, grains, and stored food are considered responsible for "grocer's itch." *T. siro,* or a similar species, causes "vanillism" in workers handling vanilla pods, a subspecies of *T. longior;* "copra itch" in persons handling copra; and *Rhizoglyphus parasiticus,* "coolie itch," in tea plantations in India. It is doubtful if these mites cause other than transitory intestinal symptoms, although they are found in the feces. When inhaled they produce a pneumonitis with associated eosinophilia that is known as acariasis.

Treatment. Various soothing lotions may be used for the cutaneous lesions caused by chicken, rat, and mouse mites. For grain and food mites, local applications of mild antiseptics relieve the annoying pruritus and prevent secondary infection. Menthol-phenol paste or soothing lotions afford relief for tyroglyphic infestations, but the affected parts should be thoroughly cleansed and Lindane ointment also applied. Pneumonitis due to mites may be treated with carbarsone.

ORDER ARANEIDA: SPIDERS

Many species of spiders use venom to paralyze their prey. Man rarely suffers, since the common spiders are seldom able to penetrate the skin, or, if successful, produce but a mild local erythema. A few species, however, cause serious symptoms.

The unsegmented body consists of a cephalothorax, with four pairs of legs, which is separated by a slender constriction from the hairy sacculated abdomen. The mouth parts include a pair of poison jaws or chelicerae, through the tips of which venom from paired glands in the cephalothorax is discharged.

Life Cycle. Spiders spin their webs in all manner of recesses or out-of-the way places, both inside and outside human habitations. They trap flies and other insects in the web, paralyze them with venom, and suck the body juices. Spiders develop by incomplete metamorphosis. The eggs are laid in masses, usually encased in a cocoon in which the young remain for long periods. The spiderlings pass through eight to nine molts before becoming mature adults.

Spiders Injurious to Man

A number of species throughout the world produce systemic poisoning by their bites. The large, hairy, ferocious-looking tarantulas, the "banana spiders," although sometimes capable of killing small animals, inflict only slight, or at most painful, injury to man. The small spiders of the genus *Latrodectus* (Fig. 135), however, possess a potent venom that may produce serious symptoms. Various species of this genus are found in Europe, Australia, New Zealand, the Philippines, Africa, the West Indies, and South and North America.

Lactrodectus mactans.   The black widow, *Latrodectus mactans,* sometimes called the hour-glass, shoe-button, or po-ko-moo spider, is the most dangerous species in the United States, where cases of spider bite with death have been reported. It ranges from southern Canada to Chile and is most abundant in the far western and southern sections. The female, 13 mm, considerably larger than the male, 6 mm, has a dark brown or black thorax and legs, and a jet black abdomen with a characteristic orange-red spot in the form of an hourglass on the ventral surface. The spider infests lumber heaps, rail fences, stumps, undersides of privy seats, outbuildings, cracks in basements, and even houses. It avoids strong light and usually bites only when disturbed. During the summer the female lays several masses of 100 to 600 eggs in a cocoon attached to her web. The young spiderlings hatch in 2 to 4 weeks and become adults the next spring.

PATHOGENICITY.   The nonhemolytic venom of *L. mactans* is probably a tox-albumin that acts as a peripheral neurotoxin. The symptoms vary with the location and the amount of venom. The bite is accompanied with a sharp smarting pain. The site, most frequently on the buttocks or genitalia of males, shows a bluish-red spot with a white areola and sometimes an urticarial rash. Systemic symptoms follow a uniform course, corresponding to the stages of lymphatic absorption. vascular dissemination, and elimination of the toxin. At first there are throbbing, lancinating pains, and numbness in the affected part. Then pains of increasing intensity spread over the abdomen, chest, back, and extremities with rigidity and spasticity of the muscles, which may simulate the acute abdomen of perforated gastric ulcer or appendicitis.

The patient becomes dizzy, weak, thirsty, and nauseated, and shows symptoms of shock. Elimination of the toxin is characterized by recovery from shock, di-

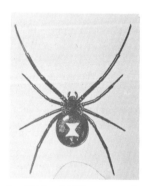

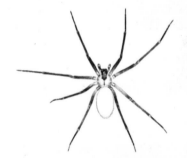

LATRODECTUS   MACTANS

BLACK   WIDOW SPIDER

VENTRAL   VIEW
NOTE "HOURGLASS" ON ABDOMEN

LOXOSCELES   RECLUSA

BROWN   SPIDER

DORSAL   VIEW
NOTE "VIOLIN" ON CEPHALOTHORAX

Fig. 135. Spiders poisonous for man. Natural size.

minished muscular pains, and residual fever and toxic nephritis. The mortality is low, chiefly among children. Death may result from respiratory or circulatory failure.

TREATMENT.   The following treatment for the bite of the black widow spider, *Latrodectus mactans,* is representative for all the poisonous species, except for specific antivenin. If the bite is on the extremities, a tourniquet should be applied and cryotherapy administered to prevent the systemic dissemination of the poison; an attempt should be made to remove the venom by suction from the incised wound. Relief of pain is afforded by rest in bed, hot baths, and morphine. Shock may be combatted by intravenous administration of 10 ml of 10 percent calcium gluconate or 10 percent magnesium sulfate combined with 5 percent glucose. Cortisone has been reported to give some relief. The intramuscular injection of *L. mactans* antivenin, if available, usually gives relief within 30 minutes.* The injection may be repeated in 1 to 2 hours, if necessary.

CONTROL.   DDT, Chlordane, and Dieldrin have been used with some success in outdoor privies, a favorite habitat of *L. mactans.* Children should be taught to be careful in localities frequented by this spider.

NECROTIC ARACHNIDISM

The bites of the small brown spider *Loxosceles laeta* of South America and *Loxosceles reclusus* of Central United States produce necrotic cutaneous lesions (Fig. 136). Within an hour after the bite a painful edema develops, and soon large areas of the skin are involved. As the edema subsides gangrene develops and later, with the detachment of the eschar, deep ulcerations remain (Fig. 136). Occasionally, the toxin of *L. laeta* causes a systemic involvement characterized by hematuria (Fig. 137), anemia, high fever, convulsions, and cyanosis, which may terminate fatally. The early administration of corticosteroids, of questionable value, is recommended for therapy. Recovery from loxoscelism gives a solid immunity.

ORDER SCORPIONIDA: SCORPIONS

Scorpions are elongated terrestrial arachnids with large pedipalps terminating in stout claws, a nonsegmented cephalothorax with four pairs of legs, and an elongated abdomen. The caudal extremity bears a hooked stinger for the discharge of venom (Fig. 138).

Scorpions, nocturnal in their activities, lie under rocks, logs, or other protective coverings. They may invade human habitations especially during the rainy season in the tropics. They seize their prey, usually spiders and insects, in their claws and by a backward-downward thrust of the tail-like abdomen insert the stinger with the paralyzing venom. They are viviparous, and the young are carried for some time on the back of the female. There are numerous species of scorpions throughout the world.

The small species either are not able to penetrate the skin of man or merely cause minor stings. The large venomous scorpions are species of *Buthus* in northern Africa and southern Europe, and *Centruroides* in Mexico and Arizona. Man is

---

* Antivenin (*Lactrodectus mactans*) Lyovac, Merck Sharp and Dohme, West Point, Pa.

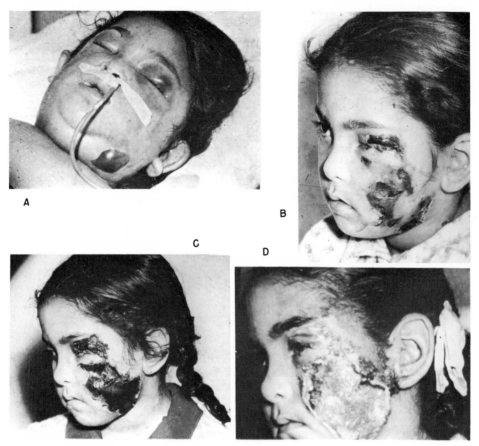

Fig. 136. Necrotic arachnidism. A, 8 hours; B, 6 days; C, 23 days; D, 40 days. (Courtesy of Dept. of Parasitology, School of Medicine, University of Chile.)

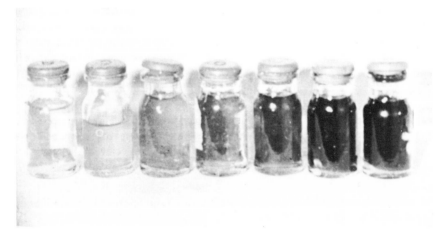

Fig. 137. Urine from patient bitten by *Loxosceles.* Note increasing amount of hemoglobinuria. (Courtesy of Dept. of Parasitology, School of Medicine, University of Chile.)

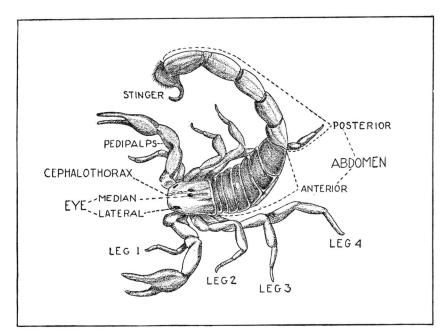

Fig. 138. Schematic representation of scorpion with arched abdomen.

usually stung when his bare hands or feet unexpectedly come in contact with scorpions that are concealed in clothing, shoes, or other hiding places. Serious, and even fatal, systemic reactions, especially in children, have been reported. The mortality in children under 5 years of age is reported as high in India and Egypt. Scorpion venom is a toxalbumin that produces paralysis, nervous disturbances, convulsions, and pulmonary disorders. The local symptoms are relatively mild, but extremely painful. Systemically, there is a radiating burning sensation and a rapid onset of general numbness, muscular twitching, and itching. In severe cases there are muscular spasms and convulsions resembling strychnine poisoning and symptoms of shock. Fatal cases show accelerated respiration and pulmonary edema.

Treatment.   A tourniquet should be applied immediately and the venom removed by suction from wounds made by the stingers of the large scorpions. Pain may be relieved by local applications of ice packs, ethyl chloride spray, ammonia, analgesics, or injections of novocaine or epinephrine in the vicinity of the wound. Systemic treatment is designed to combat shock and pulmonary edema. Cortisone has been reported to be useful. In severe cases, antivenin, if available, should be given.

Control.   Attempts to reduce the scorpion population have not proved particularly successful. For houses and their vicinity, the spraying with 0.5 percent Dieldrin or a mixture of 10 percent DDT, 2 percent Chlordane, and 0.2 percent pyrethrum in a light oil base has been recommended.

ORDER PENTASTOMIDA: TONGUE WORM

The species of medical interest in these degenerate worm-like arthropods belong to the genera *Linguatula* and *Armillifer*.

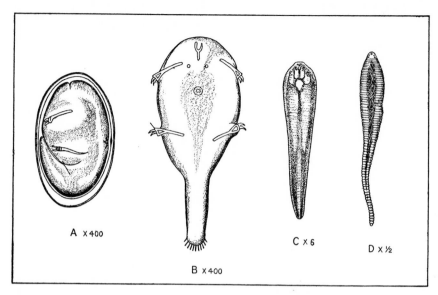

Fig. 139. *Linguatula serrata.* A, embryonate ovum; B, acariform embryo; C, nymph; D, adult. (A and B redrawn from Leuckart, 1860; C adapted from Darling and Clark, 1912; D adapted from various sources.)

The adult and nymphal stages of *L. serrata* (Fig. 139) are found in the nose and paranasal sinuses of dogs and other carnivora, and larvae and encapsulated nymphs in herbivorous animals. Human infection with the adult is rare, but a number of larval infections have been reported in Europe, Africa, and South and Central America. The eggs, when ingested by a mammalian host, hatch into four-legged larvae that pass through the intestinal wall and encyst in the liver, lungs, spleen, mesenteric glands, eye, and other organs.

A. armillatus of Africa, *A. moniliformis* of Asia, and possibly other species of this genus have been found in man. They are distinguished from *Linguatula serrata* by their cylindrical ringed bodies that resemble a string of beads. The adult is a parasite of pythons and other snakes. The nymphs are found in primates and various wild and domesticated mammals. Human infection with the larvae and nymphs is fairly common in Africa, particularly in the Republic of the Congo. The nymphs are found in the liver, intestinal mucosa, peritoneal cavity, lungs, and conjunctiva. Boiling or filtering drinking water should prevent infection by eliminating infective eggs.

TECHNICAL METHODS FOR THE DIAGNOSIS AND TREATMENT OF PARASITIC DISEASES

17

Diagnosis of Parasitic Diseases

It must be remembered that inhabitants of the tropics may have not only parasitic and the so-called tropical diseases, but also any of the numerous cosmopolitan diseases. Thus, a young missionary from Africa with a high fever, considerable weight loss, an enlarged liver, and a high alkaline phosphatase level had widespread carcinomatosis, and not malaria or African sleeping sickness. A Puerto Rican youth with a slight fever and weight loss was suffering from tuberculosis, and the few *S. mansoni* eggs in his stool did not point to his chief problem. Not infrequently the findings of a few helminth eggs or protozoan cysts is given so much diagnostic prominence that the real cause of the patient's illness is overlooked.

Many parasitic infections are asymptomatic or produce only mild symptoms; hence, one must develop a high index of suspicion. Routine blood and stool examinations will uncover many unsuspected infections. It is obvious that a busy clinician will not do his own laboratory examinations; but he should know their pitfalls and accuracy. Most important, the physician should know what specimen to collect, the value of purged stools in amebiasis, the uselessness of stool examination in enterobiasis, and the necessity for repeated stool examination in amebiasis and schistosomiasis.

Recently, several instances of fatal overwhelming infections with *Strongyloides* have been reported. One patient had several hospital admissions with chief complaints of diarrhea, dysentery, and abdominal pain. Operations were performed several times, yet no stools were examined for eggs or parasites. A toothpick, glass slide, feces the size of a small rice grain, a microscope, and a suspicious medical student or intern could have made the diagnosis. The patient's eosinophilia ranged from 1 to 9 percent.

Eosinophilia is given great importance in the medical mind as a sure indication of a parasitic infection. Infections with parasitic worms and protozoa *may* have associated eosinophila, which varies considerably depending on the reaction of the patient. Eosinophilia is usually more marked in recent than in chronic infections. Numerous other diseases have associated eosinophilia, as is indicated below.

Parasitic Diseases
Nematoda
  Trichinosis
  Trichuriasis

Hookworm
Filariasis
Strongyloidiasis
Enterobiasis

Ascariasis
Visceral larva migrans (*Toxocara*)
Cestoda
 Diphyllobothrium—rarely
 Taenia
 Hymenolepis
 Echinococcus
Trematoda
 Schistosomiasis
 Clonorchiasis
 Fasciolopsiasis
Protozoa
 Amebiasis
 Amebic abscess of liver
 Malaria
 Trypanosomiasis, African
 Leishmaniasis
Allergic Conditions
 Serum disease
 Hay fever
 Migraine
 Asthma
 Angioneurotic edema
 Skin diseases
  Pemphigus
  Psoriasis
  Eczema
  Dermatitis herpetiformis
  Urticaria
Bacterial Diseases
 Convalescence from infections (good sign)
 Scarlet fever

Gonorrhea
Impetigo
Rheumatic fever—chorea
Osteomyelitis
Filterable Virus Disease
 Herpes zoster
 Lymphogranuloma
 Measles convalescence
Tumors
 Tumors of lungs & peritoneum
 Carcinoma (rectal)
 Sarcoma
 Hodgkins disease
Blood Diseases
 Chronic myeloid leukemia
 Polycythemia
 Leukemia, eosinophilic
 Lymphosarcoma
Miscellaneous
 Antibiotic therapy
 Agammaglobulinemia
 Splenic extirpation
 Ingestion of raw meats (liver)
 Ulcerative intestinal diseases, proctitis
 Digitalis therapy
 Insulin therapy
 Starvation
 Pernicious anemia, at beginning & remissions during liver therapy
 Nephrosis & nephritis
 Lead poisoning
 Arsenic poisoning
 Periarteritis nodosa
 Dermatomyositis

A low total white blood cell count suggests visceral leishmaniasis, and a high count may help us distinguish between viral hepatitis and protozoal and helminth liver invasion. Liver function tests are of some value both in the diagnosis of parasitic diseases and in their exclusion from the diagnosis.

The geographic distribution of parasitic infections is varied, and knowledge of their distribution is of great value in knowing what to look for in a patient. The patient with urologic problems who had been living in New Jersey all of her life with no history of foreign travel, could not have had *Schistosoma haematobium*. It is true she was experiencing urinary discomfort and passing red blood cells in her urine. Desquamated epithelial cells were mistaken for the terminal-spined *S. haematobium* eggs. On the other hand, a Yemeni gentleman who had lived in Portland, Maine, from 1919 to 1944, was found to have far-advanced liver damage with marked ascites. He had lived in Yemen until he was 14, then spent 5 years in the British Navy prior to taking up residence in Portland. Eleven consecutive daily stools were examined before schistosome eggs were found in his stool. His early

Arabian habitat, fortunately, encouraged the medical resident to continue stool examinations.

Although the geographic distribution of parasites aids us in diagnosis by directing our attention toward certain possibilities, the world is so vast and careful surveys so limited that one may be the first to find the first case from a region. A number of years ago a missionary, Miss B. from Portuguese Angola, appeared at the New York City Tropical Disease Clinic with extensive skin lesions (Fig. 55). Scrapings of the lesions revealed *Onchocerca* microfilariae. Miss B. then asked us if by any chance this parasite could be responsible for the gradual loss of sight of her fellow missionary who had accompanied her and was in the waiting room. Poor Miss M.'s vision was 20/400, and in spite of repeated visits to ophthalmologists in Canada and the United States, nothing had been achieved. It was onchocerciasis; a nodule containing numerous adult worms was removed from her head, and she was treated with Hetrazan with considerable improvement in her vision. The area where these two missionaries served was in a supposedly *Onchocerca*-free area; at least it had not been reported there. This solved the eye difficulties of a number of the missionaries, as a skin survey of the area showed the parasite to be quite prevalent. New, and even more extensive distribution of parasites is being reported: a focus of *S. mansoni* in the Dominican Republic, *S. japonicum* in Thailand, and visceral larva migrans from many areas.

Parasitic infections may have relatively long incubation periods and this must be recognized in history-taking: malaria 1 year, strongyloidiasis 36 years, schistosomiasis 25 years, and echinococcosis 9 years.

Food habits, lack of shoes, swimming or other exposure to fresh water, and insect bites are helpful in ruling out or in, parasitic infections. The aunt who visited her farmer-nephew in Cuba and gave a history of many mosquito bites and a nephew who was experiencing chills and fever, had reason to be sick and to have a good supply of *Plasmodium vivax* in her blood. Her first diagnosis was influenza.

The clinical picture of parasitic infections is varied, as would be expected from the many mechanisms by which they injure man. Tissue invasion and destruction may produce fever, headache, pain, chills, nausea, and vomiting. Pressure of growing parasites gives rise to pain, and in the brain to various motor and sensory abnormalities. Parasites may obstruct the intestine, bile ducts, lymph channels, and capillaries of the brain, and cause serious and bizarre symptoms. Extensive anemia may be produced by red cell destruction, hemorrhage, ingestion or action on the hemopoietic tissues, and migration of parasites or their eggs.

To the physician, the usual site of the parasite in the host is necessary information, but we must not forget the parasitic peregrinations which lead to exotic signs and symptoms. Several years ago, an upstate New York physician called long distance and asked about the treatment of schistosomiasis. We gave him the desired information, thinking that he had under his care one of the ubiquitous Puerto Ricans. On asking if his patient was from that island, we learned that the patient was an elderly woman who had resided in New York State all of her life except for a short excursion to Hawaii several years before. On the removal of her gallbladder a small mass was noted on the upper intestinal wall, which on sectioning contained a parasite which they diagnosed as a *Schistosoma*. Her stool was negative for eggs. As this patient had never visited a recognized endemic area of schistosomiasis, we requested a section of the material for study and suggested that antimony therapy for schistosomiasis be withheld. Careful study of the sections gave the diagnosis of *Fasciola*. This wayward worm was causing its host no recognizable symptoms and, because of its encysted position, no eggs found their way into the patient's stool. *Fasciola* is not uncommon in Hawaii, a delicious water-cress salad being the source of infection.

DIRECT IDENTIFICATION OF PARASITES

The successful identification of parasites requires experience in the differential characteristics of the various species of parasites, their cysts, eggs, and larvae, as well as familiarity with the pseudoparasitic forms and artifacts that may be mistaken for parasites.

Pseudoparasites.   In the feces, a variety of objects may be mistaken for intestinal protozoa and helminthic eggs, and free-living nonparasitic or nonpathogenic animals may be confused with the pathogenic. The free-living protozoa, known as coprozoic species, either reach the feces after its passage from the human body or are swallowed and pass unchanged through the alimentary tract. A safe rule to follow is that motile trophozoites in old feces, or in specimens kept warm and moist, belong to coprozoic species. A single, egg-like artifact in the stool of a patient with pernicious anemia is given undue prominence in the diagnosis of a diphyllobothriasis anemia. Blood platelets above or with superimposed red blood cells in patients with fever become malaria parasites. A patient with fever of undiagnosed lymphoma origin was given unwarranted hope by an intern for this reason. All diagnosis by the enthusiastic and partially tutored should be checked by experts. Stools that have lain around the patient's home for a day or two, insecurely covered, may present bizarre and wonderful artifacts that crawl or are wafted into the specimen. Fly maggots and other arthropods are common.

Some of the animal and plant cells and artifacts that may be mistaken for intestinal protozoa or helminthic eggs by the inexperienced observer are shown in Figure 142. The intestinal yeasts and fungi furnish perhaps the greatest source of confusion. *Blastocystis hominis* (Fig. 140, 18), a harmless intestinal commensal 10 to 15 μ, is frequently mistaken for protozoan cysts with its spherical central mass, thick outer protoplasm, and thin cell membrane. Vegetable cells may be differentiated by their thick cellulose walls and striations, and pollen grains by their capsular markings, micropyles, and coloring. Epithelial and squamous cells, leukocytes, and particularly large endothelial macrophages may be mistaken for protozoa. Air bubbles, oil and fat globules, mucus, and starch granules have been mistaken for protozoan cysts.

Parasites.   The intestinal and atrial protozoa are identified by the morphology of their trophozoites and cysts, and those of the blood and tissues by their characteristic intra- and extracellular forms and, occasionally, by their spores. Helminthic parasites are identified by the morphology of the adult, egg, and larva (Fig. 141).

SEROLOGIC, CUTANEOUS, AND CHEMICAL DIAGNOSIS

Although various serologic tests are of considerable value in the diagnosis of parasitic infections, owing to the difficulty in preparing antigens the tests are seldom readily available to the practicing physician.

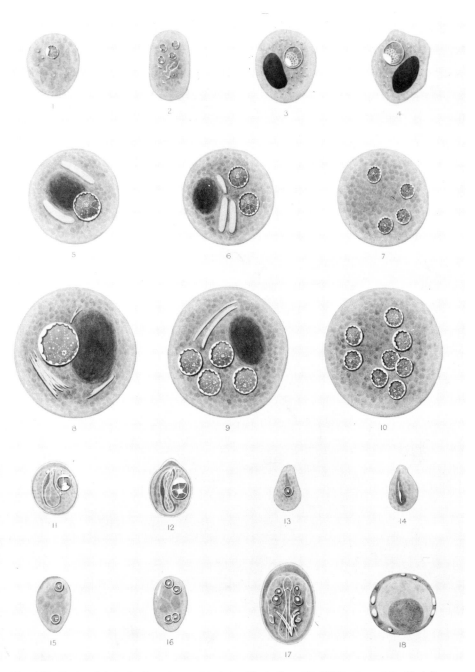

Fig. 140. Cysts of intestinal protozoa treated with iodine (X 2000). 1 and 2, *Endolimax nana;* 3 and 4, *Iodamoeba bütschlii;* 5, 6 and 7, *Entamoeba histolytica;* 8, 9 and 10, *Entamoeba coli;* 11 and 12, *Chilomastix mesnili;* 13 and 14, *Embadomonas intestinalis;* 15 and 16, *Enteromonas hominis;* 17, *Giardia lamblia;* 18, *Blastocystis hominis,* a yeast resembling a protozoan cyst.

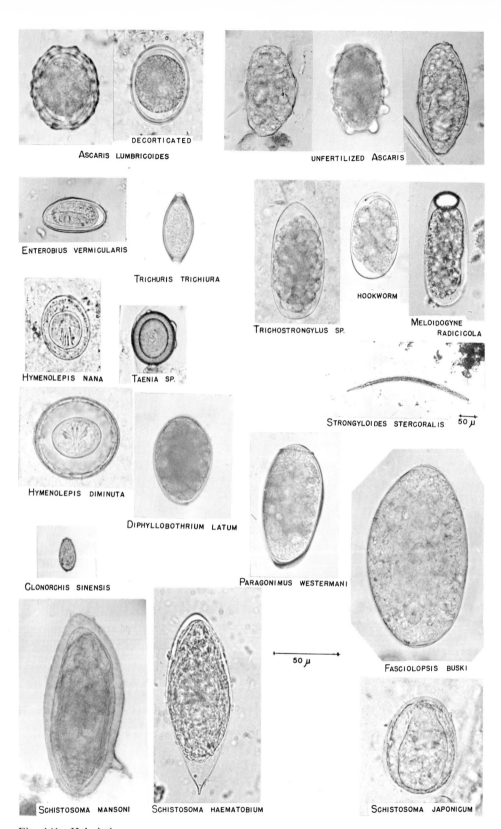

DECORTICATED

ASCARIS LUMBRICOIDES

UNFERTILIZED ASCARIS

ENTEROBIUS VERMICULARIS

TRICHURIS TRICHIURA

TRICHOSTRONGYLUS SP.

HOOKWORM

MELOIDOGYNE RADICICOLA

HYMENOLEPIS NANA

TAENIA SP.

STRONGYLOIDES STERCORALIS

50 μ

HYMENOLEPIS DIMINUTA

DIPHYLLOBOTHRIUM LATUM

CLONORCHIS SINENSIS

PARAGONIMUS WESTERMANI

50 μ

FASCIOLOPSIS BUSKI

SCHISTOSOMA MANSONI

SCHISTOSOMA HAEMATOBIUM

SCHISTOSOMA JAPONICUM

Fig. 141   Helminth eggs.

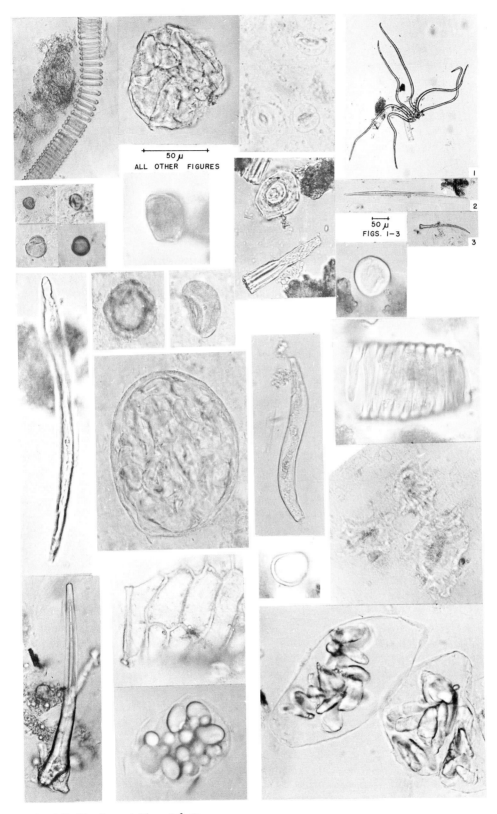

ALL OTHER FIGURES

50 μ

50 μ
FIGS. 1–3

Fig. 142. Fecal vegetable artefacts.

315

Parasites and their products act as antigens, which, when parenterally introduced into the body of the host, evoke the production of antibodies. The concept of
specificity applies to the formation of antibodies; a particular antigen produces
antibodies that react only with that antigen. Such antibodies remain in the tissue
cells or enter the circulation, where they constitute part of the serum globulin. The
detection of these antibodies constitutes serologic and cutaneous diagnosis. Antibody production is not of high order in most parasitic diseases. The parasites that
invade the tissues produce the most pronounced immunologic response. Ectoparasites or helminths of the intestinal canal usually do not evoke an appreciable
elaboration of antibodies. The intestinal helminths that produce antibodies either
invade the host during their larval stages or have sufficient contact with the tissues
to permit the absorption of their products or secretions. Specific humoral antibodies
in the blood serum of the host may be demonstrated in vitro by serologic procedures, such as agglutinative, precipitative, lytic, complement-fixing, and hemag-
glutinating tests, and fluorescent antibody studies; supersensitivity may be shown
by intracutaneous tests, and changes in the proteins of the blood serum may be
detected with nonspecific chemical flocculative tests. These tests are used for
diagnosis of parasitic infections.

The serologic and cutaneous tests tend to be specific for individual or for
closely allied groups of parasites, while the flocculative chemical tests are nonspecific. Their success depends upon the technic employed, the efficiency of the
antigen, and the presence of detectable antibodies in the host. They have not been
successful uniformly in the diagnosis of parasitic infections because of unsatisfactory antigens, insufficient antibody formation, and group- or cross-reactions in related species. Antibodies usually are not present in detectable concentration until
after the second or third week of infection.

The blood serum of the patient is usually used for serologic tests, the cerebrospinal fluid less frequently. The blood serum should be relatively fresh, sterile,
free from hemoglobin, and should be held in the refrigerator.

The serologic technics and the intracutaneous test are outlined in standard
textbooks on laboratory methods. Other tests such as slide flocculation, circumlarval precipitate, Sabin-Feldman dye test, and nonspecific chemical flocculation,
are also used for the diagnosis of parasitic diseases. In a few instances they are
the only available definitive laboratory procedure, as the parasite may not give
off forms that are present in the stool, urine, or blood, or they may be present in
minimal numbers. Serologic and skin tests may therefore be found especially useful in:

1. Nematode infections: *Trichinella spiralis, Angiostrongylus,* visceral larva migrans, filarial infections

2. Trematode infections: *Paragonimus westermani, Schistosoma* infections.

3. Cestode infections: *Echinococcus* and cystercercosis

4. Protozoan infections: Visceral leishmaniasis, Chagas' disease, toxoplasmosis,
intestinal and hepatic amebiasis.

Slide Flocculation Test.   This modification of the precipitation test, based on
the technic of the Kline slide test for syphilis, employs alkaline aqueous solutions
of dried antigens that have the power to coat cholesterol or bentonite crystals and
to act as specific and sensitizing antigens. The test is used for the diagnosis of
trichinosis and schistosomiasis.

SEROLOGIC DIAGNOSIS OF PARASITIC DISEASES

TESTS / DISEASES	Complement Fixation	Precipitin	Hemagglutination	Inert Particle Flocculation	Fluorescent Antibody	Methylene Blue Dye	Intradermal
Invasive Amebiasis (intestinal - hepatic)	o	*	*				
Toxoplasmosis	+		+		*	*	
Echinococcosis	+		*	+			+
Chagas' Disease	*		*				
Trichinosis	+			*			+
Schistosomiasis	+	o		o	o		o
Filariasis			o	o			
Visceral Larva Migrans			o	o			
Malaria			o		o		
Cysticercosis			+				
Pneumocystosis	o						

* Test highly recommended

\+ Test reliable

o Test of limited clinical usefulness

Circumlarval Precipitate Test. In this modification of the precipitation test, a living larva or a small adult worm is brought into contact with immune serum in a sealed hanging-drop suspension. Precipitates form about the mouth and sometimes about the vulva and anus after 24 hours incubation at 37° C. It has been suggested that these precipitates form when the secretions and excretions of the worms come in contact with the antibodies in the immune serum. Sometimes the larvae are immobilized and killed. The test has been used for trichinosis. A similar reaction has been noted with the cercariae and eggs of schistosomes.

Sabin-Feldman Dye Test. The Sabin-Feldman dye test is useful for the diagnosis of toxoplasmosis. Since living toxoplasmas incubated in immune serums, like lysed bacteria, lose their affinity for dyes and become less refractile with granular cytoplasm, this test is considered to be a manifestation of incomplete toxoplasmolysis. The serum of the suspected person, if it contains antibodies, will prevent the subsequent staining of the cytoplasm with alkaline methylene blue. A complement-like accessory factor present in some normal human serums is required for the reaction. Since this specialized test requires living organisms, it is not performed by the ordinary diagnostic laboratory.

Intracutaneous Test.   The intracutaneous test has proved of diagnostic value in certain parasitic diseases, chiefly when other diagnostic methods are ineffective. A small amount of an aqueous solution or suspension of an antigen derived from a parasite is injected intracutaneously on the volar surface of the forearm. Measures for guarding against pseudoreactions include the determination of abnormal skin sensitiveness and dermagraphism by the stroke test with a blunt metal probe, and control injections of extraneous foreign proteins or other substances in the antigen. Interpretations of the significance of their immediate and delayed reactions vary with the individual parasitic infection.

IMMEDIATE REACTION.   A wheal of variable size, showing pseudopodia and surrounded by an area of erythema, is formed at the site of the intracutaneous injection, reaches its maximum in from 10 to 20 minutes, and usually begins to disappear within 60 minutes. Occasionally, smaller wheals appear a short distance from the primary wheal and later merge with it. Measurement of the size of the wheal including pseudopodia is helpful in distinguishing between positive and negative reactions. The variable results of different observers may be due to different linear standards.

DELAYED REACTION.   A local inflammatory reaction with pruritus may occur at the site of the injection in 8 to 24 hours. Superficially, there is an area of erythema with subadjacent induration due to interstitial edema, capillary dilation, and cellular infiltration. The indurated area often has a definite edge, and intense reactions may simulate erysipelas or cellulitis. Intense itching of the local area is a frequent complaint. The erythema may fade within 12 hours or persist for several days.

Nonspecific Chemical Flocculation Tests.   Several nonspecific flocculation tests, which are based upon the disequilibrium of the serum proteins, particularly increased euglobulin, have been used in the diagnosis of protozoan infections. Although these tests have no specific relation to the causative organisms, they have a practical diagnostic value, at least as screening tests. Among these tests are: (1) Henry's melano-flocculation test for malaria, (2) protein tyrosin test for malaria, (3) Chopra's antimony test for kala-azar, (4) Sia's euglobulin precipitation test for kala-azar, and (5) Napier's aldehyde (formol-gel) test for kala-azar. Napier's test has been extensively used in the diagnosis of kala-azar and is probably the most satisfactory of these tests. It is not specific for kala-azar, since positive reactions may occur also in those with tuberculosis, trypanosomiasis, malaria, and schistosomiasis. The test is performed by adding a drop of commercial formalin to 1 ml of the patient's serum. If positive, the serum assumes within 30 minutes an opaque jelly-like consistency.

18

Technical Diagnostic Methods

In a small textbook it is only possible to describe a few simple technical methods which are most practical and commonly used.

The identification of parasites depends upon the proper preparation of material for their microscopic study both in the living state and in stained preparations. The warm stage is an aid in examining the vegetative forms of protozoa. It is advantageous to know the approximate size of the various parasites, but individual variation precludes the differentiation of species by size alone. Whenever practical, material should be examined in the fresh state and in as natural a medium as possible. Fixed material is more convenient to transport, does not deteriorate, and can be examined at leisure, but the immediate examination of fresh material is often essential.

Collection of Material for Examination

Feces. Feces should be collected in a clean, dry container free from urine. Feces from patients receiving barium, bismuth, oil, or antibiotics are unsatisfactory for the identification of protozoa. Feces should be examined *before* administration of barium or bismuth or not until 1 week after their use. A formed specimen may be examined for protozoan cysts, but a liquid specimen, either diarrheic or after a saline purge (Page 31, *Diagnosis* for *E. histolytica*), is more satisfactory for identification of trophozoites. A liquid or semiliquid specimen should be examined immediately, or it must be preserved. Thin fecal smears or small bulk specimens of liquid stools may be preserved with the MIF fixative stain (see below) or polyvinyl alcohol in Schaudinn's solution (see below) for later examination. Adult *Ascaris,* pieces of *D. latum* strobila, and proglottides of *T. saginata* and *T. solium* may be passed in the feces. Adult pinworms may be seen on the outside of the stool or, occasionally, in a diarrheic specimen.

Most helminth eggs are identifiable for days after the passage of the stool.

At times duodenal contents will reveal *Giardia, Strongyloides* larvae, and *Clonorchis* eggs, when they are undetected in the feces. Specimens obtained by duodenal drainage should be allowed to settle or be centrifuged, and the sediment examined in a direct smear.

The sigmoidoscope is useful not only for visualization of the lower bowel, but is also of value for biopsies or collecting aspirated material for microscopic examination or cultures, for amebiasis, balantidiasis, or schistosomiasis. Material from sigmoidoscopy should be placed in a very small amount of normal saline in a small tube; the sediment should be examined. Cotton-tipped swabs are useless for obtain-

319

ing specimens of ameba trophozoites. Perianal swabs are used for the collection of eggs of *Enterobius* and *Taenia.* The most effective of these technics is the Graham Scotch tape swab. In this technic, a strip of ¾-inch Scotch tape is attached to the under side of a microscope slide, brought over the edge to the top —extending three-fourths the length of the slide—then the end turned under for a tab. This slide is then attached to a tongue depressor at 1 inch from its end (Fig. 46). After use, the Scotch tape is smoothed onto the slide, and examined under low power and reduced light. The preparation may be cleared by placing a drop of toluol between the slide and tape. A drop of iodine in xylol, which gives a stained background for the eggs, as well as clearing, is preferred by some workers. Eggs and, occasionally, whole pinworms may be detected this way.

Private and Public Laboratory Facilities

Examination of specimens for parasites may be done in private or hospital laboratories. Public health departments of the larger cities offer laboratory service, and all state health departments have such service available: They supply specimen containers and mailing tubes, which are available through the local health department. State and city health departments supply physicians with a list of laboratory services available to them, and instructions for collecting and mailing specimens. Special serologic tests may be available at the National Communicable Diseases Center of the U. S. Public Health Service, Atlanta, Ga. Often, investigators who are developing a new laboratory diagnostic test welcome serum from patients with the suspected disease.

Preparation of Specimens from Feces for Examination

Adult Helminths. Adult worms recovered from the feces are washed in warm sodium chloride solution with prolonged shaking to promote relaxation, and then are examined fresh or are killed by fixing solutions for preservation in toto or for sectioning. For large nematodes, 5 to 10 percent formalin at 80° C with a small amount of glycerol makes a good fixative and preservative. Specimens may be left in the formalin or stored in 70 percent alcohol after transfer through graded alcohols. Small nematodes may be fixed in warm 70 percent alcohol and preserved in the same solution. Trematodes and the proglottides of cestodes may be examined by pressing them between slides or after relaxation by chilling in a refrigerator.

Proglottides may be cleared somewhat by mounting in 5 percent acetic acid to dissolve the calcareous corpuscles or by the gradual addition of glycerine. They may also be cleared after a brief preservation in 70 percent alcohol by immersion in carbolxylol (75 percent carbolic acid, 25 percent xylol), or dehydration in 95 percent alcohol, 100 percent alcohol, and immersion in oil of wintergreen. If the uterus of the proglottid is empty of eggs, making identification difficult, a method for demonstration of the branches of the uterus is to inject India ink into the central uterine stem using a 1- to 2-ml hypodermic syringe with a ¾-inch, 25-gauge needle. After injection, wash off excess ink on surface and press proglottid between slides. This is very satisfactory with fresh or relaxed proglottides, but may also be used on proglottides which have been brought into the laboratory already fixed in alcohol.

Search for the small scolices, scarcely larger than a pinhead, is a tedious but necessary task in checking the results of anthelmintic treatment of tapeworms. All post-treatment stools should be collected and washed through a 20-mesh screen.

Cysts and Eggs in Unconcentrated Feces. The examination for protozoan trophozoites and cysts and for helminth eggs and larvae may be made with fresh material or with fixed stained preparations. In fluid and semifluid feces, select the bloody mucus or tiny specks of tissue, and in formed feces scrape material from the surface in several parts of the fecal mass.

UNSTAINED PREPARATIONS. A small quantity of the selected fresh material is placed on a warm slide with a toothpick, applicator, or platinum wire; thoroughly emulsified in one or two drops of warm physiologic sodium chloride solution; and mounted with a coverglass. A satisfactory preparation should have a slightly opaque density but should be sufficiently thin to allow newspaper print to be legible through it. Examine first with the low-power 16-mm objective and then study suspicious objects or selected fields with the high-power 4-mm objective. Trophozoites and cysts of protozoa and helminth eggs and larvae appear in their natural shapes and colors. It is advantageous in searching for motile trophozoites to use a warm stage. For helminth eggs, success depends upon freeing the eggs from fecal debris. At least three films should be examined before negative results are reported. Concentration methods are necessary in light infections.

IODINE AND SUPRAVITAL STAINING. The treatment of fresh coverglass mounts with iodine or supravital staining aids in the differentiation of protozoa. The iodine mount, which may be made on the same slide as the plain mount, is useful for the examination of cysts and eggs, but the trophozoites are killed. The chromatin material of amebic cysts stands out in relief against the yellow-brown cytoplasm, the nuclear structures are differentiated, and the glycogen masses stain a mahogany brown (Fig. 140). Iodine solutions of various strengths have been used. Equal quantities of 1 percent isotonic eosin solution and 0.2 percent brilliant cresyl blue added to a coverglass preparation of feces provide a satisfactory vital stain, the active trophozoites appearing as clear, translucent, shiny, pale, blue-green objects against a pink background.

FIXATION AND STAINING. The merthiolate-iodine-formaldehyde (MIF) fixative stain is a valuable asset in preserving specimens of feces containing intestinal protozoa and helminth eggs intact for later laboratory examination. It is useful in preserving specimens in survey studies, in mailing fecal material to the laboratory, and in collecting large samples for teaching purposes or for concentration procedures. The ordinary loss and deterioration of organisms in stools that are allowed to stand may be prevented by placing the fecal specimens in the fixative within 5 minutes after passage. The fixative stain consists of two solutions, which are only combined just previous to the preservation of the feces.

Merthiolate-formaldehyde

Tincture of merthiolate No. 99, Lilly (1:1,000)	200 ml
Formaldehyde, U.S.P.	25 ml
Glycerol	5 ml
Distilled water	250 ml

Lugol's iodine

Iodine	5 g
Potassium iodide	10 g
Distilled water	100 ml

For bulk feces the solutions are mixed in the proportion of 9.4 ml MF and 0.6 ml Lugol's for each gram of feces, and in proportionate volumes for lesser amounts. The fecal material is added with an applicator and mixed thoroughly. The preserved material will keep for a year in tight-fitting bottles. Screw-top vials are convenient. The Lugol's solution should not be over 3 weeks old; if over 1 week, increase by 25 percent, and over 2 weeks by 50 percent. For examination, remove a drop of the surface layer of the sedimented feces to a glass slide, mix the particles of feces, and apply a coverglass. The staining reaction comprises an initial iodine staining phase and a subsequent eosin stage that gradually replaces the iodine. Trophozoites stain immediately, but cysts respond more slowly. For flotation concentration, the supernatant fluid in the vial containing the bulk preparation is replaced with a brine solution and the usual procedure followed. For fresh fecal specimens brought to the laboratory, a drop of distilled water is placed on a slide and an equal amount of MIF solution is added; a small fleck of feces is thoroughly mixed, and the preparation is mounted with a coverglass for examination.

PERMANENT AND PRESERVED MOUNTS.   Permanent mounts permit species differentiation through detailed study of structures and ensure material for demonstration or reference. This method requires fixation and staining. The method of choice is wet fixation, which causes less distortion of the parasites than dry fixation. The thin moist undried smear on a coverglass or slide is immersed in the fixing solution. Material that contains no albuminous matter should be mixed with serum or smeared upon a slide coated with egg albumen in order to make it adhere. Schaudinn's sublimate solution and its various modifications are satisfactory fixatives. They are described in standard laboratory textbooks.

Polyvinyl Alcohol Fixation.   Polyvinyl alcohol added to Schaudinn's solution is a good fixative, adhesive, and preservative for protozoa in dysenteric feces and other liquid material. The powdered polyvinyl alcohol should be added with continuous stirring to the solution at 75° C. It remains satisfactory for use for several months.

Schaudinn's fluid (2 parts saturated aqueous solution of $HgCl_2$ to 1 part 95 percent ethyl alcohol)	93.5 ml
Glycerol	1.5 ml
Glacial acetic acid	5.0 ml
Polyvinyl alcohol, powdered	5.0 g

1. One part of the fecal suspension may be mixed with three parts of the fixing solution in a vial. Smears may be prepared immediately or months later by spreading a drop or two of the mixture on a slide.

2. Dry thoroughly at 37° C overnight.

3. Relatively thin rectangular smears should be made to prevent wrinkling.

4. The films may be stained by the long or rapid Heidenhain iron-hematoxylin procedures. Before staining, the dried films should be placed in 70 percent alcohol containing iodine to remove the mercuric chloride.

Permanent Stains.   There are many methods of staining fecal smears. Those that produce the best results are usually the longest and most complicated. The iron-hematoxylin method with its numerous modifications to increase the rapidity of the process is the classic method of staining protozoa in fixed preparations. Both the long and rapid methods are described in standard laboratory textbooks.

Lawless' permanent mount stain provides a rapid method of staining trophozoites and cysts, the protozoa appearing blue to purplish. The fixative stain remains stable for 6 months, if kept in tightly stoppered brown bottles.

Saturated solution of mercuric chloride in water	594 ml
Alcohol, 95%	296 ml
Glacial acetic acid	50 ml
Acetone	50 ml
Formaldehyde, U.S.P.	10 ml
Acid fuchsin	1.25 g
Fast green FCF	0.50 g

1. Transfer staining solution with pipet in sufficient quantity to cover the moist fecal film.
2. Heat over flame to steaming but do not boil.
3. Wash gently in tap water and drain.
4. Pass through 50 and 70% alcohols, 30 seconds each; and through 95 and 100%, 15 seconds each.
5. Clear in xylol for 1 minute and mount in balsam or clarite.

Wheatley's modification of Gomori's trichrome stain gives a rapid method for staining of intestinal protozoa.

Stain

Chromotrope 2R	0.6 g
Light green SF	0.3 g
Phosphotungstic acid	0.7 g
Glacial acetic acid	1 ml
Distilled water	100 ml

The acetic acid is added to the dry ingredients, allowed to stand 15 to 30 minutes, then distilled water is added. Good stain is purple in color.

Procedure
1. Place thin, moist fecal smear in Schaudinn's fixative for 10 minutes.
2. 70% alcohol with iodine (amber color) 2 minutes
3. 70% alcohol, 2 changes, 2 minutes each
4. 50% alcohol, 2 minutes
5. Rinse in tap water
6. Stain 8 to 15 minutes
7. 90% alcohol with 1% acetic acid—10 to 20 seconds
8. 100% alcohol, rinsed twice
9. Xylol, 1 minute or dip until clear
10. Mount with synthetic mounting medium: Permount or Harleco synthetic resin.

Concentration Methods for Protozoan Cysts and Helminth Eggs and Larvae. Concentration methods fall into two main classes: (1) sedimentation and (2) flotation, each with a number of technics. In both types a preliminary straining of the feces through wire mesh or cheese cloth, to remove bulky material and coarse particles, is advisable.

SEDIMENTATION.   Sedimentation is less efficient than flotation for the concentration of protozoan cysts and many eggs, but is more satisfactory for schistosomal and operculated eggs. Simple sedimentation in tall glass cylinders with settling, decantation, and replacement with wash water, although time-consuming, causes no distortion of the eggs and, if prolonged, permits the hatching of miracidia. Centrifugal concentration, either with water or chemicals, is more efficient than simple sedimentation.

Water Centrifugal Concentration.   Cysts and eggs are concentrated uninjured by chemicals by the water centrifugal method, which is particularly suitable for schistosomal and operculated eggs, and of value for *Ascaris* and hookworm eggs and *Strongyloides* larvae in light infections. The degree of concentration, however, is not great.

FLOTATION.   The flotation technics for the concentration of cysts and eggs are based on the differences in specific gravity of certain chemical solutions (1.120 to 1.210) and of helminth eggs and larvae and protozoan cysts (1.050 to 1.150). Sugar, sodium chloride, or zinc sulfate solutions are employed chiefly. The eggs and cysts float to the surface in the heavier solutions, while fecal material sinks gradually to the bottom. Flotation is superior to sedimentation for concentrating cysts and eggs other than operculated, schistosomal, and infertile *Ascaris* eggs. Zinc sulfate flotation is used most frequently and is preferable to sugar, calcium chloride, or brine flotation. The optimal time for examination of specimens from chemical solutions is 5 to 20 minutes, since the cysts tend to disintegrate after 30 minutes.

Zinc Sulfate Centrifugal Flotation Technic.   This valuable method of concentrating cysts and eggs employs a zinc sulfate solution of specific gravity 1.180, which is made by dissolving 331 g of granular $ZnSO_4 \cdot 7H_2O$, U.S.P., in 1,000 ml of water and adjusting to exact specific gravity using a hydrometer. For formalized feces, a solution of higher specific gravity, 1.200, should be used. It is considered about 80 percent effective in detecting eggs and cysts in light infections. It destroys trophozoites, but does not impair the morphology of cysts for an hour, although immediate examination is advisable.

1.   A fine suspension is made by comminuting 1 g of freshly passed feces in about 10 ml of lukewarm tap water.

2.   In order to remove the coarse particles, the suspension is strained through one layer of wet cheesecloth in a funnel into a small test tube, 100 by 13 mm. This step may be omitted without material loss.

3.   The suspension is centrifuged for 1 minute for 2,300 rpm. The supernatant fluid is poured off, about 2 ml of water is added, the sediment is broken up by shaking or tapping, and additional water is added to fill the tube.

4.   The washing and centrifuging is repeated until the supernatant fluid is fairly clear. Usually it is necessary to do this three times.

5.   The last supernatant fluid is poured off, about 2 ml of zinc sulfate of specific gravity 1.180 is added, the sediment is broken up, and sufficient additional zinc sulfate to fill the tube to the rim is added.

6.   A coverglass is placed over the top of the tube, which is centrifuged again for 1 minute at 2,300 rpm.

7.   The coverglass is removed and mounted on a clean slide in a drop of Lugol's iodine solution for microscopic examination.

Method of Counting Eggs.   In surveys of infected populations, it is sometimes desirable to determine the intensity of infection by obtaining the approximate number of eggs. The daily output of eggs varies, requiring counts on several specimens; cycles occur in egg production; the effects of the consistency of the stool, diet, faulty digestion, and other factors are unknown; and the output per worm may vary in different hosts. In general, the output per day is more dependable than the number of eggs per gram of feces. Egg counts before treatment may determine the desirability of treatment and those after may determine its success.

STOLL'S EGG-COUNTING TECHNIC. The technic is a dilution, rather than a concentration, method. Stoll displacement flasks graduated at 56 and 60 ml, and egg count pipets graduated at 0.075 ml and 0.15 ml, are available.

Procedure

1. Fill the Stoll flask to the 56-ml mark with N/10 sodium hydroxide.

2. Using an applicator stick, add sufficient feces to raise the fluid level to the 60-ml mark (i.e., 4 ml of feces).

3. Add 15 to 20 glass beads (3 mm diameter), stopper tightly with rubber stopper, and shake from time to time. It is best to prepare the flasks in the afternoon and allow them to sit overnight. On the following morning, examine the bottom of the flask to be sure no lumps of feces remain unbroken.

4. When the feces have completely disintegrated, shake for 1 minute and *immediately* remove 0.075 ml with a Stoll pipet and place on a slide (1½ by 3 inch slides are easier to use) covering it with a 22-mm square coverslip.

5. Count the eggs with a 10 power eyepiece and 10X objective, first examining any liquid around the edges of the coverglass and then systematically examining the whole slide.

Computations

To compute the number of eggs passed per day:

Make counts on 2 drops of 0.075 ml each, total of 0.15 ml.

Original fecal dilution is 4 ml in 60 ml, or 1 to 15.

Hence, to compute the number of eggs in 1 ml of feces, multiply the number of eggs found by 100.

To compute the number of worms present:

Assume 100 g feces daily human (adult).

Therefore, the total number of eggs passed per day may be obtained by multiplying the total found in 0.15 ml by 10,000.

Determine the number of female worms present by dividing the total number of eggs passed per day by number of eggs passed by a female worm per day.

Approximation of the total number of worms may be obtained by assuming an equal number of males.

Female *Necator* passes approximately 9,000 eggs per day.

Female *Ascaris* passes approximately 200,000 eggs per day.

Female *Trichuris* passes approximately 5,000 eggs per day.

TECHNICAL METHODS FOR EXAMINATION OF PARASITES FROM BLOOD

Preparation of Blood Films. The preparation of good blood films is important for the differentiation of parasites, especially the protozoa.

FRESH WET FILM. The fresh wet film is useful for the detection of trypanosomes and microfilariae.

THIN DRY FILM.   The stained thin dry film permits the study of the morphology of the parasite and the condition of the blood corpuscles. It provides a more reliable morphologic differentiation of protozoan parasites and their relation to the blood cells than does the thick film. The technic of making the thin film, either on a coverglass or slide, is the same as in hematologic studies.

THICK DRY FILM.   The dehemoglobinized thick film, which yields a much higher concentration of parasites than the thin film, is useful when parasites are few or thin films are negative. It is of particular value for the detection of plasmodia in malarial surveys and in patients with chronic infections or under antimalarial therapy. It is also of value in detecting trypanosomes, leishmaniae, and microfilariae. The thick film is not a thick drop, but a smear spread at a thickness of 50 μ or less, so that it is sufficiently transparent for microscopic examination when the hemaglobin is removed.

The technic of preparing the thick film is as follows:

1.   A large drop of blood is spread quickly and evenly on a clean slide in a film about 10 mm in diameter with the corner of a slide, needle, toothpick, or applicator, or by slowly rotating the slide. If the blood has been obtained with a capillary pipet a film of any desired size and thickness may be made.

2.   Allow the film to dry, protected from dust, for 1½ hours in an incubator at 37° C or overnight at room temperature to cause it to adhere to the slide. Both thick and thin films may be mounted on the same slide in examining blood for malarial parasites.

These slides may be stained in either of two ways:

1.   The thick drop may be laked in distilled water until the color of the hemoglobin has disappeared, dried, and the whole slide stained with Wright's stain as for routine blood smears.

2.   The thin smear may be fixed with methyl alcohol, dried, and the whole slide stained with dilute Giemsa stain. A 2 percent Giemsa stain in buffered water pH 7.0 for 45 mniutes and rinsed in buffered water has proved very satisfactory.

Knott Technic for Concentration of Microfilariae

1.   Draw 1 ml of blood from the vein and immediately expel this blood into a centrifuge tube containing 10 ml of 2 percent formalin solution.

2.   The blood and formalin solution are thoroughly mixed by inverting the tube and shaking it. The solution kills the microfilariae, which die in a stretched-out attitude; it also lakes the red blood cells.

3.   a. Allow the tube to stand for 12 to 24 hours; the sediment will collect in the tip.

   or

   b. Centrifuge the material for 5 to 10 minutes and throw the microfilariae and other solid blood constituents to the tip of the tube.

4.   Decant the supernatant fluid.

5.   With a long capillary pipet draw up the sediment from the bottom of the tube and spread it over a glass slide, uniformly covering an area approximately 2 by 5 cm.

6.   Examination

   a. If one wishes an immediate diagnosis, the slide can be examined wet for microfilariae.

   or

b. Allow the slide to dry overnight and stain with Giemsa for 45 minutes (1 part concentrated Giemsa to 50 parts buffered water pH 7.2). Destain 10 to 15 minutes in water, pH approximately 7.2 Allow to dry and examine.

TECHNICAL METHODS FOR EXAMINATION OF PARASITES FROM TISSUES AND BODY FLUIDS

Protozoa and helminths, particularly larvae, may be found in various organs and tissues of the body, as well as in the blood.

Hepatic puncture is useful in the diagnosis of visceral leishmaniasis. Liver biopsy may reveal *Toxocara* larvae and schistosomal worms and eggs.

The bone marrow may be examined in trypanosomiasis and malaria when the blood is negative. In visceral leishmaniasis it is less valuable but less dangerous for diagnosis than splenic or hepatic puncture. Specimens are usually obtained by puncturing the sternum, crest of the ilium, vertebral processes, trochanter, or tibia.

The lymph nodes may be examined for the diagnosis of trypanosomiasis, leishmaniasis, toxoplasmosis, and filariasis either by puncture or by biopsy.

Material for examination may be obtained from mucocutaneous lesions by scraping, aspiration, or biopsy. Scrapings or sections may be taken from the dermal lesions of post-kala-azar leishmaniasis. Material may be obtained from the ulcer or nodule of oriental sore by puncturing the indurated margin of the lesion with a sterile hypodermic needle or by passing a sterile capillary tube through an incision into the tissues at the base of the ulcer and aspirating gently. Stained films or cultures are made from the aspirated material. Similar methods are used for the early lesions of American leishmaniasis; however, for the advanced mucosal lesions, biopsy of the infected tissues is necessary. *L. donovani* may be present on the nasal mucosa from which it may be removed with swabs.

The migratory larvae of *Ancylostoma braziliense, A. caninum, Strongyloides stercoralis,* or *Gnathostoma spinigerum* may be found in skin.

Onchocerca volvulus may be found in subcutaneous nodules; *Dracunculus medinensis* may be removed from its subcutaneous canal by traction or surgical incision. *Loa loa* may be removed surgically from its migratory tract, often about the head and eye; and, rarely, *Gongylonema pulchrum* may be located in the subcutaneous tissue of the buccal mucosa.

Rectal snips for schistosomiasis may be made through a proctoscope; and a piece of rectal mucosa from the region of Houston's valve, 2 by 2 by 1 mm, may be extracted with a sharp scoop. The material is examined microscopically by compression between slides after submergence in water for 30 minutes. Viable eggs have active flame cells.

Diphyllobothriid spargana are obtained from the skin, and subcutaneous, and deeper tissues. The cysticerci of *Taenia solium* may be found in muscles and subcutaneous tissues by biopsy or by roentgen rays. The hydatid cysts of *Echinococcus granulosus,* usually in the liver, lungs and other organs, very rarely may be present in the muscles.

Cerebrospinal Fluid. The cerebrospinal fluid is examined after centrifuging for trypanosomes, toxoplasma, and, rarely, trichinae.

Sputum. The eggs of *Paragonimus westermani* are commonly found in the brown-flecked sputum of infected persons. Occasionally, the larvae of *Strongyloides stercoralis* and, more rarely, those of *Ascaris lumbricoides* and the hookworms, may be coughed up during their pulmonary migration. In pulmonary echinococcosis, the contents of the hydatid cyst may be evacuated in the sputum.

A small amount of sputum is transferred to a slide with a toothpick and examined under a coverglass. The sputum may be mixed with an equal amount of 3 percent sodium hydroxide and, after standing, centrifuged; the sediment is examined microscopically.

The identification of parasites in the cerebrospinal, pleural, pericardial, peritoneal, hydrocele, and joint fluids; urine; and sputum is usually confined to the microscopic examination of the centrifuged sediment in wet coverglass preparations or in stained films. The physiologic character of the various fluids may modify the procedure.

Staining of Parasites from Tissues.   The methods of staining smears containing parasites from tissues and body fluids are similar to those used for blood films.

CULTURAL METHODS FOR PROTOZOA

Entamoeba Histolytica.   *E. histolytica* grows readily under partial anaerobiosis in nutrient mediums containing bacteria and rice flour, although strains may show growth idiosyncrasies. The other intestinal amebas may grow, at least for a few generations, on such noncellular mediums. Boeck and Drbohlav's diphasic medium, as modified by Dobell and Laidlaw, and Cleveland and Collier's medium are commonly used for diagnosis.

Leishmania.   The several species of human leishmaniae vary in their ability to grow on various mediums. To prevent bacterial contamination from the inoculated material, 500 units of penicillin may be used in each tube. The Novy, MacNeal, and Nicolle (NNN) medium is the oldest and most commonly used diagnostic medium for leishmanias and *T. cruzi*.

Cellular Media.   Tissue cultures and the chick embryo have been used for the cultivation of *E. histolytica, Trypanosoma cruzi* and other trypanosomes, Leishmanias, *Toxoplasma gondii,* and avian and simian plasmodia. The standard methods of tissue culture with embryonic chicken and mammalian explants are employed.

19

Treatment of Parasitic Diseases

READ THE DIRECTIONS IN THE DRUG PACKAGE!

Treatment of the infected patient includes medical and surgical measures, a hygienic regimen to build up general resistance, and the use of specific chemotherapeutic agents. General medical treatment, largely supportive and symptomatic, is designed to maintain or increase the resistance of the patient. It includes rest in bed during the acute stages, reduction of fever, maintenance of fluid equilibrium, opiates and sedatives to reduce intestinal peristalsis and give repose, a bland nutritive diet of proper vitamin content, and treatment of complications and intercurrent diseases. Iron may be necessary for anemic patients. In certain parasitic diseases, operation may be indicated, which can range from the minor extraction of the capitulum of a tick to the major removal of an hydatid cyst.

The physician should be familiar with the parasiticidal action and toxic properties of the common chemotherapeutic agents, so that he may select appropriate drugs. Before starting treatment the parasite should be identified, its location in the host determined, the intensity of the infection estimated, and the amount of damage approximated. Successful chemotherapy depends upon the use of a drug that has a minimal toxic effect on the host and a maximal action on the parasite. Success depends also upon its administration and dosage, auxiliary therapeutic preparation and after-care of the patient, and additional procedures to prevent reinfection. The physical condition of the patient and the impairment of vital organs by other diseases may contraindicate the use of certain drugs.

Prepurgation with sodium sulfate tends to eliminate the mucus and fecal debris that protect the parasite, but sometimes the increased peristalsis may accelerate the passage of the drug through the intestinal tract. Postpurgation aids in the removal of killed or anesthetized worms from the intestine. The sodium sulfate, 30 g for an adult and 2 g for each 10 pounds of weight in children, is dissolved in a glass of water. Contraindications for purgation are signs of intestinal obstruction, appendicitis, debilitation, and pregnancy. Drugs are administered orally, intravenously, and/or intramuscularly, depending upon the nature of the drug and the condition of the patient. Also, some may be used in enemas or applied to local lesions.

For helminths in the lower intestinal tract, it may be desirable to administer the drug in a protective enteric coating to prevent its premature absorption.

The dosage for children may be calculated in proportion to the weight of the child or by certain empirical rules, although children usually tolerate proportionately greater amounts than adults. Clark's rule is to multiply the average adult dose by the weight of the child in pounds and divide by 150. Fried's rule for infants is to divide the age in months by 150 and multiply by the adult dose.

The first problem is who should be treated: the patient with a hookworm infection with 10 worms? One with an asymptomatic *Giardia* infection? A patient passing an occasional *S. mansoni* egg? In general, if we have a safe, effective chemotherapeutic agent, all infected individuals should be treated. A few hookworms may consume little blood, but they consume it 365 days a year, including Sundays and holidays, as long as 14 years. Until a parasite is shown to be beneficial to man, there is no reason to give it housing and hospitality, and to permit it to continue its asexual or sexual orgy. In areas where reinfection is certain, usually only patients with heavy infections or whose health is threatened are treated.

The object of therapy is to cure the patient, which involves the elimination of the parasite. In infections with such parasites as hookworm and *Schistosoma,* elimination of 95 percent of the parasites may lead to the disappearance of the patient's signs and symptoms. In parasitic infections where there is a multiplication or addition of the parasite in the host, as in amebiasis and malaria, elimination of the parasite must be complete. As we reduce the host's parasite load, careful laboratory search, using proper technics on adequate specimens at proper intervals, must be made. It may be necessary to wait weeks or months for the parasite to reappear in diagnosable numbers.

Patients with multiple parasitic infections present interesting therapeutic problems, especially as to the order in which the several infections should be treated. If one of the infections is especially painful or threatens life, it should be treated first —and vigorously. The order of treatment of patients with several chronic infections depends upon several factors. In general, short oral courses of therapy are given before long courses of therapy involving injection. If one of the infections is hookworm, which responds dramatically to a single dose of tetrachlorethylene or Alcopara, this infection might well be treated before a 40-day course of therapy for schistosomiasis was instituted. Many patients defect before the completion of long series of injections and hence do not have the benefit of needed shorter oral therapy for other parasites. Often several drugs may be given concurrently. One must take care, however, that their side effects and toxicities are not additive.

Chemotherapy can be a useful diagnostic tool when clinical diagnosis is impossible and when laboratory tests are unavailable or questionable; thus, hepatic amebiasis responds clinically and diagnostically to therapy.

READ THE DIRECTIONS ON THE DRUG PACKAGE!

A number of chemotherapeutic agents that are not readily available commercially, or are not approved by the Food and Drug Administration, due to the infrequency of the need of them in the United States are available through:

> Epidemic Intelligence Service
> Parasitic Diseases Section
> Epidemiology Program
> National Communicable Diseases Center
> Atlanta, Ga. 30333
> Day telephone: 404—633-3311 Ext. 3676 & 3677

Among these drugs are:

Pentamidine isethionate (Lomidine) for *Pneumocystis carinii* and early stages of *Trypanosoma gambiense* infections

Niclosamide (Yomesan) for *Taenia saginata, Hymenolepis nana,* and *Dipylidium caninum* infections

Parenteral chloroquine and parenteral quinine for pernicious *Plasmodium falciparum* infections

Bithional for the treatment of *Paragonimus westermani* infections.

Index